Also by Marcia Zimmerman

The A.D.D. Nutrition Solution

Eat Your Colors

Marcia Zimmerman, C.N.

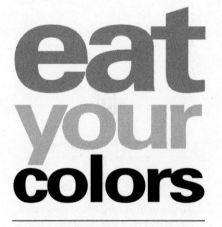

Maximize Your Health
by Eating the Right Foods
for Your Body Type

AN OWL BOOK

HENRY HOLT AND COMPANY • NEW YORK

The information in this book is for educational purposes only.
It is not intended to substitute for the advice of a health care
professional. Consult your health care provider if you have
a serious condition before using the suggestions in this book.

Henry Holt and Company, LLC
Publishers since 1866
115 West 18th Street
New York, New York 10011

Henry Holt® is a registered trademark
of Henry Holt and Company, LLC.

Library of Congress Cataloging-in-Publication Data
Zimmerman, Marcia.
  Eat your colors: maximize your health by eating the right foods
for your body type / Marcia Zimmerman.
    p. cm.
  "An Owl book."
  Includes index.
  ISBN 0-8050-6728-0 (pbk.)
    1. Nutrition. 2. Functional foods. 3. Natural foods.
  4. Diet therapy.   I. Title.

RA784.Z53 2001
613.2—dc21   2001016917

Henry Holt books are available for special promotions
and premiums. For details contact: Director, Special Markets.

First Edition 2001

Designed by Victoria Hartman

Printed in the United States of America

1 3 5 7 9 10 8 6 4 2

Contents

Part Three

Foods for Your Color Meal Plans

Part Four

Harmonize Your Colors

Introduction

Eat Your Colors is a book about the healing power of nutraceuticals, foods that have medical-health benefits, including prevention and treatment of disease. Nutraceuticals are a popular subject today, having captured the attention of scientific investigators and a public that has grown increasingly interested in the disease-preventive power of food. Yet choosing the right foods has never been more complicated. We have been inundated with complex and often conflicting reports on what foods we should eat. Low-fat diets rich in carbohydrates compete against the claims of high-fat, low-carbohydrate diets. And a recent finding that high-fiber diets offer no protection against colon cancer has consumers tossing out high-fiber cereals in favor of less fibrous old favorites. Experts continue to offer us contradictory reports on the potential benefits or danger, as the case may be, posed by specific foods such as eggs, nuts, and margarine. Meanwhile, others offer diet plans that are complex, difficult to follow, and hard to understand.

There have been many books and articles written about nutraceuticals discussing the specific benefits to be gained from eating a particular group of foods. Yet, none have provided specific instructions for readers to get the greatest benefit from these special foods. Instead, they've merely listed the foods and explained their benefits, leaving the reader to figure out which are most appropriate for his or her individual need and how much of each food must be consumed to reap the health benefits. Are some of these foods more important than others for you? How do you match the most appropriate nutraceutical foods with your personal health concerns?

Food has a powerful effect on the mind, emotions, and physical and immune responses of the body. The effect a particular food will have on an individual depends on many factors, one of which is your body type. "One man's food can be another man's poison"—so the saying goes. It expresses the fact that food and drug effects upon the body differ greatly between individuals. *Eat Your Colors* will explain why some foods don't seem to agree with you while others will heighten your awareness and energy levels. *Eat Your Colors* will show you how to take advantage of the latest scientific information and avoid foods that are wrong for your type while eating foods that will help balance your physical and mental energy.

Eat Your Colors offers a nutrition solution that is easy to understand, easy to follow, and easy to stick to. It contains sensible and time-tested dietary wisdom that will be a constant in this turbulent world of changing nutrition information. *Eat Your Colors* is a book that teaches you how to access the healing power of nutraceuticals. It is the very first book to provide detailed nutraceutical eating plans based on three color types—Red, Yellow, and Green. It uses the power of Ayurvedic medicine to identify your body type by color and then provide you with a color-coded plan that will bring you optimal health, energy, and longevity. It takes the mystery and complication out of nutraceuticals by using the simple language of color to match appropriate foods with your color.

Eat Your Colors provides a questionnaire based on physical and psychological characteristics, lifestyle, and family history that will allow you to determine your primary color. *Eat Your Colors* gives detailed and scientifically based information on six food colors. Three of them are fruit and vegetable colors: shades of red, yellow, and blue/green. The other three are complementary food colors; white, tan, and brown. These colors include cereal grains, legumes, animal foods, nuts, seeds, and oils. Your primary colors, red, yellow, and blue/green, will become the basis of your nutraceutical eating plan, while your complementary colors will provide supporting nutraceutical foods. *Eat Your Colors* thus provides you with a personalized color palette of therapeutic foods for health maintenance and disease prevention.

In addition to the detailed diet plans given for your type, a special section addresses "what if" situations. These are simple suggestions on how to eat your color foods without disrupting the eating habits of others. It tells you what to do when eating foods that are "off color" and how to navigate menu choices when dining out. *Eat Your Colors* also discusses what illnesses your color type is most prone to, and explains what specific foods and nutrients can be used to prevent these conditions.

Eat Your Colors unravels the mystery of nutraceuticals and will help you make life-changing food decisions for the twenty-first century.

Marcia Zimmerman
Alameda, California
August 2000

part one

Nutraceuticals and Ancient Healing Arts

❖

Let food be your medicine and medicine
be your food.
—Hippocrates

1

What Is a Nutraceutical?

The term "nutraceutical" was unknown until the mid-1970s when Stephen DeFelice, M.D., created the term to identify a broad class of health-promoting nutrients. The term nutraceutical was chosen to embrace the concept that a specific subclass of nutrients has pharmaceutical-like effects on the body. By classifying these important compounds, Dr. DeFelice and others hoped to highlight the importance of these newly discovered nutrients. Dr. DeFelice also established New Jersey's Foundation for Innovation in Medicine to promote the fledgling branch of nutraceutical medicine and encourage research on the specific actions and health benefits of this class of nutrients. Now, nearly twenty-five years later, there are several subdivisions of nutraceuticals—*vitamins, minerals, semi-vitamins, peptides, phytochemicals,* and *zoochemicals.*

> ❖ We're asking, is there a way that we can delay the onset of diseases, maybe reduce the symptoms and improve the quality of life through better nutrition? We believe that [nutraceuticals are] a viable scientific and business proposition.
> —Diana Twyman, Monsanto Corp., 2/4/98

Since its beginning the nutraceutical wave has been gaining momentum as research continues to reveal how these potent chemicals prevent disease. Americans have been willing to take health matters into their own hands and today nearly half take dietary supplements. Many also believe in nutraceutical benefits. Food manufacturers have been eager to tap into the wave of interest in nutraceuticals by offering a proliferation of "designer" or "functional" foods that promise solutions to consumer health concerns. These foods are chemically enhanced with nutraceuticals and offer the promise of preventing cancer, lowering risk of cardiovascular disease or improving brain function. They include products such as:

- Potato chips that enhance memory
- New Age drinks that improve your love life
- A candy bar that reduces hot flashes
- A cookie that helps you bulk up and lean out
- Margarine that cuts cholesterol
- Meat alternatives that cut cancer risk

You may have already heard of some of these products, or seen them on your supermarket shelves. *Functional* or *designer foods* represent a revolution in the food industry: a prescription for health that blurs the line between food and medicine. Food manufacturers are excited about these products because they appeal to a better educated public—one that is growing older, richer, and more willing to self-medicate with foods and supplements. These medicinal foods command premium prices, too—enticing food and pharmaceutical companies to pump up even more products with disease-fighting nutrients. And despite a few pitfalls in product development and higher consumer cost, this market for nutraceutical/functional foods is booming. By the end of the twentieth century, sales had topped $15 billion and future potential is projected by some to reach a staggering $250 billion, half of current food industry sales!

> ❖ The market for functional foods is now about $15 billion a year and is likely to grow more than 10 percent annually well into the twenty-first century.
> —Clare M. Hasler, Ph.D., Director, Functional Foods for Health Program, University of Illinois at Urbana-Champaign

> ❖ The hottest thing in the food biz these days is groceries with health powers, stuff that does more than just keep us from starving.
> —Daniel Q. Haney, Associated Press, 11/21/99

Food manufacturers have been quick to pick up on these new marketing opportunities. At the end of 1999 Quaker Oats company announced its intention to develop and market a new line of designer foods in a joint venture with Swiss pharmaceutical giant Novartis. Quaker's new products will tout government-approved health claims that these foods are better for you than older familiar brands. Who are the consumers most likely to buy medicinal foods?

According to the International Food Information Council, two-thirds of Americans ready to buy such foods for their health are over forty-five years old, mostly college educated and earn more than $50,000 per year. Many have shopped in health and natural food stores, prompting grocers to feature health food displays and products in mainstream supermarkets in an attempt to appeal to these customers.

It's extremely difficult, however, for mainstream grocers to educate shoppers on the benefits of costlier functional foods. What has been successful in natural foods markets doesn't necessarily translate into mainstream grocery marketing. Grocers are beginning to figure this out and some are committed to educating their customers with special signage, nutrition information, and recipes. We have a long way to go before functional foods are fully integrated into mainstream grocery shopping. That makes the information in this book vitally important.

> ❖ Consumers began seeking a more proactive strategy for "improving health through foods, switching from simply avoiding unhealthy food ingredients and balancing one's diet to seeking out foods and ingredients that offer a demonstrated health benefit or 'positive eating.'"
> —Dr. Elizabeth Sloan, President, Applied Biometrics, 4/1/00

Are Designer Foods Good for You?

Have you been confused about the health benefits in these new foods? Do they offer *real* health benefits supported by the scientific literature and touted by the press? Unfortunately, just adding a phytochemical to a food doesn't inevitably make it better, especially if the phytochemical being added doesn't naturally occur in the food selected. For example, unhealthy foods like potato chips, crackers, cookies, or candy are ideal for delivering phytochemicals because they are popular choices among consumers. But adding a phytochemical doesn't overcome the nutritional deficits in such foods. By contrast, foods that *naturally* contain phytochemicals offer greater health benefits because they contain groups of nutrients that complement and support one another. This is what nature intended and what scientists have found out through trial and error.

The quest to prove the anticancer benefits of carotenoids is a striking example of how nature has taught us this lesson. The scientific process is based upon identifying and proving a single substance is responsible for an observed effect. Beta carotene, the orange pigment in fruits and vegetables, has been thought to be a protective factor in preventing lung cancer. This belief was based upon several trials that found an inverse correlation between consumption of orange fruits and vegetables and lung cancer. Scientific investigators wanted to prove beta carotene can reduce the risk of lung cancer among people at high risk for the disease. The Carotenoid and Retinol Efficacy Trial (CARET) included two large groups of people—approximately 40,000 individuals—who were given a combination of beta carotene and vitamin A as preventive agents against lung cancer. A significant amount of dietary beta carotene is normally converted into vitamin A, yet the cancer protective benefits stem from the carotene, not its vitamin product. By adding vitamin A, the scientists hoped to maintain high levels of beta carotene and thwart its conversion into the vitamin.

Both studies were halted at the end of 1995 after it was discovered the supplements appeared to offer no benefit and might actually be harming the participants. As it turned out, the large daily doses given—50,000 International Units of beta carotene plus 25,000 IU of vitamin A—likely crowded out other helpful carotenoids in the tissues of study participants. Previous studies that had reported cancer-preventing benefits from eating carotenoid-rich foods contained a mixture of carotenoids. Consequently, the CARET study may have been doomed from the beginning since cancer prevention appears to flow from several classes of naturally occurring nutrients, not single isolated ones. Beta carotene is just one of a class of six hundred known carotenoids—none of the others were included in the CARET study.

We have learned from this that foods naturally rich in a variety of phytochemicals appear to be much more effective than foods that have been supplemented with only one or two. You can enjoy the benefits of phytochemical-enhanced foods as long as you don't substitute them for a healthy diet—preferably one that is customized for you.

Shopping for designer foods with added phytochemicals unnecessarily complicates your food-buying decisions and leaves you vulnerable to the whims of food marketers. What happens when your favorite cholesterol-fighting cookie is no longer available? And how do you identify which phytochemicals will be most beneficial for you? Most important, if you rely exclusively on designer foods for disease prevention, you will be missing out on most of the other phytochemicals you need.

Eat Your Colors Meal Plans Provide Better Total Nutrition than Designer Foods

You don't *need* to buy expensive designer foods or read complicated scientific information to benefit from the many positive effects of nutraceuticals. All you need to do is apply the customized eating plan provided in *Eat Your Colors*. This book presents a new, unique way of thinking about food and offers detailed scientific information identifying phytochemicals and explaining how they work to prevent disease.

Nutrition has been an integral part of the healing arts for centuries, and color was one way healers could identify which foods were beneficial for specific ailments. They did not have the means (or concern) for determining the chemical nature of foods, or why they worked. Incredibly, what these ancient healers found by trial and error then applied over the centuries, today's scientists are now validating using modern methods. The color of foods tells you which are good for your type and will help you prevent diseases most common in your type. To the scientist, color indicates which phytochemicals are likely present and what he or she should analyze for. The modern story of nutraceuticals plays out in the pages of this book, and it validates the need to apply what you read in *Eat Your Colors*.

Back to the Beginning

Hippocrates was a Greek physician who lived between 460 B.C. and 377 B.C. He is credited with influencing the development of ideals and the ethics code for physicians and has been named the father of modern medicine for this reason. Hippocrates, reportedly influenced by Hindu medicine, and the physicians who followed him regarded the body as a whole and treated diseases accordingly. One could not heal a diseased part of the body without treating the whole patient within the context of his or her diet and total environment.

"Let food be your medicine and medicine be your food." By the time Hippocrates uttered those words in the fourth century B.C., selecting foods for their specific healing properties had already been practiced for nearly two thousand years. Hippocrates and ancient healers who preceded him would wonder at our penchant for isolating certain disease-fighting food chemicals and then adding them to totally unrelated foods, to yield *functional* foods! To them all foods were functional—containing innate attributes that could alter the course of disease. Selecting foods most appropriate for the individual constituted the early practice of nutritional medicine.

Now, let's learn how these ancient healers matched appropriate foods with the individual and why they used body typing as an integral part of medical practice.

2

The Ancient Wisdom of *Eat Your Colors*

The idea of developing an eating strategy based on your constitutional or body type is not a new one. Body-typing systems have been practiced in India, Egypt, China, Japan, and Tibet for thousands of years. All ancient healers saw humans as part of the universe, resonating with its energetic principles. They based their spiritual, psychological, and medical systems on the natural world and man's place within the cosmos. The ancient systems regarded the individual as an extension of the great elements of the universe— air, earth, fire, ether (space or the void), and water. Just as nature keeps these elements in balance within the macrocosm, they must also be kept in balance within the microcosm—the human body. This may seem a little strange to our Western way of thinking, but it provides a simple and effective model for a better understanding of who we are.

> ❖ Ayurveda is a way of life, a way of cooperating with Nature and living in harmony with Her. Health in Ayurveda means harmony, and there is really no end to the degree of harmony you can achieve if you set yourself to the task.
> —Dr. Robert Svoboda, Ayurvedic physician

The Natural World and Medicine

The oldest continuously used healing system known to man is Ayurveda. The word Ayurveda means "knowledge of life" and this medical system was a dominant force in the development of all other medical systems throughout the world.

Ayurveda was developed in India and has been refined for over five thousand years. According to Vedic thinking, there are three fundamental forces within the universe—the creative, preservative, and transformative forces. These forces are also manifest within the body and are expressed as our basic constitution. The Ayurvedic constitution-based system grouped people according to their physical and psychological characteristics. Individuals sharing the same constitutional type would have corresponding strengths and weaknesses, and could be expected to respond in like manner to environmental challenges. Uniform treatment strategies based on this belief were designed for each type.

For thousands of years the teachings of Indian healers were passed orally from generation to generation. Several hundred years ago, physicians began keeping detailed records of what they observed, and eventually these records made up a significant body of medical information called the *Materia Medica*. This medical book defined patterns of disease and appropriate treatments. The oldest written accounts were recorded and modified between the eighth and third centuries B.C. Ancient Ayurveda, as these teachings have come to be called, was further modified during the intervening years into modern Ayurveda. We will now take some of the principles of modern Ayurveda and explain how they relate to your body type.

Ayurveda and Constitutional Typing

Ayurveda has identified three fundamental *forces* in nature. The first is the *creative force* that is evident when new life springs forth. The second is the *preservative force* that stores all the things necessary for birth. The third force is *transformative*, that which turns the preservative force into the creative force, as seen in new life. Humans are part of nature and as such also contain these three forces. In Ayurveda they are known as *doshas*. These natural forces must be kept in balance regardless of whether we're talking about the external world or that within our bodies. According to Dr. Robert Svoboda, a well-known Ayurvedic physician, the word *dosha* means "things which can go out of whack." Thus dosha expresses the ever-changing balance between the body's creative, preservative, and transformative processes. All the social, environmental, and cultural factors one is exposed to will affect the balance between the three doshas. Yet, while each of us is a unique combination of all three doshas, one of them will predominate. This is our constitutional type. Each person's dominant force or constitutional type was present at birth—determined by his or her parents' genes and constant throughout life. Does the creative force within you dominate the forces of transformation and preservation? Or, does either of the other two dominate? Once you have discovered which force dominates—your constitutional type—you will be able to understand why your body responds the way it does. You will be able to detect subtle changes in your response to the changing environment around you and take the necessary steps to restore your balance.

Balance between the three constitutional, or body, types has been recognized by Ayurvedic healers as essential for the maintenance of good health and freedom from disease. Over time, they developed elaborate systems around the types and this became the body of medical knowledge that was passed from generation to generation. The recommendations of traditional healers included lifestyle changes, spiritual and physical exercises, and a selection of specific foods, herbs, and spices. The practice of traditional medicine embodying constitutional typing is still practiced in China and India, alongside modern allopathic medicine. Modern Ayurveda is an increasingly popular medical system and is widely practiced in the United States and other Western countries.

> ❖ Although centuries old, the concept of individual constitution is a new concept for the Western mind, a new way for all of us to understand our "relationship" with Nature. Ayurveda is above all meant for all people who by harmonizing themselves seek to act as harmonizing forces in the universe.
>
> —Dr. Robert Svoboda

We now need to link each of the doshas, or forces, with a natural element that is a physical expression of that dosha. Later on, we will learn to recognize physical symptoms within our body that indicate which of our forces is out of balance—in other words, what's out of whack.

Constitutional Types and Their Link to the Natural World

The physical phenomena of the universe, including its natural elements, have been closely associated with body types throughout the history of Ayurveda. As noted at the beginning of this chapter, the five natural elements according to Ayurveda are earth, water, air, ether, and fire. According to physical laws, the first three—earth, water, and air—embody the three chemical states of matter. Earth, the most solid element, contains densely packed molecules with little movement. Therefore, it contains potential or stored energy but little kinetic or moving energy. Water molecules are less tightly packed and possess greater kinetic energy. They flow to fill their container, taking on the container's shape in the process. Air or gas molecules move most freely and are highest in kinetic energy. They bounce from place to place and have no visible or specific shape. This led early scientists to assume air molecules had little or no substance.

Now, what about the two remaining elements, fire and ether?

Fire is pure transforming energy that can turn solids to liquids and liquids to gases. The energy of fire, as everyone knows, is very hot and intense, and you will find these characteristics expressed in one of the three body types. Ether represents the void or space in which the other elements are free to take form. It contains no substance, shape, or energy but provides the invisible support for natural expression.

The three body types are physical expressions of these five elements, each type being a condensation of one or two elements. The elements are useful models to express our natural characteristics. Are you a fiery, intense kind of person who likes to get things done (transform)? Or, are you one who prefers stability (earth) and is slow to move like water? Are you a creative, airy type who has a hard time containing your natural enthusiasm? Our physical, emotional, and mental characteristics are the expression of the elements closely associated with our body type. Therefore your body type embraces both a natural element and a universal force. In Sanskrit, the language of Ayurveda, the three types are known as *Vata, Pitta,* and *Kapha.* The elements and forces associated with them are air/ether (creative), fire/water (transformative), and water/earth (preservative).

Vata manifests ether and air, and the characteristics of this type are closely associated with our concept of these elements. *Vata* is kinetic energy or movement, and physical symptoms commonly seen in this type are of an "airy" or "windy" nature. Vata types tend to have "internal wind"—expressed as intestinal gas when eating the wrong foods. They are also sensitive to "wind" or cold in the joints, and arthritis and stiffness are common problems. Vata types are creative and imaginative. They are also prone to nervousness and stiff aching joints.

Kapha embodies the elements of earth and water, and this type has the tendency to retain fluids and easily becomes congested with an excess of mucus. Kapha types move slowly, are apt to have a sluggish metabolism and have difficulty maintaining ideal weight. They are well-balanced, stable individuals who seek to preserve the status quo. They form long-term relationships and are a stabilizing influence in society.

Pitta is associated with fire and water. These individuals retain body heat, are always thirsty, sweat a lot, and tend to overeat. They complain of gastric upset, hyperacidity, and may experience a burning sensation when passing stools after eating the wrong foods. Pitta types are transformative and are good at getting ideas into action. They excel at organization and management.

Each body type will have a tendency toward a particular set of symptoms associated with its element. The characteristics of each type will be fully explored in chapter 3. The characteristics and associated symptoms will be used in the questionnaire in chapter 4 to help you identify your type. I will explore conditions that evolve from these symptoms more fully in chapter 16.

The Attributes of the Body Types

In addition, each type has inherent qualities or attributes that further characterize it and help us identify which one predominates in us. The attributes are paired characteristics: dry/wet, cold/hot, rough/smooth, sticky/clear, light/heavy, mobile/stable, hard/soft, liquid/solid, and gross/subtle. You will find questions about your attributes in the body-type questionnaire. Most important, the attributes are the basis for treatment of conditions. If you're cold, add heat. If dryness is present, use moisture. If sticky mucus is present, use foods and herbs to clarify and expel it. By familiarizing ourselves with the attributes for all the types, we can learn to recognize what's out of balance and take steps to relieve it before it becomes a serious problem. Many people can identify their inherent weaknesses. These are the unpleasant symptoms that frequently plague us. Fatigue after eating, interrupted sleep, nasal and throat catarrh (mucus) and lethargy are all symptoms of imbalance. Until now, we didn't know the cause or how to alleviate them. We also have conditions that only affect us from time to time. By knowing the attributes, you will be able to pick the appropriate strategy to overcome them. For example, you may be a dry Vata person but you catch a cold and have lots of congestion and mucus. Excess wetness is a Kapha symptom and so you adopt a Kapha diet until you recover. You are still a Vata type but your condition is Kapha. The wisdom of Ayurveda will teach you how to overcome your most common complaints and balance your type.

Constitutional Types and Color

This is a book about color—yours and that of the foods you should eat. Incredibly, Ayurveda has provided us with a color scheme based on our constitutional or body type. Therefore, I have chosen to use color to identify the body types in this book. Color will help you easily relate to your type and help associate the Ayurvedic body typing system into our Western way of thinking, particularly concerning the phytochemical content of foods. By knowing your color, you will be able to match it with appropriate-colored foods and get the phytochemicals most needed to keep you in balance. This is the basic plan for *Eat Your Colors*.

The color of Vata, pale yellow, is strongly associated with its attributes of lightness, dryness, and mobility. The color red gives us a mental image of fire and its heat and intensity, the attributes of Pitta. Blue-green, the color of water and the element associated with Kapha, is the ideal color for this type. From now on, I will refer to each of these types by their color. Now, let's show why a change of diet is the easiest and most useful way to stay healthy, and why diet is the factor that can most easily be controlled or adjusted in treating every individual.

Vata = Yellow
Pitta = Red
Kapha = Green

Using Food as Medicine

Diet has always been the basic component in Ayurvedic treatment strategies, and it will be the most important tool you can use in maintaining your own health. Ayurvedic and other traditional healers made their recommendations based on the constitutional type of the person being treated and relied on the innate healing intelligence of the body to overcome disease. They painstakingly categorized every food, herb, and spice according to the effect each had on the individual constitutional type. The dietary concepts and colors that were associated with each type are the basis for *Eat Your Colors* eating plans. Once you know your color, you can easily select foods that match your color. You will also learn to identify foods by their taste.

Foods were identified by ancient healers as one or a combination of six tastes: *sweet, salty, sour, bitter, astringent,* and *pungent.* The tastes were determined by rolling the food over the tongue and describing the resulting sensation. Among the tastes, we most often eat foods that are sweet, salty, or sour. These tastes predominate in Western diets and are found in snack foods, dairy products, meat, most seasonings, and sweeteners. By consuming an excess of these three tastes we are eating an unbalanced diet. Fruits, vegetables, and many culinary herbs and spices contain bitter, astringent, and pungent tastes and these are the foods we need to increase. They are also the most colorful foods and the ones I will concentrate on in the *Eat Your Colors* plans. Each type will have a specific color category of foods to choose from. Foods in your color category contain the healing phytochemicals—those right for your type.

Making some simple substitutions in your selection of foods will provide you with more nutritious foods. For example, most people choose iceberg lettuce, which is sweet, over darker bitter greens such as arugula, dandelion greens, endive, or romaine. Yet the darker bitter ones contain a wider range of phytochemicals with healing properties. Your daily food choices can be healthier if you make wiser choices based on what you learn in this book. There are even healthier choices for foods we don't consider especially healthy—like chocolate. Pure chocolate is a bitter food and one that has gotten a lot of press because of its antioxidants. In most chocolate confections the healthy bitter principle has been diluted by the addition of cocoa fat, sugar, and milk products that make up most of the weight of the finished product. Consuming chocolate with all these other unhealthy ingredients won't do you much good. However, if you are a chocolate aficionado, I suggest you choose products that are less processed and as bitter and dark as you can tolerate. Better still, choose bitter foods and herbs right for your color that will boost your digestive capacity.

Astringent foods are known for their distinctive "bite." The astringent principles are in the skin of most fruit. Those that are astringent, such as apples, grapes, berries, mangos, peaches, and cherries, have sweet-tasting flesh. Astringent vegetables such as the greens listed above often have a bitter aftertaste when they're chewed and swallowed. This doesn't win them any popularity contests among most Americans! While astringent foods may challenge our taste buds, they have strong medicinal properties that involve tissue contraction, elimination of swelling, and strengthening of blood vessels.

Pungent foods are aromatic. We experience this taste as much with our sense of smell as with our sense of taste. Many culinary spices and medicinal herbs are pungent. The pleasant aroma of cloves, cinnamon, curry, mustard, and hot peppers is familiar to most. Sea vegetables (seaweed), artichokes, beets, bell peppers, onions, radishes, turnips, and watercress are pungent vegetables. The pungency of onion and garlic is certainly apparent when they are cut or chopped. Pungent foods and herbs activate detoxification enzymes in the body. These enzymes expel poisons from the system and quench free radicals.

Eat Your Colors uses the sense of taste to identify foods that are best for your type. Yellows choose foods that taste salty, sweet, or sour. These include yellow and orange fruits, and vegetables rich in carotenoids. Reds choose foods that are sweet, bitter, or astringent, including red or purple fruits, and vegetables rich in polyphenols. Greens choose sour, astringent, and pungent foods, including cruciferous vegetables and dark leafy greens. You'll get more detailed information on tastes for your type in chapters 5–10. Using taste is an easy-to-grasp part of the *Eat Your Colors* system and will put you in tune with what your body is telling you. The more body signals you can learn to read, the more efficient you will become at maintaining your own health.

The body types are responsible for all physiological functions and they regulate bodily processes. Although one type will predominate—your color—the other two are also present. Your personal palette will provide foods that match your color and foods that complement it. You will learn to recognize when your colors are out of balance and make appropriate corrections with foods and supplements.

And so we go back to the beginning—the way nature intended. Keeping the body in harmony with its internal and external environment became and still is the central theme for Ayurvedic physicians. Great emphasis has always been placed on constitution in Ayurvedic medicine and its practitioners have been careful to treat their patients without aggravating their basic constitutional type. *Eat Your Colors* embodies the spirit of Ayurveda, teaching you how to keep yourself in balance and respond appropriately to life's challenges by modifying your eating habits.

3

What Defines Your Color?

We have seen how body typing was important in the Ayurvedic medical system and how it was the basis for a valid treatment strategy. Hippocrates reportedly borrowed from the Vedas in forming his humoral theory of four types—phlegm, black bile, yellow bile, and blood. He called his types "humors" and used them to describe physical and personality traits. He believed the predominance of one humor over the others determined one's physical characteristics and personality—reminiscent of the Ayurvedic system. These terms and their association with personality types persisted well into the Middle Ages. We still find the terms he used around today. *Sanguine* refers to the reddish color and passionate hot nature of the blood type. *Bilious* (yellow bile) describes a yellowish green color of bile and a disposition that is peevish and ill-humored. A person who is calm and has an unemotional temperament is described as *phlegmatic*. The humoral theory and its emphasis on body chemistry as the major factor in determining temperament has survived in some form for more than 2,500 years. As time passed, the psychological association of body typing assumed greater importance than physical associations. With the advent of modern psychology, body typing became even more popular. People today continue to be interested in body typing as a means of better understanding who they are.

Body Type and Personality

Several interpretations of body type, also known as somatotype, have been proposed in the last hundred years. Ernst Kretschmer, a German psychiatrist, formulated a morphological or body-type theory. He published his theory *Physique and Character* in 1921. Kretschmer's theory was popular in Germany through the 1940s but was not accepted much outside the country. In 1940, William H. Sheldon proposed a different morphological theory, three soma-totypes that grouped people according to their physical and personality traits. Dr. Sheldon named the types *endomorph, mesomorph,* and *ectomorph.* According to this classification system, endomorphs are good-natured people with a large round body and an excellent digestive capacity. Meso-morphs are muscular with a squarish frame. They love adventure, like to dominate, are assertive and bold. Ectomorphs are tall and thin, flat-chested, and tend to be introverted, creative, and anxious. The three body types bear some striking similarities to the Ayurvedic model. However, Sheldon's system places much more emphasis on psychological traits than Ayurveda. More-over, it only serves to classify people without offering any nutrition solution to overcoming their innate weakness. Although widely embraced at the time, Sheldon's theory has fallen into disrepute.

Body Typing and Diet

In 1996, Peter D'Adamo published the popular book *Eat Right 4 Your Type.* Dr. D'Adamo's system is based on blood type and how the four types—O, A, B, and AB—evolved as early man migrated from Africa across Asia, and Europe. This theory is intriguing in that it regards blood type as resulting from evolutionary change. It is a better system than those that preceded it because it links diet with blood type. And it is a step in the right direction in that it recommends diets appropriate for each type. However, using blood types as a basis for food selection lacks the substance and validation of the Ayurvedic system.

Body Typing and Athletics

Body type may be useful in athletics as a determinant of exercise capability. William Bolonchuk, Ph.D., and colleagues at the U.S. Agricultural Research Service investigated the metabolic responses to exercise of tall, thin men and those who were more muscular or even mildly overweight. Not surprisingly, they found that while the tall, thin people were able to do as much work as their more muscular colleagues, they were not as efficient at extracting oxy-gen from air. It took more inhalation and exhalation of air to derive the same volume of oxygen and they accumulated more lactic acid in their muscles. The investigators attributed this to lower muscle mass in the lean men and thus fewer energy-producing components. This work is an example of valida-tion by modern science of the Ayurvedic model. There is a physiological basis for the observation that tall, lean individuals do not handle exercise in the same way as heavier counterparts. While more muscular men excel at power and strength activities, lean individuals do better at endurance sports.

It seems we never tire of our quest to discover who we are, why we excel at some things, and why we react to our environment the way we do. Ayurveda provides the answers to these questions. Let's see what Ayurveda teaches about each body type.

The Three Types: Case Histories

Yellow

Sue is a typical Yellow type—tall with a slender build—one of the lucky ones who never have a weight problem. In fact, she has trouble keeping weight on, and efforts to put on muscle weight have not been successful. Although generally pleased with her slim build, Sue has always been critical of her overly large joints which seemed to be a mismatch for her otherwise lithe body. Sue is a high-energy person, moving about quickly, often flitting from one place to another as if she were a butterfly. When she speaks, her voice comes in quick bursts and she has difficulty staying with one topic. If she speaks for extended periods of time, her voice weakens, making it difficult to continue.

Sue's skin is clear with a tendency toward dryness, especially during the winter months when her cuticles crack and her heels become extremely rough. Sue's hair is straight, dark, and thin with a tendency to break easily. Her brown eyes are set close together with a gaze that frequently appears unattached.

Sue's appetite tends to vary from day to day and she is a fanatic and picky eater, preferring health drinks and plain vegetarian fare. Yet despite healthful eating habits, Sue is bothered by frequent discomfort after meals. On occasion her sleep is interrupted by intestinal gas and she has had problems with constipation since childhood. She has depended on laxatives much of her life.

Sue is a nervous type who tends to be anxious and fearful. Seemingly trivial matters can cause her much distress and she seems unable to put them out of mind. She loses considerable sleep while trying to work through them. Now at midlife, Sue has started to complain of stiffness and aching in her joints and is afraid she is "falling apart." It started with one knee joint making noise when she walked. Her chiropractor attributed her creaking joints and increasing stiffness to biomechanical problems. He discovered that Sue's left leg is a little shorter than her right and this was putting undue stress on the latter. Years of wear and tear from running had taken their toll and he advised against engaging in any high-impact aerobics.

Sue has also battled muscle cramping in her feet and also across her shoulders. She has experienced some irregularity in heartbeat, especially when she's tired or stressed. However, her physician decided the symptoms were not a cause for concern, after he did a complete workup. He did advise her to cut back on caffeinated beverages and this alleviated the problem.

She owns her own retail business but leaves the management of her store to an employee. She has built a good business through involvement in the community. As her community service duties have increased, she has been less involved in the day-to-day running of her store. Yet, her business is profitable enough to permit Sue frequent travel around the world. She prefers to visit exotic places such as the rain forest and obscure South Sea islands.

I am going to describe the Yellow constitutional characteristics now and you will see why Sue typifies this type.

Characteristics of the Yellow (Air/Ether) Type

Physical—The Yellow body type is lean, tends to be flat-chested and not muscular. Joints may appear large in proportion to their long, lean frame. Yellow types are constantly in motion, although their quick movement tends to be awkward and uncoordinated. They don't have a lot of stamina and their constant motion wears them out. If they engage in sports, they are most likely to prefer endurance sports, although they don't have the energy reserves to compete effectively in distance events.

Yellows tend to have dry skin that is rough and cracks easily. They may have a few prominent dark moles. Their hair also tends toward dryness and is difficult to manage. Nails are brittle, break easily, and are often bitten. Yellow types complain of being cold and their hands and feet are usually cold. The noses of Yellows are often either bent (hooked) or turned up at the end. A deviated septum is common among Yellows. They usually have crooked teeth and the two halves of their bodies may be mismatched—limbs being longer on one side or feet that are different sizes.

Dietary Habits—Yellow types love change and their eating habits reflect this. Their appetite varies from day to day and so does their digestion. It's important for these types to eat substantial foods that help anchor them energetically. Yellows are fast metabolizers in that calories are burned quickly and weight gain may be difficult. They get dizzy and spacy in between meals and must eat quickly to restore energy levels. This tendency is most pronounced when they drink a lot of caffeine and eat sugary foods. These nervous fidgety types overeat when pressured—either trying to meet tight deadlines or engaged in too many exciting activities. Such overindulgence often meets with digestive problems, gas, and constipation. If Yellows do gain weight, it's around their belly and this may be the only part of their physique that doesn't look thin.

This type does best with warm foods and beverages, unless the weather is extremely hot. The best tastes for them are sweet foods that support their body's demand for energy; sour foods that aid digestion; and salty foods that help their bodies retain moisture. Yellows are the only types that can eat beef, but this depends on how efficient their digestion is. They're OK with chicken, especially dark meat, but may have problems with turkey, which is drier. Yellows can eat almost any fruit except the red/purple ones (apples, rhubarb, raspberries, pomegranate, Satsuma plums, and raw tomatoes). They have problems digesting foods that cause gas, such as green peppers, raw onions, raw garlic, beans, peanuts, and cabbage, or that are dry and crunchy such as cereals, popcorn, crusty breads, crackers, and chips. Most Yellows tend to be constipated—often alternating between loose and hard stools.

Brain and Nervous System—Yellow types have sensitive nervous systems and when they eat the wrong foods, they get nervous, agitated, irritable, depressed, and have difficulty sleeping. They also don't respond well to excessive use of stimulants such as caffeine, and alcohol wires them, rather than having the expected sedating effects. Yellows often suffer from central nervous system problems such as headaches, sharp pains or cramps in the solar plexus, neck and shoulder pain, joint pain, lower back pain, arthritis, neuralgia, sciatica, and insomnia. They can also develop heart murmurs, arrhythmia, angina, and high blood pressure—all the result of overstimulation of the central nervous system.

Yellow types are creative but have difficulty staying with tasks long enough to complete them. They are quick to learn, have very creative minds, but have difficulty remembering things. Even dreams are difficult for them to remember. Yellow types love to chatter happily away and will converse with themselves if no one else is around. They even talk in their sleep and are prone to waking in the middle of the night with wonderful and creative schemes. It seems their brains are constantly busy—even as they sleep. A recurring theme for Yellows' dreams is flying or soaring. If speaking is part of their career, they need training to keep thoughts flowing smoothly and give a cogent delivery. Voice training also teaches them how to keep from straining their vocal cords. Otherwise, they tend to tire and lose their voices when speaking for prolonged periods of time.

Psychological and Spiritual—Yellows bore easily and are always looking for new adventures. They love to travel, move from place to place, and frequently rearrange furniture in their home. They usually take on more than they can handle and then worry about missed deadlines. They have an innate fear of failure. Yellows have a tendency to harbor a poor self-image and be self-deprecating. They love to be involved in groups but are not interested in being in charge. They often have difficulty with relationships and don't seem to retain long-term friendships.

Yellows have a deep sense of spirituality and love to explore the deeper meaning of life. They inspire others, yet crave solitude. This type easily achieves deep spiritual understanding. However, the exercise of religious beliefs changes quite often and Yellows may even experiment with extreme sects.

Lifestyle—Yellows don't like authority or rules, preferring to make their own. They like having their own business but are not good money managers. Therefore they will likely run into trouble if not partnered with someone who manages the business for them. Professions in which Yellows do well include international affairs, political consultant, foreign minister, interpreter/translator, teacher, lecturer, author, law enforcement, musician, philosopher, counselor, monk, clergy, union leader, inventor, and artist.

Yellows love the sun and prefer warmer climates. They respond well to massage therapy and visiting a spa gives them a new lease on life. Exercise is difficult for Yellows because of their inconsistent energy levels. However, yoga, tai chi, and chi gong are excellent choices. Yellows should not exercise vigorously, but many do, believing it is good for them.

The most difficult time of year for the Yellow type is fall, and this is when health challenges are most likely to occur. Yellow types are prone to sleep problems between 2 and 6 A.M. and are likely to feel fatigued between 2 and 6 P.M. Accordingly, they should not plan tasks that require intense concentration during the afternoon hours. They generally like to rise very early and go to bed before 10 P.M.

Red

Pete is of medium height, well built, and very fit. His skin is light, freckled, prone to sunburn and his thinning hair is light reddish brown and somewhat oily. He has large expressive hazel eyes that focus sharply. Pete has always preferred cooler climates since he seems to be hot all the time. His skin is sensitive and he burns easily. As a teenager, Pete had acne problems, and he still breaks out in rashes when encountering allergens.

Pete has a hearty appetite and needs to eat on time. He gets irritable and grouchy when meals are late. He always eats breakfast, usually oatmeal or some other grain, before he goes to work. Pete also loves to cook and throws himself into elaborate multicourse meal preparation. He doesn't tolerate interference when he's working in the kitchen. It seems he is totally engaged in food preparation as an expression of both his skill and artistic nature. He specializes in preparing Asian and Indian dishes and has become an expert at combining the exotic flavors of these cuisines. He likes to serve something sweet after meals, but it's generally light and fairly simple.

Pete has excellent energy levels and exercises daily, running at least five miles. He loves to work and spends long hours at his job as a division manager of a large international company. He is well liked, has been promoted often, and is on the fast track in advancing through his company. He has good organizational skills and is fair-minded with his subordinates, although he won't tolerate substandard performance. He is known for his rectitude and can be quite unforgiving of others who display less upstanding character. Pete has a sharp intellect and an excellent memory. He enjoys teaching others but has little patience for those who are slow or unwilling to learn.

He has always done well in physical skills, concentrating on those that require artistic talent. As a child, he won competitions in model building and as a young adult enjoyed stage set construction, welding, and woodworking. Pete is intensely competitive, directing his energies toward completing projects at work and at home. When pushed, he can be extremely blunt and argumentative. He has a quick temper, which he has learned to keep under wraps. No one misses the fact, however, that he is angry.

Now, let's see how Pete's characteristics categorize him as a Red type.

Characteristics of the Red (Fire/Water) Type

Physical—Red types are of medium build, with a well-proportioned body and athletic appearance if they are fit. They are well-coordinated, decisive, and purposeful in movement. Their hair is fine, often reddish or copper-hued with a tendency toward premature graying or balding. People with red in their hair have strong Red tendencies even if they are primarily Yellow or Green types. Red types have soft warm skin, blush easily, and have rosy cheeks or a ruddy complexion. They have lots of freckles and several moles. Their skin is oily or they may have oily patches in their complexion. Their skin is sensitive, burns easily, and breaks out in acne or impetigo. They perspire a lot, even when the weather is cold. Their eyes are usually gray, green, or copper/brown and large with intense or sharp visage. Their nails are soft, flexible, and well formed. The noses of Reds are straight and sharp, often with a reddened tip.

Dietary Habits—Reds have a strong, steady metabolism and consistent energy levels. They have great stamina, good appetites, and strong digestion. They gain and lose weight easily and excess weight accumulates evenly on their body. They prefer cold drinks, carbohydrate foods (grains, cereals, bread, beans, pasta, root vegetables) for sustained energy, and bitter vegetables such as arugula, collards, dandelion greens, endive, kale, and sprouts that improve digestion. They also do well with astringent foods, including cruciferous vegetables, green beans, parsnips, potatoes, spinach, squash, and sweet potatoes. The best fruits are red/purple (apples, rhubarb, raspberries, pomegranate, Satsuma plums), all berries, melons, avocados, coconut, dates, figs, grapes, pears, and prunes. Cod, haddock, and whitefish are good for Reds, but pork and red meat other than lamb increase their naturally hot constitution. They also do well with poultry. Beans and most grains, except buckwheat, rye, soy, and brown rice, are good for Reds and they do best on a mostly vegetarian diet.

Brain and Nervous System—Reds have great mental energy and can easily process new information and act upon it—displaying high levels of intelligence. They plan and oversee projects with efficiency and like to be in charge, leaving the implementation to others. They have a heightened sense of competitiveness and can be aggressive, bossy, and fanatical. They are quick to anger and may have hot explosive tempers, although most have learned to control their emotions. They are often impatient with others who don't measure up to their standards or are slow to grasp concepts.

Red types have excellent memories and remember details others have long forgotten. They can harbor a grudge for a long time and, when wronged, don't immediately get mad, they just wait to get even. Some Reds love to stir up trouble or precipitate a crisis, especially if they are feeling neglected or insecure.

Psychological and Spiritual—Red types are ambitious and like to accumulate material wealth. They enjoy displaying their wealth and generally purchase the best they can afford. Reds like to hoard possessions, although they are also generous and enjoy gift-giving. They will spend money for things they consider important but are careful not to spend foolishly.

The dreams of Red types are vivid, passionate, and intense—and they dream in full color. Reds are most likely to be the dominant figures in their dreams and have good dream recall. Money matters are a common theme in their dreams. Red types are generally light sleepers and can get by on little sleep, waking refreshed and alert. Reds are good communicators, always direct and to the point. They are respected for their opinions, which are proffered generously. What they have to say is clear and focused in content. When out of balance, Reds tend to be combative, aggressive, and confrontational.

Reds can be very spiritual once they set aside their egos and learn to go with the flow. A humble compassionate spirit tames the red fire. Reds can, however, be very fanatical about their beliefs or religion.

Lifestyle—The lifestyle role of Red types is fostering progress. They are good at taking ideas and forming a plan for implementing them. They don't necessarily enjoy doing the detail work, but they are good managers and instill teamwork in subordinates. Professions for Reds include administrator, director, president, attorney, physician, career military, architect, engineer, scientist, systems manager, computer programmer, and actor. Many professional athletes are Red types. They excel in sports that demand power and stamina.

The best seasons of the year for Reds are fall, winter, and spring. Summer heat is a challenge for them and the time of year when they are most likely to experience health challenges. The most difficult time of the day for them is between 10 and 2, both A.M. and P.M. They like to stay up late at night, but should get into bed before midnight.

Typical Conditions—Reds are prone to inflammatory disorders and likely to have digestive pain and complaints. They are also prone to vascular inflammation such as systematic infections, cellulitis, phlebitis, and vasculitis. Reds tend to have gallbladder, bile and liver disorders, hyperacidity, heartburn, peptic ulcer, gastritis, impaired intestinal absorption, and digestive enzyme function. They are also prone to skin disorders (acne, psoriasis, hives, rashes), varicose veins, broken capillaries and hemorrhoids. Reds can have weak vision and get eye infections such as styes and conjunctivitis more easily than the other types. Reds tend to have loose burning stools when they have too much hot spicy food, red meat, or alcohol.

Green

Art is a typical Green type—a large man with heavy bone structure, wide shoulders and large square hands. He is not heavily muscled, but his erect posture and quiet self-assurance lend a powerful and commanding presence. Like most Green types, Art could easily gain weight, were he less physically active. Being a successful builder and lifelong outdoorsman keeps him in excellent shape. Art has thick, wavy blond hair that shows no signs of thinning despite his age, just past fifty. He has expressive blue/green eyes and soft, somewhat oily skin that tans well.

Art has a ready pleasant smile and nice, even white teeth. His overall demeanor is agreeable and he's well liked—one of those people to whom others are instinctively drawn. They feel a certain confidence in Art's physical skills and willingness to help, which has sometimes led them to take advantage of Art's good nature. He'll put up with a certain amount of this and then can be quite adamant about not providing further assistance.

Art has a good appetite and enjoys all kinds of food except dairy. He loved to drink milk as a child but found out he is allergic to it. Now he avoids all dairy products except cheese. Art can eat large amounts of food without gaining much weight because of his large frame and high activity level. He has good digestion except when he eats too much pizza or too many sweet foods. Then he is bothered by burping, belching, and heaviness soon after eating. He loves meat and poultry, preferring them barbecued. He also enjoys salads, potatoes, and vegetables. Art doesn't bother with breakfast, but depends on coffee to get going. He takes a cooler to work, usually filled with leftover meat, bread, and some fruit, which he eats at no particular time during the day. He usually works through lunch, preferring to keep a steady pace throughout the day. Despite his physical work, Art needs recreational exercise to feel his best. He tends to get moody and obstinate if he doesn't engage in one of his favorite sports at least three times a week.

Now, let's see why Art is a typical Green type.

Characteristics of the Green (Water/Earth) Type

Physical—Green types have clear, bright complexions and their skin is soft, lustrous and oily. Unlike Red types, their skin is cool to the touch and pale rather than red-tinged. Their hair can be blond, black, or light brown with blond highlights. It can be either straight or wavy and is usually quite thick. Their eyes are large and expressive, blue, green, or light brown in color. Greens have well-formed, strong fingernails and hands with square palms and short strong fingers. They are well coordinated and athletic—linebackers typify Green types. For Green water types like Art, regular mealtimes are not important and, when their diets are balanced, they have good digestion.

Dietary Habits—When Greens gain weight, it is distributed around their buttocks and thighs, as opposed to all over the body for Reds and around the middle for Yellows. Their digestion is steady and slow and they are slow metabolizers. Greens crave pungent foods to get them going. These include artichokes, beets, brussels sprouts, carrots, corn, garlic, horseradish, radishes, leeks, mushrooms, and strong spices like allspice, anise, black pepper, cayenne, cloves, mustard, and rosemary. They also do well with bitter foods such as arugula, collards, dandelion, and endive, and spices such as fenugreek, cumin, coriander, dill, peppermint, and wintergreen. Greens also tolerate coffee and tea, provided they don't drink too much of it. They tolerate alcohol better than the other types but must be careful not to drink excessively. A little red wine with dinner can help promote good digestion in Greens.

Most fruit and fruit juices other than apple don't agree with Greens and they don't handle sweet foods well at all. When out of balance, Greens can use food or drink as a source of emotional fulfillment and they may overindulge in cheese and ice cream—foods that are too sweet, heavy, and cold for them. Greens should avoid beef and pork, but they do well with poultry, lamb, organ meats, and shellfish, provided their cholesterol is normal. They should avoid eggs and dairy products.

Brain and Nervous System—Greens are naturally cautious and may seem slow to grasp concepts. However, once they learn something, they never forget it. They deliberate carefully and are good at details. They have excellent memories and are a calm stable force. Change is upsetting to Greens, and when they get out of balance, they can be stubborn, obstinate, and unyielding. Greens have strong opinions but keep them primarily to themselves. They abhor confrontation and will avoid it whenever possible. They aren't fond of talking, but when motivated to do so, clearly articulate their thoughts in a slow even pace.

Psychological and Spiritual—Greens have great patience and fortitude, although they may have difficulty getting going. They form long-lasting and stable relationships and are well liked by everyone. Greens are very fair-minded and are hard to rile up. When they feel taken advantage of they will get angry and can be a formidable foe. Greens have a steady and unshakable faith.

Dreams for Green types are not especially important and they quickly forget them. The most recurring theme is peace and calm, just a lovely experience. Dreams are uneventful and not particularly colorful. When upset over something, Greens can have dreams that are intense and emotional, so much so that sleep is disturbed. This is unusual for Greens, who love to sleep and do so deeply.

Lifestyle—Greens typify the wise seer whom others instinctively trust. They excel at detailed work and jobs that require steady, patient performance. Professions they do well at include accountant, teacher, technician, mechanic, production worker, dancer, musician, poet, gardener, curator, collector, interior decorator, negotiator, and homemaker.

Greens do best with heavy and consistent exercise. Many endurance athletes are Greens. Linebackers are often Greens. Green types like to collect possessions and they also like to hold on to their money. People who are known skinflints no doubt have considerable amounts of Green in their makeup.

The worst time of the year for Greens is winter and early spring. The time of day or night most challenging for them is 6 to 10 A.M. and P.M. Greens do best when they get up before 6 A.M. and go to bed early, between 9 and 10 P.M.

Conditions—Greens are most challenged by immune and respiratory conditions. They also have strong tendencies toward diabetes and insulin resistance disorders. If not active, these people put on a lot of weight. Obesity is a common condition among Greens. This makes them vulnerable to cardiovascular disorders as well. When overweight, they should keep an eye on changes in blood chemistry such as elevated cholesterol, triglycerides, and HDL and LDL ratios. Like Yellows, they can have cardiac arrhythmia and low back pain. Greens can develop congestive heart failure, asthma, and emphysema. Other common health problems for Green types are hay fever, food allergies, chronic sinus congestion, and belching or bloating, especially after eating the wrong foods. They may feel so tired after eating, they just want to take a nap.

You may have already identified strongly with one of these types—Yellow, Red, or Green. Now let's move on to the next chapter, which contains detailed questionnaires that should help you identify which is your primary type.

4

What Is My Type?

In this chapter, you will identify your body type: Green, Red, or Yellow. You will likely find that you're a mix of colors, not a pure body type. However, one color will predominate and that's your primary color. The other types are your complementary colors. You have inherited characteristics from both your parents, and this is what determines your type. You may also have wondered how to avoid family disease tendencies. *Eat Your Colors* will help you to clearly understand your type and how to stay healthy. You will be able to design your personal color palette, choosing your colors from the food groups discussed in Part Two.

You may find it helpful to have someone close to you help answer some of the questions since we all carry preconceived notions of who we are. You may also find the totals for all three colors are close. Having someone assist you with the test will help determine if you really are a balance of colors, which is possible, or if your answers were not accurate. It's also a good idea to have others in your family identify their colors too, so that you can more effectively plan meals. The dietary guidelines in this book have been refined over many centuries, and by following them you will experience greater energy, enjoy better stress adaptation, maintain your ideal weight, and stay healthy.

We are honoring the Ayurvedic tradition by using the *Eat Your Colors* system. By using the language of colors—primary and complementary—we are creating a model that helps us select foods that are harmonizing and balancing.

The following questions each have three possible answers: one will best describe you. Circle the letter of the answer that best describes you. You should skip any questions that don't apply. When you have answered all the questions, total the *a*'s you have circled, then repeat for circled *b*'s and *c*'s. A key at the end will identify the color for each letter. The color with the highest number of circled items is your type. The color or colors with fewer circles will be your complementary colors.

Body Type Questionnaire

Physical Characteristics:

1. Which best describes your body type?
   - ✓a. medium frame
   - b. heavy frame
   - c. lean frame

2. My body is generally
   - ✓a. well proportioned
   - b. massive
   - c. not well proportioned (e.g., legs or arms too short or too long for trunk)

3. I have
   - ✓a. medium-width shoulders and hips
   - b. wide shoulders and hips
   - c. narrow shoulders and hips

4. My bones and joints are
   - ✓a. normal in size and joints are in proportion to the rest of my frame
   - b. bones are heavy and strong with large deep-set joints
   - c. bones are light, but joints are large and prominent (finger joints are a good indicator)

5. Which of the following best describes your hands?
   - ✓a. I have medium-length fingers.
   - b. I have short, stubby fingers.
   - c. I have long, tapering fingers.

6. My teeth are
   - ✓a. even and well formed but prone to cavities
   - b. large, white and even, with few cavities
   - c. crooked or protruding, may be sensitive to hot or cold

7. Which of the following best describes your eyes?
   - ✓ a. moderate in size; penetrating blue, green, gray, or hazel in color

   b. large and luminous; light blue or light brown
   c. small and deep-set slate blue, violet, deep brown, or black

 8. How would others describe your look?
   a. sharp, focused, and intense
   ✓b. calm, expressive, loving
   c. unfocused, darting

 9. My eyes are often
   a. reddened and burning
   ✓b. clear but itchy
   c. grayish, bluish sclera (white of the eye) and scratchy

10. My nose is
   ✓a. long and straight and the tip is red
   b. short and rounded with a button tip
   c. medium in size with a deviated septum

11. How would you describe your skin?
   ✓a. My skin is sensitive and easily irritated.
   b. I have oily skin that tans well.
   c. I have dry skin that tends to be rough.

12. What is your skin color, compared to others in your family?
   ✓a. reddish with lots of freckles and moles, blushes easily
   b. light to dark with no freckles, thick skin
   c. deep color with a few moles, thin skin

13. What is the appearance of your chin and neck?
   ✓a. tapering chin, medium-length neck
   b. round full chin, folds on neck
   c. angular chin, may be too small or too large for upper jaw, long skinny
       neck

14. What color is your hair?
   a. red, strawberry blond, brown with red highlights, or prematurely gray
       or balding
   b. light brown or blond without red highlights
   ✓c. dark brown or black

15. How would you describe your hair?
   ✓a. fine, thin, and straight.

    b. oily, thick, and wavy with good luster.

    c. thin, lusterless, possibly curly or kinky

16. How would you describe your voice and the way you talk?

    a. I like to get to the point when I speak and my voice is strong.

    b. I don't like to talk and when I do I speak slowly and carefully.

    ✓c. I love to talk, although my voice weakens if I speak for long periods of time.

Psychological:

1. Which best describes your emotions?

    a. I form strong opinions and don't mind confrontation.

    ✓b. I have opinions but dislike confrontation.

    c. I am slow to form opinions and don't like to be confrontational.

2. I am apt to be

    a. impatient and quick to anger

    b. easygoing and slow to anger

    ✓c. fearful of failing, anxious

3. Which best describes your personality?

    a. strong and forceful

    b. calm, quiet, steady

    ✓c. sensitive, high-strung

4. The best thing about your personality is

    ✓a. being very practical

    b. having great fortitude and patience

    c. being flexible and changeable

5. How do you prefer to plan your time?

    ✓a. I do best following a schedule.

    b. I prefer a looser schedule.

    c. I dislike schedules.

6. How would you best describe your friendships?

    a. I form close friendships with those at work.

    ✓b. I form long-lasting friendships, not necessarily from work.

    c. I have difficulty sustaining friendships.

7. Which of these best describes how you acquire new information?

    a. I learn quickly and remember things well.

    ✓b. I learn a little more slowly but never forget.

    c. I learn very fast but have trouble remembering things.

8. Which of these best describes your learning process?
    a. I focus intently on what I'm learning and find it easy to concentrate.
    b. I stick with it until I understand; my concentration is good.
    ✓c. I have poor concentration; my mind wanders easily.

9. Which best describes how you like to work?
    a. I like to plan strategies and oversee their development.
    b. I like to carry out plans, develop keen skills.
    ✓c. I like to learn new things and form theories.

10. Which best describes your money habits?
    a. I spend money carefully, work within a budget, may enjoy bargaining.
    b. I don't like to spend money, don't need a budget.
    ✓c. I like to spend money and don't like to budget.

Metabolism:

1. How would you describe your energy levels?
    a. I have good exercise capacity and can pace myself well when I exercise.
    b. I have great stamina but I have to push to exercise.
    ✓c. I like to exercise but run out of energy quickly.

2. How would you describe your coordination and movement?
    a. I am well coordinated and move smoothly and with efficiency.
    b. I am well coordinated and move slowly and purposefully.
    ✓c. I am not particularly well coordinated and move very quickly.

3. What is your experience with weight gain or loss?
    a. I gain weight easily but I can also lose it easily.
    ✓b. I gain weight easily and have a hard time losing it.
    c. I generally stay the same weight.

4. When you gain weight, where does it tend to gather in your body?
    a. My fat distribution is even throughout my body.
    ✓b. My fat gathers around my hips and thighs.
    c. My weight gain is a "potbelly" (female) or "spare tire" (male).

5. What is your general level of activity?
    ✓a. I am moderately active.

   b. I am not active and have a tendency toward lethargy.

   c. I am very active.

6. What are your general perspiration levels?
   a. I perspire a lot even when it's cold.
   b. I have consistent levels of moderate perspiration.
   c. I rarely perspire heavily.

7. What best describes your sleep pattern?
   a. light sleeper, fall asleep easily if awakened; wake rested and need little sleep
   b. love to sleep and wake rested when I get enough sleep
   c. trouble falling asleep and can't go back to sleep if awakened; wake up tired

8. Which of these statements best describes your dreams?
   a. Very intense, often violent and occur in vivid colors; I have good dream recall.
   b. Very pleasant and uneventful; I seldom try to remember them.
   c. Erratic, may include flying or soaring; I have difficulty remembering them.

9. Which of these describes your menstrual cycles? (women only)
   a. regular, prolonged with heavy bleeding
   b. regular but light pale blood
   c. irregular and light

10. What are your PMS symptoms? (women only)
   a. very light cramping, irritability
   b. no cramping, some bloating and water retention
   c. intense cramping, diarrhea or nausea

Appetite and Digestion:

1. Which of the following best describes your appetite?
   a. I have a good appetite and tend to overeat.
   b. I enjoy food but can easily skip meals.
   c. The amount I eat varies from day to day, but I feel weak if I don't eat often.

2. What are your breakfast eating habits?
   a. I do best with a light breakfast.

    b. Skipping breakfast is easy for me.

    c. I function best when I have eaten a good breakfast.

3. Do you ever fast?
    a. I can fast, but I'm apt to be grouchy. ✓
    b. Fasting is easy for me.
    c. Fasting is difficult for me.

4. How much liquid do you typically consume?
    a. I drink a lot of liquids.
    ✓ b. I drink very little.
    c. My drinking habits are erratic.

5. What are your general eating habits?
    a. I eat quickly and often more than I should.
    ✓ b. I eat slowly and moderate-sized servings.
    c. I usually eat on the run and often can't finish what's on my plate.

6. Which of the following best describes your digestive process?
    a. I have at least one bowel movement daily.
    ✓ b. I have good digestion and regular bowel habits.
    c. I am frequently constipated, or alternate with loose stools.

7. When experiencing indigestion, which area of your body is uncomfortable?
    a. the middle, just beneath my ribs
    ✓ b. upper part, under my ribs
    c. around my navel and lower

8. At what temperature do you prefer your foods and beverages?
    a. cool beverages and warm, not hot food
    ✓ b. both hot and cold food and beverages
    c. hot food and beverages

9. What is your frequency of urination?
    a. very frequent
    ✓ b. moderate
    c. not much and tend to hold it

10. What season of the year is most challenging for you?
    ✓ a. summer
    b. winter
    c. autumn

Career:

11. Circle the career(s) that apply to you.

Type A *(loves to foster progress)*	Type B *(likes technical skills)*	Type C *(champions causes)*
administrator, director, president, designer, architect, engineer, scientist, manager, actor, doctor, media personality, pilot, career military, banker	chef, healer, task force member, accountant, technician, programmer, mechanic, production worker, dancer, negotiator, gardener, interior decorator, counselor, curator, collector, customer service, sales, construction	teacher, philosopher, musician, lecturer, law enforcement, international liaison, foreign minister, communicator, political consultant, religious, monk, minister, charity organizer, inventor, artist, writer

Conditions:

12. Circle any of the following characteristics that apply to you:

Group A
1. bruise easily
2. rapid or irregular heartbeat
3. high blood pressure
4. anemia
5. astigmatism, cataracts, glaucoma

Group B
1. frequent respiratory infections
2. lower back pain
3. chronic sinusitis
4. frequent colds or flu
5. poor sense of taste

Group C
1. receding gums
2. scoliosis or crooked limbs
3. frequent muscle cramps in legs or feet

4. frequent tension in neck and shoulders

5. nervous, high-strung

13. Circle any of the conditions for which you have a family history (mother, father, sister, brother, grandparents). These conditions may also be present in you.

Group A

1. heart disease
2. hepatitis
3. gallstones
4. leukemia
5. skin cancer
6. acne, boils, dermatitis
7. eye diseases; styes, conjunctivitis, "dry" eye
8. depression

Group B

1. diabetes
2. obesity
3. congestive heart failure
4. emphysema
5. hay fever or chronic sinusitis
6. pneumonia
7. gastric ulcers
8. asthma

Group C

1. food allergies
2. arthritis
3. diseases of the colon like irritable bowel syndrome, diverticulitis, colon cancer
4. anxiety disorder
5. sore throat, tonsillitis, strep throat
6. hypertension, arrhythmia
7. incontinence
8. erectile dysfunction, low sperm count

Scoring: Count up the number of *a*'s, *b*'s, and *c*'s you circled. For the conditions section, count the number of items you circled under *a*, *b*, or *c*, and add them to your score. Your totals for each letter will tell you your color: *A* corresponds with Red, *B* with Green, and *C* with Yellow. The highest total will indicate your primary color. One color may predominate (a very high total for one color) or, like most people, you will have one or two scores close in value. The relative values of the totals will indicate your particular blend of colors.

Now that you know your type, let's move on to Part Two, where you will learn which foods are your color. I am going to return to the language of science I introduced in Chapter 1. I will explain how the phytochemicals in each of the six food groups work in your body and why you should eat them.

Foods and Phytochemicals: Why You Should Eat Your Colors

❖

Right now, the only thing that's saving us
from scurvy is the french fry!
—Paul Lachance, Ph.D.,
professor of food science,
Rutgers University

5

Yellow Foods

You may be accustomed to choosing brightly colored fruits and vegetables for their visual appeal and using them to create meals that are more appetizing. But did you know that the colors—various shades of yellow, orange, green and red—are due to plant pigments, and that these pigments are not just ordinary colors, but powerful disease-fighting phytochemicals? The colors come from a large family of natural plant compounds called terpenes whose best-known members are carotenoids and vitamin E. Carotenoid-rich fruits and vegetables are visually appealing, and they are what originally inspired the concept of *Eat Your Colors*.

If you are a Yellow type or Yellow combination type, yellow, orange, green, and red are your primary colors and you should eat at least one food from each of these groups every day. Carotenoids are some of the most powerful disease-preventing agents known and they are the primary colors for Yellow types. There is a wide variety to choose from: yellow and orange squash, carrots, sweet potatoes, yams, all tropical fruits, all citrus fruits, most yellow/green and all red vegetables, to name just a few. The darker green carotenoids are also good for Green types, while those that are orange/red are best for Red types. A complete guide for who should eat which carotenoid is given at the end of this chapter.

What Are Carotenoids?

Carotenoids are fat-soluble compounds that occur in a wide variety of plants that protect them from sun damage (photooxidation) and aid in attracting birds and insects for pollination. Some animals, notably birds with bright yellow, red, and green plumage, get their coloration from the carotenoids in their diet. Female birds seem to be drawn to the more brightly colored males. Studies have shown that those males have had a better diet, are healthier, and will thus produce better offspring. In humans, the biologically active carotenoids we get from our diet also determine our overall health. The carotenoids are concentrated in the membranes surrounding cells and their internal components. From this strategic location carotenoids can impact numerous cellular events and affect the health of the whole body.

According to U.S. Department of Agriculture data, approximately seven hundred different carotenoids and their metabolites have been identified. Fifty to sixty commonly occur in the modern diet, and twenty-two of them, plus their biologically active forms, have been found in human serum. Approximately 10 percent of the carotenoids, namely alpha, beta and gamma carotenes, are converted within the body into vitamin A or retinol.

Color and Chemistry of Carotenoids

Carotenoids can be grouped by their colors: orange, yellow/green, and red. The human eye sees these colors because carotenoid molecules absorb high-energy blue and violet light from the visible spectrum. Orange carotenoids are the best known, the primary one being beta carotene. Most orange fruits and vegetables contain alpha and gamma carotene along with beta carotene. These are the only carotenoids that the body converts into vitamin A. Beta carotene is the primary vegetable source of the vitamin, but alpha and gamma carotenes are also good sources.

Carotenoids come in several chemical forms that determine their biological activity and though their biochemical actions are being increasingly understood, there is still much to learn about how they function. These are some of the things that have been discovered about carotenoids.

Carotenoids Work as a Team

Scientists have found that while the various chemical forms of carotenoids have different biological activity, they appear to work most effectively as a team. That's why scientists at the National Cancer Institute found that beta carotene supplements did not prevent lung cancer among smokers. Studies that have shown cancer preventive effects used carotenoid-rich foods instead of a supplement containing just one carotenoid. The bottom line is, you must *eat your colors*. You can certainly add vitamin and mineral supplements in moderation, but they are no substitute for a good diet. As nature intended, all carotenoid-rich fruits and vegetables contain several of these colorful phytochemicals and they are fundamental for life. To better understand how these carotenoid phytochemicals work, researchers have focused primarily on their antioxidant properties.

How Carotenoids Function as Antioxidants

Carotenoids, being fat soluble, protect the fatty membranes that envelop cells and their internal compartments. They occupy a niche similar to vitamin E and protect the vitamin from excessive free radical destruction. Although vitamin E is the dominant free radical scavenger within cellular membranes, it donates one of its own electrons to a free radical, temporarily deactivating the free radical but leaving the vitamin unstable. Carotenoids attack free radicals using a different method that keeps vitamin E intact and blocks further free radical mischief. Instead of donating electrons, carotenoids grab and hold on to free radicals, by attaching the free radical to the carotenoid backbone. They can also absorb the energy from free radicals, making them less harmful.

Using these two methods, carotenoids make an important contribution to reducing cellular aging and promotion of disease. There is a hierarchy in free radical scavenging ability among the carotenoids, depending on the tissue involved. For example, lycopene is more reactive against ultraviolet light (UV radiation) in skin tissue than beta carotene, but the latter more effectively protects the cornea from UV radiation.

Carotenoid Activity

Beta carotene is the most active of these pro-vitamins and, at one time, it was assumed this was its chief role. Once the antioxidant activities of the carotenoids were discovered, scientists assumed that since beta carotene was the most active pro-vitamin it must also be the most active antioxidant. However, in many tissues, the beta carotene is eclipsed by other carotenoids in antioxidant power. Others, such as lycopene and astaxanthin, are better trappers and scavengers of oxyradicals (free radicals containing oxygen). Singlet oxygen, superoxide, hydroxyl, and peroxyl radicals are examples of oxyradicals. These free radicals are capable of interacting with the unsaturated fatty acids in cell membranes and their intercellular components. They also attack any fatty acids circulating within body fluids such as blood, lymph, and tissue fluid. Oxyradicals steal electrons from the fatty acids, turning them into unstable molecules and setting up an oxidative chain of events that can potentially destroy large numbers of cells. Oxidative damage is considered to be the primary cause of accelerated aging, cancer, and most other chronic diseases. Carotenoids trap oxyradicals as described above and prevent them from attacking the fatty acids in cellular membranes and fatty acid complexes circulating in body fluids. Scientists have discovered that alpha carotene, gamma carotene, lycopene, and astaxanthin have even greater antioxidant activities than beta carotene in many tissues. Moreover, scientists are finding that the chemical structure and tissue location of individual carotenoids largely determine their function.

Functions of Carotenoids by Color

The *Orange Carotenoids* (alpha, beta, gamma, and zeta carotene). Orange carotenoids are the most prevalent in nature and the most diverse in activity within the human body. In addition to supplying vitamin A (except zeta carotene), the orange carotenoids prevent degradation of biological membranes, surrounding all cells and their intercellular components. One of the most important cellular structures that benefits from the protectiveness of orange carotenoids is DNA. Orange carotenoids block free radicals from entering cells and they also prevent oxidative damage to the DNA molecule. DNA is the mastermind for all metabolic functions, and it carries our genetic blueprint. DNA stamps other molecules with specific instructions for building biological systems. Therefore, any alteration in DNA structure produces "funny molecules" that don't function correctly and eventually cause a breakdown of body systems. Carotenes also increase cellular production of proteins that repair oxidized DNA. Red carotenoids often team up with the orange ones to enhance antioxidant effects, and most red fruits and vegetables contain hefty amounts of the orange carotenoids as well. Dietary supplements of mixed carotenoids containing orange and red pigments are most effective in preventing damage to DNA and repairing strand breaks that do appear. These effects appear to be further enhanced when zinc and nicotinamide (vitamin B$_3$) are added.

Orange carotenoids are effective chemopreventive (cancer preventive) agents. There are several ways they act, one being to improve the process of cell-to-cell communication. Membrane proteins regulate this intercellular "cross-talk," and they are encoded by genes. A specific gene called connexin 43 is one that has been identified that prevents distortion of messages being passed between cells. Distortion of signals between cells is one way cancer cells are formed, and by preserving the integrity of intercellular communication, carotenoids are making an important contribution to cancer prevention.

Cells that have lost their ability to communicate and have become dysfunctional will self-destruct. This process of self-killing is known as *apoptosis* and is one of the body's most effective methods for removing old or poorly functioning cells. Canthaxanthin has induced apoptosis in human cancer cell cultures and may have similar effects in the body. Canthaxanthin naturally occurs with other orange carotenoids and supplies an added benefit from eating these foods. Dietary supplements of canthaxanthin alone are not recommended because they may cause kidney damage in susceptible individuals.

Alpha carotene may be a better cancer preventive agent than beta carotene. Japanese researchers compared the effects of these two orange carotenoids on three types of cancer, liver, lung and skin, both in cell culture and animals. Alpha carotene was more potent in arresting all three cancers than beta carotene. Italian researchers confirmed the findings on alpha carotene and prevention of skin cancer in cultured cells. Studies such as these underscore the importance of supplying a broad range of carotenoids including alpha carotene as naturally found in foods.

Orange carotenoids protect against cardiovascular disease in several ways. Researchers from the National Center for Chronic Disease Prevention and Health Promotion in Atlanta analyzed data from 11,327 men and women looking for an association between vitamin and carotenoid intake and the chest pain known as angina pectoris. They found that orange carotenoids were strongly associated with a reduced risk of angina. However, vitamins A, C, E, and B_{12}, serum and red blood cell folate did not appear to offer protection against the disease.

Orange and red carotenoids are effective in reducing sun damage to skin, and some people have used large amounts of beta carotene supplements in the hope of enhancing skin color. However, using beta carotene, or any other carotenoid, alone is not as protective as using a mixture of orange and red carotenoids. Adding vitamin E also reduces UV-induced skin damage. Recent examination of data collected from the Physician's Health Study in 1982 found no protective benefits against nonmelanoma skin cancer among physicians who took a beta carotene supplement (50 mg/day) for twelve years. Studies using multicarotene supplements plus vitamin E may provide evidence of greater protective benefit against skin cancer, but until such evidence emerges, it's best to eat these colors rather than relying on dietary supplements.

Researchers have also suggested orange carotenoids may modulate immune response. Evidence from animal studies showed that carotenoids significantly enhanced the release of immune-stimulating complexes, interleukin-1 (IL-1) and tumor necrosis factor-alpha (TNF-α). However, stronger immune-regulating effects by red carotenoids in comparison to the orange ones have been reported.

The *Yellow/Green Carotenoids* (lutein, zeaxanthin, alpha and beta cryptoxanthin). Cataracts are a worldwide problem, accounting for half of the 30 to 50 million cases of blindness currently diagnosed. In the United States, age-related macular degeneration (AMD) outranks cataract as the leading cause of blindness, largely due to correction of cataracts by surgery. Approximately 1.3 million of these surgeries, which substitute a synthetic lens for the cloudy one, are performed annually in the United States.

The macula is an area of intense yellow pigment in the center of the retina. Light shines through and is concentrated on the macula. Analysis of the macula has shown that it is extremely high in two yellow carotenoid pigments: zeaxanthin and, to a lesser degree, lutein. Incredibly, levels of these two carotenoids in the macula exceed those of any other carotenoid in body tissues by close to 100 times. However, autopsied AMD eyes were found to have 30 percent less zeaxanthin and lutein than normal eyes. It is believed that these yellow pigments absorb and reduce the intensity of blue light hitting the retina, thus preventing it from damaging macular cells. In the lens of the eye, lutein and zeaxanthin prevent photooxidation and help prevent cataract formation. These are the only carotenoids found in the eye and they are believed to play a vital role in preventing cataracts, macular degeneration, and perhaps other degenerative retinal disorders.

It has been known for some time that people who eat dark green vegetables such as spinach, kale, and collards have increased levels of lutein and zeaxanthin in their serum and that this has been associated with reduced incidence of cataracts and AMD. Recent analysis has shown that while darker greens are a good source of lutein, they contain very little zeaxanthin, which appears to be the more important of the two in preventing these eye conditions. A team of British scientists analyzed egg yolk and thirty-three fruits and vegetables for lutein and zeaxanthin content. They found that yellow, yellow/green, and orange foods are the richest source of both carotenoids that make up between 40 and 50 percent of the total carotenoids in these foods. Included are egg yolks, yellow corn, kiwi fruit, orange sweet peppers, grapes, spinach, orange juice, zucchini and other kinds of squash. Since zeaxanthin is more concentrated than lutein in the eye, eating the brighter colors may offer better eye protection.

Cataracts are extremely common in people over age seventy-five, with seven out of eight Americans being afflicted. But you can improve your chances against getting cataracts by eating at least three daily servings of fruits and vegetables rich in lutein and zeaxanthin. Harvard University scientists made this determination after analyzing data from two large epidemiological studies involving 110,000 men and women. A research team at the Human Nutrition Research Center on Aging at Tufts University in Boston took a closer look at levels of carotenoids, vitamin C, and vitamin E and incidence of cataracts. In this study, the plasma carotenoid levels and carotenoid nutrient intake levels were measured among seventy-seven patients with cataracts against thirty-five people without cataracts who served as controls.

Not surprisingly, those who had eaten fewer than three servings of fruits and vegetables per day had lower amounts of carotenoids and vitamins in their serum and a higher incidence of cataracts. In a subsequent study, the Tufts team studied the effects of a diet rich in carotenoids in preventing AMD as well as cataracts. The researchers made a strong case for consuming carotenoids, particularly xanthophylls like lutein and zeaxanthin, to protect against these debilitating conditions. Many foods rich in xanthophylls are also good sources of vitamin C. A number of the studies mentioned above have also identified vitamin C as important in cataract prevention.

Lutein has also been found to be an effective cancer preventive. In a February 2000 article published in the *American Journal of Clinical Nutrition,* Martha Slattery and her colleagues from the University of Utah Medical School reported a 17 percent lower incidence of colon cancer among those who ate a diet containing lutein-rich fruits and vegetables. Although levels of other carotenoids, including alpha carotene, beta carotene, lycopene, zeaxanthin and beta cryptoxanthin, were tallied, lutein was found to offer the greatest protection. The major food sources of lutein identified by Dr. Slattery and her team were kale, spinach, broccoli, lettuce, tomatoes, oranges and orange juice, celery, and greens. No association was found between consumption of beta carotene–rich foods such as apricots, carrots, mangos, melons, peaches, nectarines, and pumpkin.

The *Red Carotenoids* (lycopene and astaxanthin). The red carotenoids are non-pro-vitamin A carotenoids with potent antioxidant activity. Lycopene accounts for about 50 percent of total carotenoids in human serum and is concentrated in the testes, adrenal glands, and prostate gland. A comparison of lycopene content has shown a 20 percent greater concentration in adrenals and prostates as compared to adipose (fat) tissue. Moreover, several research teams from around the world have shown that lycopene is well absorbed and is active in tissues.

Dietary consumption of lycopene has been associated with a lower risk of several cancers, including prostate cancer. Harvard University researchers compared carotenoid and vitamin A levels in benign and cancerous prostate tissue from 25 men with prostate cancer. They found that there was a strong correlation between tissue levels of lycopene in both cancerous and benign tissue from the same individual. Men who had the lowest levels also had the most aggressive cancers. Alpha carotene, lutein, alpha cryptoxanthin, zeaxanthin, and beta-cryptoxanthin, all of which are found in prostate tissue, did not appear to be correlated with occurrence of cancer.

A research team at Northwestern University Medical School in Chicago analyzed retained plasma samples from healthy men enrolled in the 1982 Physician's Health Study for several major antioxidants including lycopene. Lycopene was the only antioxidant found at significantly lower mean levels in the men who developed prostate cancer, as compared to those who did not, although beta carotene appeared to enhance the effects of lycopene. The researchers concluded that eating lycopene-rich foods such as tomato products might reduce the occurrence or progression of prostate cancer.

Consumption of tomato-based products has been associated with decreased risk of several cancers. The evidence for a benefit was strongest for cancers of the prostate, lung, and stomach. Other cancers that may be prevented by lycopene are breast, cervical, colon, endometrium, esophagus, lung, oral cavity, pancreas, stomach, and rectum.

Lycopene has also been reported to prevent several chronic diseases, among them cardiovascular disease (CVD). Low-density lipoprotein (LDL) is a kind of cholesterol that is considered the "bad" kind, primarily because it promotes oxidative damage to arterial walls that results in lesion formation. Once lesions form, calcium and other materials accumulate to form a *plaque.* As plaques grow, vessel walls become thicker and blood flow is restricted. In the heart, blood flow may be so reduced that a heart attack occurs. In a large European study that compared carotenoid levels among patients from ten different countries, it was found that lycopene was the most protective against acute myocardial infarction (heart attack).

LDL cholesterol contains a large percentage of fatty components that are easily oxidized by free radicals and is a major factor in initiating plaque formation. Beta carotene may be more effective in blocking LDL oxidation than lycopene. However, lycopene has been found to reduce serum LDL and total cholesterol levels. In one study, cholesterol production was reduced by 14 percent. High doses (60 mg/day) of lycopene supplements taken for three months were needed to achieve these results.

Lycopene is the red pigment that gives tomatoes and other fruits and vegetables their color. Tomatoes are the food source highest in lycopene, but other good sources are pink grapefruit, watermelon, and blood oranges. The form of lycopene changes in cooked or pureed tomatoes, and appears to be better utilized in those forms than in raw tomatoes, as evidenced by higher blood levels in human volunteers. Dietary supplements of lycopene from tomato seeds are also very effective and several studies used the supplements to study lycopene effects. Supplements containing 5 mg of lycopene may be the best way to provide this valuable carotenoid, especially for Red types who should not eat tomato products. I will go over this in detail in chapter 16.

Astaxanthin could well be the most significant carotenoid "find" of the twenty-first century. It is the red pigment concentrated in aquatic creatures and not found in significant amounts in humans. Found in phytoplankton, zooplankton, marine animals, fish, and some waterfowl, astaxanthin is the most powerful antioxidant carotenoid known. This has led scientists to suggest that the high concentration of astaxanthin in aquatic plants and animals is associated with its superior ability to prevent UV photooxidation and may protect them from UV radiation when they grow, swim, or feed near the water's surface. Astaxanthin's presence in these animals is apparent in the red color of their flesh (salmon, trout, crab, shrimp) and feathers (flamingos). Aquatic birds also concentrate astaxanthin in their eyes to protect the retina from photooxidation by UV light, which is intensified by reflection from water. Since we eat mostly land-based plants and animals, the amount of astaxanthin normally found in our bodies is minimal.

The power of astaxanthin against oxygen free radicals has been estimated by some researchers to be ten times that of other carotenoids and one hundred times more effective in trapping these radicals than vitamin E. This has led one investigator, Dr. Wataru Miki from the Suntory Institute for Bioorganic Research in Osaka, Japan, to dub astaxanthin "super vitamin E." A particularly intriguing aspect of astaxanthin's power is that it settles itself into cellular membranes by spanning the intramembrane space and attaching to both sides of the membrane. In this position it can readily trap oxyradicals approaching either from the top or bottom of the membrane. Once trapped, the oxyradicals are incorporated into the chemical structure of astaxanthin, to be released when another appropriate antioxidant is available. The membrane span formed by astaxanthin has the additional function of giving greater stability to the entire membrane complex.

Like its carotenoid cousins, astaxanthin is an anticancer agent through its antioxidant properties and interaction with proteins and lipids. In one animal study, the anticancer effects of astaxanthin, canthaxanthin, and beta carotene were compared. The animals were fed a supplement of one of the carotenoids and then inoculated with mammary cancer cells. Astaxanthin was reported to be the most effective carotenoid in reducing the number of mammary tumors that occurred. The highest doses of astaxanthin given the mice appeared to produce the best results. Several other studies have reported anticancer effects due to astaxanthin blocking oxidation of lipids in membranes and body fluids.

The immune system is an intricate regulatory network that provides protection against disease-causing organisms, tumor growth, and autoimmune overreactivity. Astaxanthin appears to be a more effective anti-inflammatory agent than other carotenoids. Several years of study on the way astaxanthin activates immunity have been done by researchers at the School of Medicine, University of Minnesota. These scientists have determined that astaxanthin does not provide immune modulation through any of the well-known carotenoid functions (pro-vitamin A activity, antioxidant activity, or gap-junctional enhancement). Rather, it seems to boost production of thymic cells (T-cells) and increase antibody production. Japanese researchers also reported that astaxanthin significantly activated cytokine release from T-cells. Cytokines are proteins that activate other immune cells and modulate immune response.

Astaxanthin supplements have been found by Dr. Curt Malmsten and his Swedish colleagues to result in a threefold improvement in strength and endurance among healthy young male athletes receiving an astaxanthin supplement (4 mg daily). The men receiving a placebo and who served as controls did not experience a significant level of improvement. Exercise increases metabolism and produces greater numbers of oxidative radicals as a natural by-product. As these radicals accumulate, muscles fatigue and exercise capacity is reduced. The antioxidant capacity of astaxanthin quickly eliminates these free radicals so that work capacity is increased.

This work has important anti-aging implications. Mitochondria are the energy-producing organelles within every cell, and oxygen is the fuel mitochondria use to produce energy. Oxyradicals are inevitably produced as by-products of energy yielding processes. Astaxanthin and to a lesser degree other carotenoids and vitamin E protect lipids (fatty acids) in mitochondrial membranes from oxidative damage. Comparing the relative oxyradical quenching capacity of several carotenoids, Danish scientists showed that the more stable a carotenoid was, the more it suppressed lipid peroxidation. In this study, astaxanthin was the most stable, and therefore the most successful at inhibiting lipid peroxidation. As for vitamin E, Japanese scientists demonstrated that astaxanthin protected rat liver mitochondrial membranes from oxyradicals 100–500 times more effectively than vitamin E.

Astaxanthin is a relatively small molecule that is fat soluble like other carotenoids. However, astaxanthin differs from the others in that it has water-friendly properties that enable it to easily unload trapped radicals to vitamin C, for elimination from the body. Astaxanthin can cross the highly selective blood brain barrier where it may function as the most effective brain antioxidant. This is extremely important because oxidative damage is considered to be a major factor in degeneration of brain cells. In addition, astaxanthin is well absorbed into the light-sensitive tissues of the eyes and can prevent photooxidation. Presumably, that's why waterfowl concentrate this powerful carotenoid in their eyes. Astaxanthin has enormous implications for ameliorating diseases of the eyes, brain, and central nervous system.

Summary of Carotenoid Functions

Carotenoids are *chemopreventive*, or anti-cancer agents. This means that they protect normal cell growth and cellular reproduction, and block tumor growth. They help cells communicate with one another and assist in cellular differentiation. Carotenoids also stimulate immune surveillance, the system that recognizes and destroys anything foreign to the body including bacteria, viruses, and tumors. Thus carotenoids help protect against the common cold, flu, various infections, and even some cancers. Other anti-cancer activities of carotenes are induction of genes that repair DNA, suppression of genes that cause tumor growth (oncogenes), and activation of those that prevent spread of cancer (anti-metastasis). Carotenes also appear to reduce the risk of cardiovascular disease by slowing vessel lesion formation and preventing LDL cholesterol oxidation. Nature provides carotene-rich foods during all seasons of the year. Amazingly, the carotenes that are best for your type will occur in the season when your health may be most challenged. Let's see how each of the colors is associated with a specific phytochemical.

Why Carotenoid Foods Should Be Part of Your Daily Eating Plan

The carotenoid foods are essential to maintaining good health and preventing chronic disease. As part of your *Eat Your Colors* daily plan, you should choose at least one carotenoid in each category—yellow/orange, yellow/red, and yellow/green—that is right for your color.

It may seem strange that although these foods are all carotenoids, some are better for each color type. The selections have been made because traditional healers have made these distinctions. In Part One, we saw how the Ayurvedic and other traditional systems classified foods according to their energetic principles. Foods rich in carotenoids contain different blends of the individual carotenoids, as we have seen. From a chemical standpoint, these differences determine the molecular energy of the food and its effect on an individual. While modern physical chemistry explains these subtle differences, ancient healers picked up on them through careful observation of how individual foods affected each body type.

Carotenoid Pigments (Phytochemicals) and Their Actions

Carotenoids include a range of phytochemicals from A to Z. That is, alpha carotene to zeaxanthin, each accumulating in specific tissues of the body. We have seen that astaxanthin, lutein, and zeaxanthin occupy individual compartments within the eye. On the other hand, lycopene concentrates in the skin, lungs, and prostate gland. Following is a summary table of the most important carotenoids, what each does and which foods contain them.

Summary of Carotene and Terpene Phytochemicals

Foods	Carotenoids	What They Do
Yellow		Pro-vitamin A activity
mango	alpha cryptoxanthin	(alpha, beta, gamma
papaya	beta cryptoxanthin	carotenes).
peaches	lutein	Cell differentiation agents.
prunes	zeaxanthin	Oxygen free-radical scavengers.
acorn squash	limonene	Protect DNA from oxidative
yellow summer squash	alpha carotene	damage.
winter squash	epsilon carotene	Repair DNA.
passion fruit	carotenoid epoxides	Intercellular communication.
yellow sweet peppers	neoxanthin	Immune modulation.
white grapefruit	neochrome	
lemons	violaxanthin	
oranges	auroxanthin	
pomelo	lutein epoxides	
tangerines		
Orange		Same as above
apricots	alpha carotene	
asparagus	beta carotene	
cantaloupe	gamma carotene	
carrots	beta cryptoxanthin	
mangos		
passion fruit		
orange sweet peppers		
pumpkin		
sweet potato		
winter squash		
Red		Quenchers of singlet oxygen
pink grapefruit	lycopene	radicals.
red hot and sweet peppers	zeta carotene	Protect white blood cells.
tomato, fresh	phytofluene	May help prevent colon, breast,
tomatoes, cooked, sauces	phytoene	lung, prostate, skin cancers.
watermelon		May reduce angina pectoris.
crab, lobster, salmon and other		May protect brain, retina,
red-fleshed fish	astaxanthin	nervous system.
Yellow/Green		Prevent photooxidation.
avocado	lutein	Protect macula in the eye.
green beans	zeaxanthin	Prevent age-related macular
broccoli	alpha cryptoxanthin	degeneration, retinal damage.
brussels sprouts	beta cryptoxanthin	
cabbage	neoxanthin	
collards	violaxanthin	
sweet corn	lutein epoxides	
kale	chlorophyll	
kiwi		

romaine lettuce
dark green leafy lettuce
muskmelon (honeydew)
okra
green peas
spinach
summer squash
tangerines
turnip greens

Monoterpenes		
citrus fruits	limonene, perillyl alcohol	Anti-cancer agents

Sources: Frederick Khachik et al. "Distribution of Carotenoids in Fruits and Vegetables as a Criterion for the Selection of Appropriate Chemopreventive Agents." *Food Factors for Cancer Prevention.* Tokyo: Springer-Verlag, 1997, pp. 204–8.

Gary Beecher, "Phytonutrients Role in Metabolism: Effects on Resistance to Degenerative Processes." *Nutrition Reviews* 57(9) (Sept. 1999 II): S3–S6.

Possible Side Effects for These Foods

Carotenoid foods are well tolerated by most people. Those who have an allergy to specific ones should avoid eating them. Carrots contain high levels of carbohydrates and diabetics may be advised to avoid them. Interestingly, diabetes is considered a Green disorder in Ayurveda and carrots are not considered good for Green types because they are too sweet and heavy.

As for Yellow types, sweet bell peppers are available in yellow, orange, red, and purple, and these colors are sweeter than green varieties. Green bell peppers are not advised for Yellows because they may cause flatulence. The other colors may be better tolerated. If you're a Yellow, you'll have to see if they work for you.

Red chili peppers are too hot for Red types and should be avoided. Raw or cooked tomatoes are not good for Reds, either. They promote acidity in the digestive system. Tomatoes are one food that presents a challenge for all types. Yellows can eat cooked tomatoes but not raw, and Greens are just the opposite. Small amounts of tomatoes in season may be OK and you should not eat fresh tomatoes during any other season. Americans love tomato products, especially ketchup, but it's wise to avoid it as much as possible. Restrict intake of tomato products, especially if you are a Red. Considering the many benefits of lycopene, this may be one carotenoid that is best supplied by taking a dietary supplement.

Grapefruit juice presents some unique problems in that it appears to interfere with several medications. Grapefruit contains a substance that blocks one of the drug-metabolizing enzymes in your liver. Consequently, the drug may accumulate to dangerously high levels. Grapefruit juice may increase the gastric irritation from aspirin and nonsteroidal anti-inflammatory drugs (NSAIDs). This is a list of medications that you should not combine with grapefruit juice.

- antihistamines
- anticoagulants (Warfarin [coumadin])
- aspirin and other NSAIDs (ibuprofen, naproxen)
- benzodiazepines (Klonopin, Xanax)
- calcium channel blockers (Procardia, Verapamil)
- cyclosporine (Sandimmune, Neoral)
- theophylline

Buying, Storing, and Cooking These Foods

Digestion and assimilation of uncooked carotenoids is partially blocked by other components in the food matrix. To increase their absorption, it is best to cook, puree, or juice them. Scientists have noted that absorption of carotenoids from food can be very low, only 1 to 2 percent, from raw vegetables such as tomatoes. The absorption of the same vegetables increases to 50 percent when they are cooked. Pureeing or chopping vegetables also increases the uptake of carotenes into the system. One research team even noted that plasma levels of lycopene were increased when volunteers drank it warmed but not when it was drunk cold. As a side note, it is possible to increase the digestive temperature of carotenoid and other foods by adding spices such as black and cayenne pepper. There will be lots more on this in the meal plans in Part Three.

The presence of bile acids and oils in the intestines at the time carotenoid foods are present also affects their uptake. That's because bile acids form transport vehicles needed to carry carotenoids across the absorptive membranes. Oils improve the solubility of carotenoids, thus assisting their transport across intestinal membranes. Dietary supplements of carotenoids are offered in oil-filled capsules for the same reason.

Which of These Fruits and Vegetables Are My Color?

These beautiful fruits and vegetables are color-coded for your type and that's why this group was chosen to set the stage for *Eat Your Colors* plans. Here are the details.

Yellows: The carotenoids are your family. You can eat all of them with few exceptions.

Your Primary Colors

Yellow/Orange Fruits and Vegetables: apricots, bananas, cantaloupe, carrots, grapefruit, lemons, limes, mangos, passion fruit, papaya, peaches, prunes (fresh, not dried), orange and yellow bell peppers, oranges, pomelo, pumpkin, sweet potato, tangerines, and winter squash

Red Fruits, Vegetables, and Seafood: pink grapefruit, red sweet peppers, tomatoes (cooked), salmon, and shellfish

Yellow/Green Fruits and Vegetables: asparagus, avocados, green beans, broccoli, collards, sweet corn, kale (cooked), kiwi, romaine and leafy lettuces, iceberg lettuce, honeydew melon, okra, spinach, summer squash, turnip greens

Your Clashing Colors

Raw tomatoes, green bell peppers, brussels sprouts, cabbage, cauliflower, green peas

Reds: Carotenoid foods are very good for you. Some you will have to avoid but they are few in number.

Your Complementary Colors

Yellow/Orange Fruits and Vegetables: apricots, cantaloupe, carrots, lemons, limes, mango, melons, oranges, passion fruit, yellow and orange sweet peppers, pumpkin, sweet potato, pears, and tangerines

Red Fruits and Vegetables: pink grapefruit, plums, pomegranate, radicchio, red sweet peppers, and watermelon

Yellow/Green Fruits and Vegetables: avocados, asparagus, broccoli, brussels sprouts, cabbage, collards, sweet corn, green beans, green leafy lettuce, honeydew melon, kale, kiwi, okra, green peas, spinach, and turnip greens

Your Clashing Colors

Bananas, papaya, peaches, raw and cooked tomatoes, chili peppers, and spinach

Greens: You also do well with most of the carotenoid fruits and vegetables, except those that contain a lot of water or have a high sugar content.

Your Complementary Colors

Yellow/Orange Fruits and Vegetables: apricots, carrots, lemons, limes, mangos, passion fruit, peaches, prunes, orange and yellow bell peppers, oranges, pomelo, and tangerines

Red Fruits, Vegetables and Seafood: red sweet peppers, red chili peppers, tomatoes (raw), salmon, and shellfish

Yellow/Green Fruits and Vegetables: asparagus, green beans, broccoli, collards, sweet corn, kale, kiwi, romaine, leafy lettuces, iceberg lettuce, okra, spinach, summer squash (zucchini), and turnip greens

Your Clashing Colors
Avocado, bananas, grapefruit, melons, papaya, plums, pumpkin, sweet potatoes, tomatoes (cooked), and winter squash

Carotenoid-rich foods are very important antioxidants, and ones that protect all of the fatty-acid components of the body. Next we will discuss the other group of important antioxidants, those that protect body fluids—blood, lymph, and tissue fluids. The antioxidants in these foods work in tandem with carotenoids to eliminate free radicals from the body.

6

Red Foods

The deep red, blue, and purple colors of fruits and vegetables come from phenolic pigments, a class of antioxidant phytochemicals with powerful protective properties. These water-soluble antioxidants complement the fat-soluble carotenoids in protecting all parts of the body. While carotenoids eliminate free radicals within cells, phenols scavenge them in body fluids.

Phenols are the most abundant antioxidants in nature—some 8,000 different ones have been described by scientists. Phenolic compounds are found in all parts of plant species, including stems, bark, vascular system, and leaves. Phenols in leaves may be hidden by chlorophyll during most seasons of the year, only to emerge in the fall as brilliant shades of red and purple.

Phenolic compounds have always been an important part of the human diet. Our hunter/gatherer ancestors esteemed berries of all kinds for their nutritional and medicinal value. Phenolic pigments paint a rainbow of colors from red to deep purple and give apples, berries, cranberries, plums, pomegranates, eggplant, and other fruits and vegetables their distinctive color. For Red types, these are one of two principal foods.

Lately, interest in the health benefits of polyphenols has increased, as their diverse antioxidant and free radical scavenging features have been discovered. Researchers have also found that vitamin C, nature's most prevalent scavenger of water-soluble free radicals, commonly occurs with phenolic compounds in fruits and vegetables. This suggests that the vitamin and phenolic compounds work as a team in scavenging free radicals and other important activities. Indeed, scientists have found the anti-cancer activities of these compounds are enhanced when both are present.

Phenolic compounds are astringent, with the degree of astringency varying from mild in berries to strong in tea tannins. Astringency is important in preserving the structure and function of all vascular tissues. Since heart and vascular system function is one of the main properties of the Red type, astringent foods are the most important for this type. (Red maintains all body functions.) Polyphenols, except for the larger tannins and ligans, are water soluble, as mentioned above. They are the primary antioxidants in body fluids including blood, lymph, tissue fluid, brain, and spinal fluids.

Phenolic compounds and vitamin C are important for Green types as well, because green maintains the structural integrity of the body. The most important structural protein in the body is collagen. Vitamin C and phenolic compounds adhere to collagen, providing its great strength and resiliency. Vitamin C is required for building collagen, and polyphenols add additional strength by reinforcing the links between collagen strands. Blood and lymph vessel walls, among other endothelial tissues, are protected by these compounds. Skin, body cavity linings, digestive and respiratory systems, organs, and the various tubes and ducts of the body are other endothelial tissues.

Phenolic compounds also chelate toxic minerals so they can be safely eliminated from the body. *Chelation* is a process whereby a mineral is completely encased by larger molecules that protect it and prevent its reactivity. Toxic minerals are devastating to the body because they displace minerals such as calcium and zinc that are needed for healthy metabolism. A few essential minerals can become highly reactive free radicals under certain conditions and phenols chelate them before they can damage tissues.

The use of phenolic compounds known as tannins dates back to 1796 and the discovery that these compounds would "tan" leather. The tannins, concentrated from oak bark, could effectively transform animal hides into impermeable non-rotting leather. Tannins stabilize the collagen strands in leather and greatly reduce the degradation normally caused by microbial and environmental factors. With the discovery of this process, one of the major non-antioxidant biological properties of large polyphenols was revealed.

Tannic acids are commonly found in foods and can give them a bitter unpalatable taste. American Indians leached tannins from acorns by boiling them before roasting and grinding them. On the other hand, smaller phenolic compounds have made an important contribution to food preparation by adding flavor. It was also discovered centuries ago that herbs and spices rich in phenolic compounds were excellent food preservatives. Rosemary, thyme, cinnamon, cloves, and turmeric are some that have been most commonly used. These herbs provided one of the most important ways of preserving foods in the days before refrigeration.

Now I will identify the individual groups of polyphenols and then discuss what each does.

Simple Polyphenols: Phenolic Acids

Phenolic acids are found in most fruits, vegetables, and herbs. Herbs owe their preservative properties to several phenolic acids, including rosemanol, rosemarinic acid, thymol, cinnamic acid, eugenol, *p*-coumaric, and caffeic acid. Rosemary has been a traditional remedy for colic and dysmenorrhea and has recently been suggested as a possible treatment for bronchial asthma, spasmotic disorders, peptic ulcer, inflammation, and atherosclerosis. It is well absorbed from the skin as well as from food and beverages. Following is a list of important phenolic acids found in berries, citrus fruits, eggplant, carrots, broccoli, cabbage, parsley, cucumbers, squash, yams, whole grains, seeds, and herbs:

cinnamic	salicylic	hydroxycinnamic
p-coumaric	gallic	piperic
caffeic	vanillic	methysticin
ferulic	anisic	dihydrokawain
isoferulic	piperonylic	kawain
ellagic	chlorogenic	tannic

Phenolic acids are excellent antioxidants and appear to play an important role in reducing the oxidative stress on the body. Remarkably, they appear to be highly specialized in how each performs its duties. Some prevent oxidation of LDL cholesterol and help prevent atherosclerosis. This effect appears to be limited to the earliest stage (initiation phase) of LDL oxidation. It's truly amazing to find out how powerful the phenolic acids in herbs and spices really are. If you'd like to see this demonstrated, purchase a loaf of herb bread containing rosemary. You'll be amazed at how long it retains its freshness!

Phenolic acids such as ferulic and isoferulic are also found in cereals and grains (see chapter 8). Gallic, ellagic, and vanillic acids are other important phenolic acids. Phenolic acids may help prevent cancer by blocking nitrosamine formation and modifying enzyme activity. *Nitrosamines* are formed from dietary nitrates and nitrites and are thought to promote cancer progression. Phenolic acids may also help prevent cancer by removing pro-oxidant minerals such as copper and iron and increasing cancer cell death. The killing activity of phenolic acids against cancer cells is helped by vitamin C. Phenolic acids in fruits, vegetables, seeds, herbs, grains, and legumes are extremely important in the antioxidant protection of the body.

Fruits are rich sources of many phenolic acids, including ellagic, malic, caffeic, chlorogenic, and coumaric. Fruits that contain these compounds are often colored red, blue and purple—the colors recommended for Red types.

Grains, legumes, herbs, and spices are also excellent sources of phenolic acids, and these foods are important for Reds, in large part because of these phytochemicals. Let's see why the phenolic phytochemicals in red fruits are so good for Reds.

Red Fruits

Scientists at Northwestern University Medical School found that ellagic acid found in red fruits can thwart cancer in several ways, all related to its unique chemical structure. The Northwestern group found that ellagic acid was effective against chemically induced cancers of the lung, liver, skin, and esophagus in animal models. While ellagic acid gives us an excellent reason to eat fruit, other compounds are also important, and some of these are unique to a specific red fruit. Let's explore some of the more outstanding red fruits and how their phytochemicals work.

Cranberry juice has become a popular beverage, and like other berry juices, it contains high levels of organic acids, primarily quinic, malic, and citric. These acids, along with the other phenolic compounds called anthocyanins, are found in all red fruits and have strong antioxidant properties. Cranberries and other red fruits are also excellent sources of fiber, which helps maintain healthy intestinal function. Fruit fiber also slows down the release of fruit sugars into the bloodstream during digestion. This helps keep blood sugar levels constant and is a major reason for eating fruit instead of just drinking the juice. Cranberries and cranberry juice have also gained popularity among consumers for the prevention of urinary tract infections (UTI).

Several researchers have reported the beneficial effects of drinking cranberry juice in the prevention of UTI. A study involving 153 elderly women was the first well-designed clinical trial on the antibacterial effects of cranberry juice. Half the women drank twelve ounces of cranberry juice cocktail daily for six months. The other half drank a beverage that tasted and looked like the cranberry cocktail and contained the same amount of vitamin C but did not contain any cranberry solids. Those who drank the cranberry juice cocktail had a 58 percent reduction in bacteria in their urine. Although these women did not have urinary tract infections, the presence of large numbers of bacteria in urine increases risk of UTI.

For several years, scientists assumed that the acidity of cranberries and their high vitamin C content were responsible for the antibacterial effects. Lending support to this theory was the observation that drinking acidic juices such as cranberry, orange, or pineapple increased urine acidity, and as acidity increased, bacterial counts dropped. Taking a cranberry juice supplement or ascorbic acid also increased urinary acidity. However, there was a piece of the puzzle missing because only cranberry juice, not the other acidic juices or vitamin C, prevented UTIs. The acidic theory was finally disproved when it was demonstrated that cranberry prevented bacteria from adhering to the cells lining the bladder. Several scientific teams further proposed that sweetening cranberry juice may partially interfere with anti-adhesion characteristics. Consequently, drinking unsweetened cranberry juice or taking dietary supplements of unsweetened cranberry juice solids hold the edge over drinking sweetened commercial juices in treating recurring UTIs.

It seems cranberries prevent other pesky bacteria from causing us harm. Eating cranberries or drinking the juice blocks the adherence of oral bacteria to plaque proteins on teeth and may be good preventive treatment against the development of dental caries. One dental study reported a 58 percent reduction in adhesion to plaque proteins by decay-causing bacteria after treatment with nonsweetened cranberry concentrate.

Cranberries may also be anti-cancer. At the Year 2000 Annual Meeting of Experimental Biology in San Diego, Dr. Najla Guthrie from the University of Western Ontario in London presented evidence that her team found breast cancer development was delayed in mice fed a cranberry-rich chow. The animals used in these experiments were bred to be naturally prone to develop breast cancer. The cranberry-eating animals developed fewer and smaller tumors than their non-cranberry-eating counterparts. The polyphenolic compounds in cranberries, other berries, and grapes have been shown to prevent other kinds of cancers in animal models and in in vitro human studies as well.

Pomegranates have been a popular food in many parts of the world and have been used to balance hormones. We now know that pomegranates contain two forms of estrogen—estrone and estradiol. The popularity of this fruit in the Middle East has prompted research into how its phytochemicals work. Two new studies were reported in 2000, suggesting that components in pomegranates prevent plaque formation in arteries. Scientists at the Technion Faculty of Medicine, Rabam Medical Center in Haifa, Israel, had a selected group of individuals drink pomegranate juice for fourteen weeks. During the trial period, the researchers assessed various risk factors that promote arterial plaque. There was a significant decrease in changes to LDL cholesterol that can lead to plaque formation, and increased antioxidant activity against LDL oxidation was found.

While the human trial was going on, mice that are especially susceptible to atherogenesis were fed pomegranate juice to assess its effects on body tissues. Macrophage activity was reduced by 90 percent, resulting in less damage to cellular membranes. *Macrophages* are large scavenging white blood cells that engulf oxidized LDL cholesterol, which is one of the body's defensive tactics.

The macrophages swell to giant proportions and begin oozing free radicals into surrounding tissues. The liberated free radicals literally dig pits into arterial walls.

In the second study, another group of researchers from the same institution used fermented pomegranate juice spiked with a concentrate of phenolic compounds extracted from pomegranate seed. They were essentially producing a powerful pomegranate wine and testing it for its antioxidant power and anti-inflammatory ability. The Israeli scientists were particularly interested in how effective the constituents in pomegranates might be as compared to those from red wine and green tea. Both of the latter have been widely studied for their ability to block pro-inflammatory eicosanoid production. *Eicosanoids* are produced from essential fatty acids and have remarkable effects as pro- and anti-inflammatory mediators. The pomegranate phenolics appeared to be just as effective as tea polyphenols and more effective than red wine phenolics in blocking inflammatory events and oxidation of membrane fatty acids. This study is particularly relevant in prevention of atherogenesis in the Middle East, where pomegranates are an important part of the diet.

Apples are an important source of protective polyphenolics in Western countries. The phrase "an apple a day helps keep the doctor away" has great importance because of the availability of apples most of the year. The juicy flesh of apples contains several important phenolic acids, including malic, ellagic, caffeic, chlorogenic, and coumaric, all with diverse disease-preventing activities. The skin of red apples contains the important flavonoid quercetin, a kind of phenolic compound (I'll explain more about flavonoids below). In total, a medium-sized apple contains approximately 290 mg of phenolic compounds.

Apples also contain fiber that may offer protection against colon cancer. Dr. Marian Eberhardt and colleagues from Cornell University tested an apple extract prepared from the apple flesh, either with or without skin, on human colon and liver cancer cells. The extract with skin inhibited growth of colon tumors by 43 percent, while the extract without skin showed a 29 percent inhibition.

Dr. Eberhardt and her colleagues also tested the apple extracts on liver cancer tumors. Tumor growth was inhibited by 57 percent with the extract containing skin and 40 percent for the extract without skin.

Apples appear to stave off lung diseases as well. At least that's what results of a five-year follow-up study on 2,512 Welshmen have shown. Welsh researchers measured several indicators of lung function in the men at the beginning and throughout the five-year period. Then they compared these indicators with the men's diets and made adjustments for exercise, smoking history, and body mass index. After processing all the data, the research team concluded that eating hard fruits, especially apples, several times a week helped maintain lung function and prevent its decline. Eating soft fruits such as citrus and vegetables was not as strongly protective.

Anthocyanidins

Anthocyanidins are a specialized group of polyphenols that primarily occur in red fruits along with ellagic and other phenolic acids. Berries contain high levels of anthocyanins, which provide the antioxidant benefits of these fruits. The specific benefits of eating berries include:

- Improving vision
- Helping to control diabetes
- Improving circulation
- Preventing cancer
- Retarding the effects of aging

Anthocyanins are plant pigments that protect many species from free radical damage. In nature, the highest amounts of anthocyanins are found in parts of the plant exposed to the harshest environmental conditions, such as leaves and bark. They are also concentrated in the skins of most red fruits. Berries are a rich source of anthocyanins and the table below lists their relative levels of proanthocyanidins. Anthocyanins take on many forms depending on the attachment of specific side chains. They have been given names to distinguish the resulting complexes; anthocyanins, anthocyanidins, and proanthocyanidins. Though I interchange the terms I am basically referring to the same group of agents.

The amount of anthocyanin pigments listed in the following table is an approximation in milligrams per 100 grams of fruit (½ cup serving). The actual content of any fruit depends on the variety, when it was picked, and the growing conditions. Testing laboratories use different testing methods and this also produces variations. Green tea was used for comparison in phenolic content, since it is a well-known source of phenolic compounds.

Anthocyanin Content of Different Fruits and Green Tea

Black Currant	37.2–61.9	Elderberry	135.0
Blueberry	25–495	Chokeberry	160.0
Boysenberry	160	Cranberry	45–100
Red Currant	10.9	Sour Cherry	——
White Currant	32.1	Apple	14.2–32.4
Marionberry	109	Plum	5.8–12.8
Black Raspberry	214–428	Pear	9.1

Red Raspberry	20–60	Peach	1–10
Strawberry	7–75	Quince	52.8–93.7
Blackberry	83–326	Green Tea	215.0

Sources: Wilska-Jeszka, J., Podsêdek, A. "Proanthocyanidins: Properties and Occurrence in Fruits." Technical University of Łódź, Poland.

Oregon Raspberry and Blackberry Commission. "Caneberries Are Healthy Fruits," *Nutraceutical Bulletin* 3 (1) (May 1999): 2–5.

Red, Blue, Black, and Purple Berries are a good source of fiber, which is considered to be a chemopreventive agent. I will discuss more on chemopreventive properties of fiber in chapter 8. Berries also contain vitamin C, which I mentioned usually occurs in foods containing anthocyanins, again highlighting the natural synergy between the vitamin and its phenolic cofactors. Berries also contain B-vitamins and minerals.

Cherries are a popular crop in Michigan and every year festivals celebrate the harvest and uses for this fruit. Locals vie for blue ribbons on cherry pie, jam, and other delectable treats. Now it seems the cherry's powerful antioxidant properties have pushed it into the limelight as an ingredient in marinades and for adding to meat before grilling. Food scientist J. Ian Gray and colleagues at Michigan State University in East Lansing have isolated a number of antioxidants from Montmorency and Balaton cherries that block formation of heterocyclic amines (HCAs). These are cancer-promoting compounds formed on well-done meat. When ground cherries (11.5% of patty weight) are added to hamburger patties before cooking, HCAs were reduced by 90 percent. This should be a boon for cooks since the cherry-laced burgers were preferred by tasters over the plain burgers. Plus, the cherries offered antioxidant and inflammatory protection from other phenolic compounds they contained. As an interesting side note, black cherries have been used as a folk remedy for arthritis for many years, presumably because of similar antioxidant and anti-inflammatory effects.

Dr. Gray and his colleagues identified another antioxidant ingredient for marinating meat that may reduce HCAs. Rosemary contains phenolic compounds that prevent formation of HCAs, and when meat is rubbed with or marinated in rosemary mixtures, HCA formation is reduced by as much as 69 percent. It appears that marinating meat, chicken, and fish with phenolic compounds found in fruit, red wine, and many herbs is an effective way to prevent formation of HCAs.

Red grapes and red wine contain several groups of phenolic compounds. The most important are proanthocyanidins, resveratrol, and ellagic acid. Proanthocyanidins are found in the membrane around grape seeds. Ellagic and chlorogenic acids occur in the grape flesh and resveratrol is concentrated in the skin. All of these compounds are powerful free radical scavengers with diverse biological effects. The interest in these compounds began with the discovery that proanthocyanidins appeared to protect the cardiovascular system.

The connection between red wine consumption and reduced incidence of cardiovascular disease has fascinated scientists for some time. Some groups have studied the antioxidant effects of phenolic acids in red wine and have found these appear to make a significant contribution to the prevention of cardiovascular disease. Other beverages that contain phenolic acids also contribute to prevention of heart disease. These include beer and red grape juice; moreover nonalcoholic wines have the same protective effects. An important subgroup of anthocyanins are the proanthocyanidins and these are the active phenolic compounds in grapes and red wine. Let's see how these compounds work.

Proanthocyanidins

The "French Paradox" describes the absence of high rates of heart disease among the French despite their eating a high-fat diet. The primary factor that distinguishes the diets of Frenchmen and Frenchwomen from those consumed in the other Western countries is their practice of drinking red wine with meals. This seeming contradiction between diet and heart disease has intrigued scientists for many years. Numerous studies have been done to determine if it is the alcohol or polyphenols in red wine that are the protective agents. While the results are equivocal, there seems to be some benefit from the alcohol in that it stimulates production of high-density lipoproteins. A more plausible explanation comes from the phenolic phytochemicals in red wine.

Both red and white wine contain these phenolic compounds. However, red wine contains much higher levels of phenolics and is considered a better source of antioxidant power than white wine. Some specific ways consuming these phytochemicals are thought to be protective include:

- Elevation of "good" HDL cholesterol and reduction of total cholesterol
- Reduced levels of atherogenic lipoproteins
- Reduction of oxidative stress
- Reduction of chronic inflammation

I must point out that while doctors believe there may be some benefit to moderate alcohol consumption, the risks of liver damage and other health concerns may override the benefits for many people. It is possible to get the phenolic compounds without drinking alcoholic beverages, since non-alcoholic wines and grape juice offer benefits similar to red wine.

Platelet stickiness (aggregation) is a contributing factor in narrowing of arteries and risk of heart attack and stroke. Researchers at the University of Wisconsin in Madison found that purple grape juice was as effective as wine in blocking platelet aggregation in dogs.

Resveratrol

This phenolic compound is found in at least seventy-two plant species, among them grapes, some berries, and some legumes including peanuts. In nature, resveratrol promotes resistance to fungal infections and provides antioxidant protection for legumes and fruits. In people, resveratrol protects the cardiovascular system by preventing damage to arterial walls and blocking adhesion of blood cells to vessel walls. Cellular adhesion is a major factor in the development of arterial plaque—ultimately resulting in atherosclerosis. Studies at the University of California at Davis and at Cornell University have suggested that resveratrol helps protect against cancer. Some of the effects that have been reported by these scientists include resveratrol acting as an anti-mutagen, dampening the initiation, promotion, and progression of cancer, and the easing of menopausal symptoms.

That resveratrol can protect against heart disease and cancer has been demonstrated through both test tube (in vitro) and animal (in vivo) testing. Scientists at the University of Illinois in Chicago found that resveratrol induces liver detoxification enzymes and reduces the growth of cancer cells. The initiation, progression, and growth of breast cancer in mice was blocked by resveratrol. It also appeared to prevent skin cancer in mice. Resveratrol is also a potent phytoestrogen; I'll discuss these later on in this chapter.

Catechins and Green Tea

Phenolic compounds called catechins, best known as the active agents in green tea, are powerful antioxidants and disease preventives. Tea drinking in China reportedly dates back to 2700 B.C. during the reign of the emperor Shen Nung. The first written record of its detoxifying effects dates from around 200 B.C. The Japanese adopted the practice of drinking tea after Buddhist monks visited China in the thirteenth century. Modern scientific investigation into the health-promoting benefits of tea began in the 1970s when it was discovered that tea seemed to protect those who drank it from cancer, heart attacks, strokes, infections, diarrhea, and dental caries. Now, more than twenty-five years later, research has shown that tea consumption may:

- enhance weight loss
- enhance immune function by reducing free radicals
- prevent cancer initiation and progression

- suppress the initiation and growth of tumors
- regulate cholesterol levels
- lower the risk of stroke
- maintain normal blood pressure and blood sugar levels
- inhibit bacterial, viral, and fungal infections
- protect the skin against UV radiation
- maintain bone mineral density
- reduce allergic reactions
- negate the effects from eating blackened meat

With so many beneficial effects reported, researchers have been extremely interested in how tea works, what the most active components are, what factors affect tea quality, and how much needs to be consumed to enjoy the benefits. Although all tea leaves come from the same plant, the chemical composition of tea depends on the climate, species of tea plant, growing and processing conditions. Green tea is made from fresh leaves that have been steamed or roasted. Black tea is made from fully fermented green tea leaves.

On average about 35 percent of green tea is solids, of which catechins account for half. Green tea also includes phenolic acids, carotenoids, chlorophyll, minerals, caffeine, theophylline, theobromine, and a unique amino acid, theanine. Black tea contains between 5 and 10 percent catechins.

How safe is it to drink large quantities of tea? This was investigated at the Food Research Laboratories, Mitsui Norin, in Japan, where it was found that no side effects occurred after feeding mice the equivalent of 50 to 100 cups per day of brewed green tea. A three-month human study there assessed the impact of taking a daily supplement of green tea extract containing 500 mg of catechins. Forty-five male and female volunteers took part, and complete blood and urine analyses plus liver enzyme functions were assessed in each volunteer. Doctors could find no disturbance in any of the functions. In fact, blood pressure, cholesterol levels, and bowel conditions were reportedly improved.

Green tea with its caffeine and polyphenols could become the next effective weight-loss ingredient. Green tea increases metabolic rate and fat burning. Ten healthy non-smoking and non-athletic men took capsules containing green tea extracts with their meals for one day and their energy output was then measured with the use of a respiratory chamber. Three different tea extracts in capsules were used. One contained caffeine and catechins, the second had caffeine but no catechins, and the third was a placebo. The men continued to eat their regular diets and rotated consumption of the three extracts so that each served as his own control. There was an average thermogenic increase of 4 percent when the men took the capsules containing both caffeine and catechins. These effects did not occur when either of the other tea extracts was taken. Green tea has inhibited several kinds of cancer in human and animal studies. Researchers from Case Western Reserve University found that green tea catechins could be effectively absorbed from the skin and may thus be effective against skin cancer. Drinking green tea, on the other hand, may protect against cancers of the lymph and prostate glands. One way the scientists found that catechins are effective against these cancers was by inducing programmed cell death or apoptosis. Another way catechins may protect against prostate cancer is by blocking androgen (male) hormone receptors on prostate tissue. Catechins appear to have similar effects against hormone-dependent breast cancers by blocking estrogen receptors in breast tissue. Drinking ten cups of brewed (2–3 minutes) green tea daily may be enough to thwart these cancers.

As for black tea, which is preferred by 80 percent of tea drinkers worldwide, British scientists have found that the tea flavonoids appear to prevent bone thinning. In a large study that measured bone density in 1,134 tea drinking women and 122 non-tea drinkers, it was found that the tea drinkers had greater bone density in their thigh bones and spinal vertebrae. Dutch researchers did a study of 3,454 individuals comparing the risk of developing atherosclerosis or narrowing of aortic arteries with black tea drinking. They found that those who drank two cups of tea daily reduced their risk by 46 percent, while those who drank four cups daily were 69 percent less likely to develop the condition. Let's move on to the next class of polyphenols, the flavonoids.

Flavonoids

Flavonoids are a large family of polyphenolic compounds, numbering over 4,000 members, widely found in fruits, vegetables, nuts, seeds, wine, and tea. It has been estimated that the typical western diet provides between 100 and 1,000 mg of flavonoids daily. These compounds are so remarkable and diverse in their health promoting activities that some scientists have proposed they be considered "natural dietary biologic response modifiers." These are agents that affect the way the body responds to environmental stressors and how it alters disease processes. The major activities of flavonoids may include modifying immune function, preventing fatty acid oxidation, preventing cancer and heart disease, alleviating allergies, and preventing viral and microbial infections. Normally, flavonoid activity is enhanced by vitamin C.

Isoflavones: Potent Phytoestrogens

Isoflavones are a distinct group of flavonoids with their own unique set of effects. They are concentrated in legumes, primarily soy, but are also found in alfalfa, kudzu, red clover, parsley, licorice root (not the candy), and grains. Soy has caught the attention of the scientific community for its ability to prevent heart disease, alleviate menstrual and menopausal symptoms, and help prevent cancer. Soy and other legumes are primary foods for Red types and important for the other types as well.

Some of the unique ways isoflavones work are worth mentioning. They bind to hormone receptors in breast and prostate tissues and block attachment of cancer-causing hormones. Receptor binding also enables isoflavones to mimic the action of estrogen. In menopausal women, isoflavones alleviate hot flashes, help prevent bone thinning, and may help delay other signs of aging. In women with premenstrual symptoms, isoflavones help to balance hormones and relieve tension. Now, let's summarize phenolic compounds, which foods contain them, and how they work.

Food	Phenolic Compounds	What They Do
Red apples, pears, plums, pomegranates, prunes	phenolic acids (citric, chlorogenic, *p*-coumaric, cinnamic, ferulic, ellagic, gallic, malic) vitamin C (estradiol, estrone, pomegranate)	*citric:* antiseptic, reduces kidney stone formation *chlorogenic:* anti-allergenic, anti-viral, anti-inflammatory *p-coumaric:* anticancer *cinnamic:* anti-fungal *ferulic:* hormone balancing, anti-spasmodic, anti-tumor *ellagic:* astringent, anti-tumor, anti-mutagen *gallic:* cancer preventive *malic:* anti-bacterial, hemopoietic *vitamin C:* antioxidant, collagen synthesis *estradiol, estrone:* phytoestrogens
Orange apricots, peaches	phenolic acids, catechins, flavonoids (kaempferol, rutin, quercetin) estrone	*catechins:* anticancer, antihistamine, antioxidant, hepatic protectant, anti-ulcer *flavonoids:* antihistamine, anti-inflammatory

Food	Phenolic Compounds	What They Do
Yellow apples, guava, pears, quince citrus	phenolic acids, kaempferol, quercetin flavonoids (hesperidin, naringin, quercetin, rutin) vitamin C	same as above
Red and Black raspberries, blackberries, boysenberries, bilberries, blueberries, gooseberries, lingonberries, marion berries, strawberries, cherries	phenolic acids, anthocyanins, flavonoids, catechins	*anthocyanins:* anti-aggregant, anti-inflammatory, prevent vessel leakage, vasodilators
Red, Purple, and Yellow grapes bilberries, rhubarb	anthocyanidins, kaempferol, quercetin (anthrones, rhubarb)	same as above *anthrones:* emetic, anti-protozoal
Green green tea, herbal teas, black tea	catechins flavonoids, organic acids	same as above
herbs soy	isoflavones (genistein, daidzein), phenolic acids	*isoflavones:* estrogenic, inhibit pro-cancer enzymes, anti-microbial
grapes red wine	resveratrol	*resveratrol:* anticancer, estrogenic, anti-fungal, reduces cholesterol

Sources: Duke, James. "Handbook of Phytochemical Constituents of GRAS Herbs and Other Economic Plants." Boca Raton, Fla.: CRC Press, 1992; "Handbook of Biologically Active Phytochemicals and Their Activities." Boca Raton, Fla.: CRC Press, 1992.

Possible Side Effects of Eating These Foods

There can be some side effects of eating these foods. Apples are well tolerated by most people, but those who have problems with flatulence may have difficulty with unpeeled apples. However, stewing or baking them usually overcomes the problem. Occasionally, an individual may be allergic to apples and apple juice. Cooking doesn't seem to alleviate allergic symptoms in sensitive individuals.

Berry allergies are much more common. Blackberries, blueberries, raspberries, and strawberries can all cause allergic reactions. In addition, pears and prunes that contain natural sulfites can cause problems for those who are extremely sensitive. Fruits that rarely cause a problem are cranberries, gooseberries, and grapes.

Rhubarb contains oxalic acid which binds dietary calcium and excretes it through urine. Those prone to calcium oxalate kidney stones should avoid using rhubarb. Other foods that also contain oxalate and should be avoided by people with this problem are raw spinach, beets, cocoa, nuts, parsley, and green or black tea.

Vitamin C–rich foods such as red fruits and citrus increase the uptake of iron. Consequently, those who have iron overload should avoid eating large amounts of these foods.

Buying, Storing, and Cooking These Foods

Fresh fruit is best purchased in season. However, apples, pears, and citrus fruits are available in most places all year. The season for berries is much shorter but most berries are available frozen or in juice so that you can enjoy them several days a week.

When you select fresh fruit, pick out those that are nearly ripe but not soft. Most fruit is shipped unripened to reduce bruising. You may have to put fruit in a special ripening container during cold weather with apples and bananas helping to ripen it. These fruits give off a gas that ripens pears, kiwi, and tropical fruits. Don't put citrus in such containers because they will mold. Citrus are best kept in a cool room and eaten within a few days of bringing them home. Avoid putting them in the refrigerator, which draws moisture from the fruit and spoils the taste. Some people purchase crates of oranges in the winter months and successfully store them for several weeks in a cool basement or garage.

Which of These Foods Is My Color?

Red Types

All red, blue, black, and purple fruits are your color. However, not many vegetables in these colors will work for you. Most of the red vegetables, such as peppers and chilis, are too hot and eggplant is too pungent. Here are the details:

Your Primary Colors

Red—all berries, plums, pomegranates, grapes, and their juices
Orange—apricots, oranges, and their juices
Yellow—pears, lemons

Green—green tea, herbal teas, limes
Other—legumes (all legumes are primary foods for Reds)

Your Clashing Colors
Red—rhubarb, red wine, tomatoes, and tomato products
Orange—peaches
Yellow—grapefruit

Yellow Types

Your Primary Colors
All of these colors: red, orange, yellow, and green

Your Clashing Colors
Eggplant, red wine

Green Types

Your Primary Colors
Red—all berries, cherries, red wine with meals on occasion
Orange—apricots, peaches, oranges
Yellow—pears, quince, lemons
Green—grapes

Your Clashing Colors
Red—cranberries, rhubarb, plums
Yellow—grapefruit

Red foods are very important in the diets of all types. They pack some of our most powerful free radical scavengers and disease fighting agents. Interestingly, some of the phytochemicals found in red foods are also found in legumes, making these foods, which I will discuss in chapter 8, primary partners for Red and Green types.

7

Green Foods

Green foods are pungent and astringent, the best tastes for Greens according to Ayurveda. Emphasizing these foods will help prevent Green disorders such as respiratory problems and obesity.

Yellow and Red types should also eat Green foods, adding them to their palette for balance. However, these types are more limited in selection. Later in this chapter I will fully discuss which foods these types should eat and why they should avoid others. For now, we will take an in-depth look at what scientists have discovered about the phytochemicals in green foods and their disease-preventing actions.

The Phytochemicals in Cruciferous Green Foods

Paul Talalay and his colleagues at Johns Hopkins University in Baltimore have been studying the disease-preventing properties of cruciferous vegetables for several years and consider them to be the most important food group in disease prevention. Broccoli, cabbage, cauliflower, and brussels sprouts are examples of cruciferous vegetables. Cruciferous vegetables belong to the family *Brassicaceae*, which also includes mustard greens and seeds. Unfortunately, vegetables in this group are among the least popular among Americans because of their pungent taste and malodor during cooking. Despite their lack of popularity at the dinner table, these vegetables have been the target of hundreds of studies throughout the world. Sharing the research limelight with *Brassicae* is another group of sulfur vegetables, members of the *Liliaceae* family, which includes asparagus, garlic, and onions.

Garlic is one of the oldest and most revered medicinal foods of all time. Onions, leeks, shallots, and chives have also had their share of glory but do not possess the notoriety or effectiveness of garlic.

The common element in these vegetables—and the root of the smell—is sulfur. It's also what makes them chemopreventive. Each vegetable within the various groups has a unique set of sulfur compounds, and each of these has a specific set of activities.

Why Sulfur Compounds Are Important

The sulfur chemical bonds are of particular importance because they effectively transform toxins and other harmful chemicals that enter the body into products that can be easily eliminated. We need these sulfur compounds to protect the body from an excess of potentially harmful active metabolites produced within our own tissues.

Sulfur-containing enzymes also process environmental toxins, medications, and chemicals in food and beverages. These substances are known as *xenobiotics*, meaning foreign to the body. Let's see how each of the sulfur vegetables can protect you from disease and which are best for your body type.

Brassicaceae Family: Crucifers and Mustards

The Latin root -*crucifer* means "bearing a cross." It was chosen to describe the flowers of *Brassicae* whose petals occur in fours in a criss-cross arrangement. You may be familiar with wild mustard that grows alongside roads. It has little yellow or white flowers with four petals arranged in a crossed configuration.

All cruciferous vegetables are characterized by a strong odor and pungency that increases with cooking or chopping. This happens because the enzyme *myrosinase*, always present in crucifers, begins breaking down the sulfur compounds. *Brassica* vegetables can be divided into two groups, the cruciferous and the mustard. All belong to the genus *Brassica* except arugula and wasabi. Here is a list of vegetables in each category:

Cruciferous Vegetables	Mustard Vegetables
Broccoli (*Brassica*)	Arugula
Broccoflower	Black Mustard Seed
Bok Choy	Canola (rapeseed)
Brussels Sprouts	Daikon
Cabbage (white, savoy, red, Napa)	Garlic Mustard (*Alliaria petiolata*)
Cauliflower	Horseradish
Collards	Mustard Greens
Kale	Radish

Kohlrabi	Wasabi
Rutabaga	Watercress
Tatsoi	
Turnip	
Watercress	

Cruciferous vegetables are the pinnacle of phytochemical research because they block many disease processes and are virtually devoid of side effects. In nature, sulfur compounds protect the plants that contain them; the strong bitter taste is an effective deterrent to being eaten by fungi, insects, or herbivores. It's not surprising that these foods are also protective in humans. *Glucobrassicin* and *glucoraphanin* are the most important sulfur compounds found in *Brassicae*. From these two parent compounds come a variety of active sulfur compounds known as biotransformation products. The process of biotransformation begins as soon as the plant cells are ruptured by chewing, chopping, or cooking. The product is a family of odorous compounds called *glucosinolates*.

Glucosinolates are found throughout the broccoli and mustard families, with highest concentrations found in cabbage and cauliflower, and smaller amounts occurring in broccoli and brussels sprouts. Approximately twelve different glucosinolates occur in crucifers, and each is further transformed into important end products. It's the biotransformation products, rather than the glucosinolates per se, that are responsible for the chemotherapeutic benefits (and odor) of this class of vegetables.

What These Compounds Do

Eating cruciferous vegetables has been associated with reduced incidence of tumors, hormone-dependent cancers, and several organ cancers, including that of the urinary bladder. Researchers from Harvard's School of Public Health conducted a large study involving 47,909 men enrolled in the Health Professionals Follow-Up Study. The scientists gathered dietary information for ten years to determine how diet affected the occurrence of bladder cancer. During this period, 252 cases of bladder cancer occurred among the test subjects. Statistical analysis showed a positive correlation between eating cruciferous vegetables and protection from bladder cancer. Among the crucifers, broccoli and cabbage appeared to confer the greatest protection. Not surprisingly, these crucifers contain the highest levels of glucosinolates. How much of these cancer-preventive compounds one gets from eating broccoli and cauliflower can vary considerably by length of storage and growing conditions. Scientists attempt to correct for these variations in a number of ways, one of which is using cruciferous sprouts.

A research team at Johns Hopkins University found that three-day-old broccoli and cauliflower sprouts contained anywhere from ten to one hundred times greater levels of the glucosinolate glucoraphanin than the mature plants.

Calcium D-glucarate is a powerful disease-fighting phytochemical enzymatically produced from the glucosinolate *sulforaphane.* In the body, calcium D-glucarate is further converted into D-glucarolactone, an important inhibitor of breast cancer. Doctors at the University of Texas's M. D. Anderson Cancer Center in Houston found that women with breast cancer had much lower serum levels of glucarate than healthy women. According to these doctors, this increased the chance their cancer could spread because these women could not effectively prevent estrogen activation of cancer processes in other body tissues.

The M. D. Anderson medical team suggested that supplementation with calcium D-glucarate could be used during hormone replacement therapy to help prevent breast cancer and might also increase the effectiveness of standard chemotherapy for breast cancer. This could be breakthrough research for thousands of women at risk for or fighting this disease.

Isothiocyanates are another unique biotransformation product from *sulforaphane,* a glucosinolate derived from glucoraphanin. Isothiocyanates, concentrated in cabbage, kale, and mustard seeds and greens, are believed to prevent lung and esophageal cancer among smokers. Several research teams from U.S. medical institutions, including John Hopkins University School of Medicine, the American Health Foundation, Ohio State University of Public Health, and the University of Minnesota Cancer Center, have reported similar results of chemopreventive effects by isothiocyanates among smokers.

Isothiocyanates also appear to goad tumor cells into self-destruction, the process known as "programmed cell death" or apoptosis. Numerous other studies have shown that isothiocyanates appear to be effective against cancers of the gastrointestinal and respiratory tracts—including mouth, pharynx and lung, plus those of the stomach, colon, and rectum.

Indole-3-carbinol (I3C) is another important cancer-preventive compound that is concentrated in broccoli, brussels sprouts, cabbage, and kale. I3C is of special research interest because like other cruciferous compounds we've discussed, it appears to block estrogen-dependent breast cancer. A research team at U.C. Berkeley, headed by Dr. Gary Firestone, has carried out several studies on the effects of I3C, including combined therapy with the drug tamoxifen. According to Dr. Firestone, a combination of I3C and tamoxifen will synergistically block the growth of estrogen-responsive breast cancer cells. Although Dr. Firestone and the other scientists mentioned above used isolated I3C, are dietary sources of I3C just as effective?

A research team from the Institute for Hormone Research in New York enrolled sixty healthy women in a three-month trial to find out if I3C could alter the production of active estrogen metabolites. The scientists divided the women into three groups: one eating a high-I3C diet containing 400 mg of I3C daily, another a high-fiber diet at 20 grams a day, and a third control group on a placebo diet. The women getting the I3C showed significantly higher levels of the cancer-protective estrogen metabolite 2-hydroxyestrone, or 2-OH E_1. Neither the high-fiber diet nor the placebo diet produced increased levels of this metabolite over baseline. Another estrogen metabolite, 16-hydroxyestrone, or 16-OH E_1, is linked to promotion of breast cancer. By promoting higher levels of the protective active estrogen metabolite, breast cancer incidence might be significantly reduced by eating cruciferous vegetables.

Possible Side Effects of These Foods

Thyroid Problems

Goitrogens are a group of naturally occurring compounds in foods that inhibit thyroid hormone synthesis. Glucosinolates are one such group of compounds and they can bind iodine when they occur in high concentrations in blood. However, eating cruciferous vegetables and other dietary goitrogens rarely reaches sufficient blood levels to cause a problem. Nevertheless, individuals who have thyroid problems or iodine deficiency should seek medical advice on whether to avoid such foods. Other foods that contain goitrogens are cassava, sorghum, corn, and millet. Cassava contains the highest levels of goitrogen, and populations that consume large amounts of this food have learned to soak, dry, and powder it to remove the goitrogens.

Pregnancy and Lactation

I will never forget my surprise when my breast-fed three-month-old son presented me with a wet diaper that smelled just like overcooked cabbage. I was a new mom, but I had a degree in biochemistry and thought I knew it all. Imagine my chagrin when I realized that the "old wives' tale" held true—that what you eat affects your breast milk. Moreover, my son had been unusually fussy, perhaps as a result of my cabbage meal, and I was forced to acknowledge that the warnings of more experienced moms were justified.

Scientists have found in animal studies that the glucosinolates from cruciferous vegetables pass the placental barrier and lactating glands; so much so, that the young are protected from developing various cancers. Human studies at the University of Minnesota School of Public Health have confirmed what I found out the hard way—moms who eat cruciferous vegetables can have colicky babies.

Does this mean that you shouldn't eat cruciferous vegetables during pregnancy and lactation? Of course not. It just means that you should follow your personal color chart more closely, providing your child with glucosinolates that your body type can process more efficiently. In my case, I shouldn't have been eating cabbage in the first place, because I'm a Yellow type and green cabbage is definitely not my color.

Drug Interactions

Fermented foods, including sauerkraut, may present some special problems for people with allergies or who are taking certain drugs. Fermentation produces high levels of tyramine, a neuropeptide that in susceptible individuals increases blood pressure and induces sweating, pounding chest, and headaches. Tyramine also enhances the effects of monamine oxidase (MAO) inhibitors such as phenelzine (Nardil) used to treat depression. Isoniazid (Rifampin) also has some MAO-inhibiting effects and people taking this drug should avoid tyramine-containing foods.

Buying, Storing, and Cooking These Foods

Cruciferous vegetables are high in vitamin C, which is reduced as the vegetables are transported and stored. Buy the freshest cruciferous vegetables you can find and don't store them in your refrigerator for more than three or four days. Better still, lightly steam them the day you bring them home and keep what you can't eat that day for snacking or future meals. As the biotransformation products are formed, vitamin C will be stabilized in the compounds formed. The vegetable should retain its bright green color and be quite crisp when pierced with a fork.

Bok choy and Napa or Chinese cabbage are delicate and should be stir-fried rather than steamed. They take only a few seconds to cook. Other kinds of cabbage can be used to make slaw, rolled around a filling and steamed, added to soups, or chopped, steamed, and served alone or with other vegetables. Cabbage makes a nice accompaniment to carotenoid-rich vegetables such as carrots. Raw kohlrabi is very good peeled, sliced, and eaten as a snack or added to salads. In fact, this is the preferred way to eat it. Cut away the leaves and stalks and eat just the base. It has a nice, clean, crisp flavor—not at all pungent. You will have to look for small, young and tender kohlrabi. The larger ones are too woody. Broccoli and cauliflower are favorites for dipping. I prefer them lightly steamed and chilled rather than raw, but suit yourself. Children often prefer them as snacks, and it's a good way to make sure they are getting this valuable food.

Eating sprouts is an excellent way to increase your intake of cruciferous vegetables. Sprouts are considered superior foods in Ayurveda because they contain highly concentrated nutrients and large amounts of enzymes that assist in the digestion and assimilation of other foods. Sprouting kits are available in most natural food stores and you will also find a wide selection of seeds available.

Which of These Vegetables Is My Color?

You may be convinced at this point that you will have to add more cruciferous vegetables and mustard to your daily food plan. But which are better for *you?*

Greens: greens are your foods! The best ones are deep green or blue/green. All of the cruciferous vegetables, mustards, radishes, and horseradish keep you in balance. You can enjoy them raw or steamed and you have the greatest variety to choose from.

Your Primary Colors
Cruciferous vegetables: broccoli, broccoflower, Chinese broccoli (rabe), brussels sprouts, cabbage (red, white, savoy), cauliflower, collards, kohlrabi, and turnips
Mustards: arugula, black and yellow mustard seeds, daikon, horseradish, mustard greens, radish, wasabi, and watercress

Your Complementary Colors
Cruciferous vegetables: all are primary
Mustards: all are primary

Your Clashing Colors
Cruciferous vegetables: rutabaga
Mustards: none

Reds do well with most cruciferous vegetables. The spiciest mustards are too hot for Reds, but the milder ones are well tolerated. Reds need especially to avoid foods such as sauerkraut, not only because it contains tyramine which raises blood pressure, but because it is vinegary and salty.

Your Primary Colors
Cruciferous vegetables: broccoli, broccoflower, bok choy, Chinese broccoli (broccoli rabe), cauliflower, collards, and kale
Mustards: arugula, watercress

Your Complementary Colors
Cruciferous vegetables: kohlrabi and rutabaga
Mustards: daikon and mustard greens

Your Clashing Colors
Cruciferous vegetables: turnips
Mustards: black and yellow mustard seeds, horseradish, radish, and wasabi

Yellows have a problem with some cruciferous vegetables because they are apt to cause intestinal gas. Most of the mustards are well tolerated. Yellows can tolerate more of these foods if they are steamed. However, it's always best to concentrate on those foods that are your primary color.

Your Primary Colors
Cruciferous vegetables: bok choy and Napa (Chinese) cabbage
Mustards: black and yellow mustard seeds, canola seeds, daikon and watercress

Your Complementary Colors
Cruciferous vegetables: broccoli, broccoflower, Chinese broccoli (rabe), and collards
Mustards: horseradish, mustard greens, radish, and wasabi

Your Clashing Colors
Cruciferous vegetables: brussels sprouts, cabbage (except Napa), cauliflower, rutabaga, and turnips
Mustards: arugula

Alliaceae Family: Onions and Garlic

The *Alliaceae* family includes vegetables of the *allium* genus; namely, onions, garlic, elephant garlic, chives, leeks, and shallots. All of these vegetables are known for their pungent taste. All one has to do is cut into them to release extremely strong vapors. Cutting unleashes a set of reactions in the bulb that produces potent phytochemicals.

The name *allium* dates back many centuries and has been attributed to many sources. Modern chemical application of the term dates back 150 years to the German scientist Wertheim's discovery that garlic's active components contain a unique hydrocarbon-sulfur bond which he named *allyl.* The sulfur compounds in garlic and other allium species are quickly transformed (within six seconds) when the bulbs are bruised, mashed or cooked. Cloves of garlic that are still covered with their protective shell have no smell. However, as soon as they are peeled or cut, they give off a strong odor, which is what your nose and eyes detect. That's because the enzyme *allinase* begins acting on the sulfur compounds, transforming them into a number of disease-preventing daughter compounds. All members of the onion and garlic family contain allin and allinase, although the levels of these compounds vary considerably. The more odorous the bulb, the more sulfur compounds it contains—and the greater its medicinal properties.

Garlic Family
Garlic (*Allium sativum*)
Elephant garlic (*Allium ampeloprasum* L.)
Bear's (wild) garlic (*Allium ursinum*)

Onion Family
Onions (*Allium cepa*)
Chives (*Allium schoenoprasum* L.)
Winter leek (*Allium porrum*)
Summer leek (*Allium ampeloprasum* L.)
Pearl onion (*Allium ophioscorodon*)
Scallion (*Allium cepa*)
Shallot (*Allium ascalonicum* L.)

The primary organosulfur phytochemicals in garlic and onions are called *thiosulfonates*, and include allylic sulfides, vinyldithiins, ajoenes, and mercaptocysteines. Other important sulfur compounds are γ-glutamylcysteines, scordinin, and several nonsulfur phytochemicals including steroids, triterpenoids, flavonoids, and fructans. Garlic has been one of the most intensely studied medicinal foods, largely because of its high sulfur content and widely recognized health benefits. Garlic contains approximately four times the amount of sulfur compounds found in broccoli and has been a dietary component of Euro-Asian and African cultures for five thousand years. Onions do not have the sulfur power of garlic, yet they also possess powerful healing effects.

Garlic and onions have been used as both food and medicine and are thought to have originated in central Asia. Early medical texts from the Middle East, India, and China all contain references to the use of garlic and onions to treat everything from poor digestion and coughs to skin conditions. Garlic was also found in the tomb of the Egyptian pharaoh Tutankhamen (d. 1352 B.C.), providing evidence it was highly regarded in Egypt as well. The Israelites are said to have used garlic during their exile in Egypt, and there is evidence they carried it with them into the Sinai Peninsula and beyond.

Garlic eventually became an important food and medicine throughout the "Fertile Crescent"—the world's richest agricultural belt—that extended into modern Israel, Jordan, Lebanon, Palestine, Turkey, Syria, and Iraq. The ideal growing conditions in this region no doubt produced garlic of superior quality, as growing conditions determine phytochemical content. From there garlic spread to Greece and Italy. Though it became an important part of culinary and medicinal practices in Italy, the Roman hierarchy are reported to have objected to the odor of garlic, relegating its use to lower-class citizens and soldiers. Roman soldiers took it with them as they marched throughout western Europe. However, by the time the Romans overran the British Isles the Celts were already using garlic. The Celts preferred to collect and use their own "wild" broad-leafed garlic, a distinct species called *Allium ursinum.* They may have convinced the Romans it was better because this garlic is popular today in Germany and other western European countries. It's also called "bear's" garlic and may have more pronounced effects in some conditions than other garlic.

What These Compounds Do

Garlic and onions have been used primarily for their cardiovascular benefits. There are several ways they may prevent cardiovascular disease, such as reducing blood fats, preventing platelets from sticking together, and as a preventive measure against age-related vascular changes. Garlic and onions are also powerful anti-inflammatory, antibacterial, and anti-viral agents.

Effects on Cholesterol—In analyzing numerous studies, doctors at New York Medical College in Valhalla, New York, reported a significant reduction in total cholesterol levels (9 percent) in patients with elevated cholesterol who received 600 to 900 mg allicin-standardized powdered garlic pills, the equivalent of a half to one clove of fresh garlic daily for eight to twenty-four weeks.

Effects on Blood Pressure—Garlic has also been found to be effective in lowering blood pressure. Australian physicians analyzed eight trials that included data on 415 hypertensive or hyperlipidemic subjects. Half of the subjects in each trial had been given garlic powder, the other half a placebo. Most of the trials ran twelve weeks and used 600 mg to 900 mg allicin-standardized garlic powder daily. The garlic-treated subjects lowered their systolic blood pressure (higher figure in blood pressure readings) by 7.7 points (mm of mercury) and their diastolic pressure (second or lower figure) by 5 points. No side effects from the garlic therapy were reported.

Effects on Blood Lipids—Fish oils are also important dietary chemicals; actually, they're zoochemicals because they're from an animal source. Canadian scientists used fish oils in combination with garlic to study fifty men with moderately high cholesterol. One-third of the men received both fish oil and garlic as supplements for twelve weeks, another third were given garlic alone, and the last third got fish oil but no garlic. The combination therapy produced the best results, lowering both triglycerides and total cholesterol. Garlic alone lowered LDL and total cholesterol, but it didn't affect triglycerides. Fish oils, on the other hand, lowered triglycerides but they actually raised LDL cholesterol, the bad kind.

Even among people with normal cholesterol levels, garlic may be good prevention. British scientists gave 68 normal volunteers either 600 mg of a standardized (1.3% allicin) garlic powder or a placebo for ten weeks. The garlic supplement reduced cholesterol levels to the low normal range and decreased triglycerides slightly.

Anti-Platelet Activity—Ajoene, a breakdown product found in crushed fresh garlic, is an effective anti-platelet compound and appears to act by altering membrane viscosity. The result is reduced "stickiness" of platelets—either to each other or to vascular walls. Sticky platelets are a major risk factor in clot formation that can result in stroke or heart attack. Onions have also been reported to possess anti-platelet activity. However, the sulfur content varies among species of onions, and only those with high sulfur content, evidenced by strong smell, are effective. Dr. Indrajit Das and colleagues at Charing Cross and Westminster Medical School in London found that in addition to anti-platelet activity, garlic has a direct effect on arterial walls. The mechanism by which this occurs is release of nitric oxide, which relaxes arterial walls.

Anti-Microbial Effects—Several studies have shown ajoene from freshly macerated garlic was effective against fungal infections including the deadly meningitis cryptococcus when the macerate was administered intravenously into infected patients.

Anticancer Effects—Doctors at Loma Linda University found that garlic was effective against cancer by blocking tumor growth, boosting anticancer immunity and deactivating cancer-causing chemical, microbial and viral toxins. These multiple effects of garlic help explain why epidemiological evidence from China suggests that regions where garlic is eaten have much lower incidence of stomach cancer as compared to regions where no garlic is consumed. Another reason why garlic may protect against developing stomach cancer is its killing effect on *Helicobacter pylori*, a primary causative agent in this cancer. Chinese doctors have found much fewer *H. pylori* bacteria in the stomach juices of garlic eating citizens.

Possible Adverse Effects of These Foods

Raw onions and garlic can produce gastric irritation and flatulence in susceptible individuals. Cooking eliminates this problem since the sulfur compounds change. Cooked garlic and onions contain converted sugars and their sulfur compounds. Peeling and slicing onions can be irritating to the mucous membranes. When the cell walls of an onion are broken, a chemical called propanethial-S-oxide is released; when it gets into your eyes, it changes into sulfuric acid, which is why you experience a burning sensation. Cutting it under running water prevents this from happening. Milder onions such as Vidalia, young torpedo reds, or Maui onions do not contain enough propanethial-S-oxide to cause a problem.

Raw garlic's potential adverse effects include minor gastric disturbances, offensive breath and body odor, and skin irritation. Garlic should not be combined with other blood-thinning and blood pressure–reducing substances because it may enhance their effects. Garlic breath is a problem for most people. Chemical analysis of garlic breath has shown that an assortment of important phytochemicals, including allyl sulfides and selenium compounds, contribute the most odor, which gradually decreases over one to three hours. Two important anticancer terpenes that do not have an odor have also been detected in garlic breath, *d*-limonene and *p*-cymene. Most people seeking the therapeutic benefits of garlic choose supplements. Onions, shallots, leeks, chives, and scallions have low-enough levels of sulfides to be somewhat less offensive, but can still leave a distinct lingering taste and odor for a short period of time after eaten raw. Herbalists suggest chewing raw parsley to help overcome the aftertaste and breath odor of onions and garlic.

Supplements of aged garlic avoid odor problems because they contain the less odorous biotransformation compounds. Though they don't offer some of the benefits that whole crushed garlic extracts do, they may work better for Red or Yellow types, who may experience stomach irritation with raw-garlic supplements.

Possible Drug Interactions—Garlic is an effective blood-thinning agent in that it reduces platelet stickiness. It may enhance the effects of platelet-inhibiting drugs such as ticlopidine (Ticlid), used to treat intermittent claudication (leg cramping and pain due to clogged veins) and prevent stroke. Garlic may also potentiate the effects of Warfarin (coumadin), an anticoagulant drug used to treat people with venous or lung blood clots. Therefore, anyone taking these medications should not use standardized garlic extracts or eat more than one clove of garlic a day.

Buying, Storing, and Cooking These Foods

Always look for firm bulbs with dry outer skins. Store them in a cool, dark place for up to a month, depending on your climate. Humidity will hasten sprouting, so refrigeration may be your only option if you live in a warm, humid climate.

Cooking garlic and onions destroys the enzyme allinase and the therapeutic sulfur compounds do not form. However, crushing or cutting the bulbs does activate allinase and the daughter compounds are formed. It's best to cut the bulbs just before cooking since the daughter compounds will quickly dissipate into the air. Only about 16 percent of the sulfur compounds remain after garlic is sautéed or stir-fried. However, this can be sufficient to reap the many benefits of garlic.

Which of These Vegetables Is My Color?

Greens

Cruciferous vegetables, asparagus, garlic, and onions are your primary foods. You can eat them raw or cooked.

Reds

Raw garlic and onions are not good for you. They are too pungent and hot for your type. You may be able to tolerate cooked onions and garlic in moderation. Avoid standardized garlic supplements. You may use steamed garlic oil capsules or a brand of deodorized garlic called Kyolic. Many Reds who have tried garlic supplements find they "repeat." If this has happened to you, just switch to the kinds I recommend in this chapter.

Yellow

Raw garlic and onions don't work for you, either. You may experience gas after eating them and some Yellow types get headaches after eating raw onions or garlic. However, you will do fine with them when they're cooked, provided you don't overdo it. You can use any garlic supplement. If your system is unusually sensitive to the pungent compounds in garlic, try switching to the kinds recommended for Red types.

In addition to the foods discussed here, a number of leafy green vegetables including collards and dandelion greens contain sulfur and are excellent disease-preventive foods. Asparagus is another sulfur-containing vegetable. Eating asparagus causes malodorous urine in many individuals. The sulfur-containing excretion compounds are S-methyl thioacrylate and S-methyl thiopropionate—harmless breakdown compounds of asparagus biotransformation products.

Now that we have examined in detail what science has revealed about the three primary colored foods—yellow, red, and green—let's move on to discussions of the three groups of complementary color foods.

8

Tan Foods

We have been concentrating on the colors of foods in the previous three chapters and learning why it's important to select foods that are your color. Most of the foods in this chapter are deep, rich shades of brown, pink, reddish brown, plus a few that are white or black. Tan or warm brown are shades that we associate with earth, and they best describe the hearty foods in this group including grains, cereals, pasta, breads, and legumes. Tan foods make up half of what we eat every day and they provide important disease-fighting phytochemicals, provided you choose whole grains over refined and processed ones.

Many people prefer products made from refined grains and flours, in part because they don't like the rough texture and nutty flavor of whole grains such as wheat, rye, and brown rice. Refined cereals and grains also taste sweeter because the noncarbohydrate parts of the grain have been removed. Yet it has been well established that eating the more highly textured, unrefined tan foods is more protective against disease. That's because various phytochemicals are lost during processing.

Science notwithstanding, you no doubt consider these foods an important part of your diet. And scientists agree that these foods should form the base of your food pyramid. These are the "substantial" and "earthy" foods we build meals around. Tan foods are your most important complementary color, and along with your primary brightly colored foods, form the basis of your *Eat Your Colors* meal plans. Tan foods supply the following phytochemicals:

- Dietary fiber, lignin, pectin, cellulose, hemi-cellulose
- Starches that resist breakdown into sugars (resistant starches)

- Phenolic compounds
- Phytic acid
- Phytosterols
- Phytoestrogens
- Saponins
- Complex carbohydrates (oligosaccharides)
- Antioxidant trace minerals: zinc, copper, manganese, selenium
- Essential B-vitamins and folic acid

Many studies have focused on the high-fiber content of these foods in disease prevention. However, some researchers suggest it's the combination of phytochemicals in whole grains and legumes that may be most protective.

Whole Grains

The term "whole grains" refers to cereal grains that have had minimal processing and contain most of the phytochemicals listed above. Nutritionists commonly refer to these foods as cereals because they are crops harvested for dry grains only. They are always cooked or processed before being eaten. The group includes rice, wheat, corn, barley, rye, oats, millet, and sorghum. All of these grains are consumed by people throughout the world. In some countries, including the United States, other grains such as amaranth, spelt, teff, and quinoa are available. Buckwheat is dried, stored, and prepared like a cereal although it is technically a seed and not a grain. Whole grains are carbohydrate-rich foods that also contain protein, essential fatty acids, and numerous vitamins and minerals. Refined or highly processed cereal grains contain few if any phytochemicals and only those vitamins and minerals that are added to "enrich" these products.

There are three general parts to a grain kernel. The bran, or outer coating, is mostly cellulose, an indigestible complex carbohydrate. Most of the B-vitamins and minerals are located under the bran layer. When the bran is removed, many of these nutrients are lost. The germ contains some starch but is primarily oils and oil-soluble vitamins such as vitamin E and tocotrienols, an important member of the vitamin E family. The largest portion of the grain, the endosperm, consists of stored starch and is the sweetest part of the grain. The endosperm also contains digestive enzymes (a kind of protein) that will break down the starch into sugars. Nature intended that the bran protect the grain when it falls to the ground and until conditions are favorable for sprouting. The germ sprouts the new plant and the endosperm provides food, vitamins, and minerals to support sprouting and initial growth of the seed. As the chlorophyll-rich stalk and leaves form, they will take over food production for the plant.

Whole Grains and Disease Prevention

Cardiovascular Disease

Two large ongoing studies, the Harvard School of Public Health male health professionals study and the Brigham and Women's Hospital nurses health study, continue to examine the role of diet and incidence of disease. Researchers have examined the protective role of whole grains against cardiovascular disease and stroke in these studies. They found that among male health professionals, those who ate the fewest higher fiber foods were at greatest risk for having a heart attack. Moreover, the heart attacks that proved fatal were associated with the lowest intakes. Among the nurses, those who ate just one or two whole grain servings a day had the lowest risk of stroke while those who ate little or none had the greatest risk. Among whole grains listed were dark bread, whole grain breakfast cereal, popcorn, cooked oatmeal, wheat germ, brown rice, bran, bulgur, kasha, and couscous.

Diabetes

Eating whole grains has also been associated with a reduced risk of Type 2 diabetes, also known as adult onset diabetes. In a six-year study of 35,988 older women in Iowa, those who had higher intakes of whole grains, total dietary fibers, and cereal fibers had much lower incidence of Type 2 diabetes, leading to the conclusion that these foods can protect against this disease in older women.

Colorectal Cancer

The scientific evidence that whole grain consumption reduces the risk of colorectal cancer has not been definitively shown. Seemingly conflicting results have been reported in the scientific literature on the role of a high-fiber diet in the prevention of recurring colonic adenomas (polyps), which are strongly associated with the risk of colon cancer. About 5 to 10 percent of precancerous colorectal polyps will become cancerous if they are not removed. Consequently, the National Cancer Institute wanted to find out if a high-fiber diet could prevent colonic adenomas, and they funded two recent studies to answer the question. The first study, the Polyp Prevention Trial, examined total daily fiber intake, including fruits and vegetables, in addition to cereals, grains, and breads among 2,079 men and women. All of the study participants had had one or more polyps removed within the preceding six months of starting the trial, which went on for four years. The study results, which showed no protective effect, surprised Dr. Arthur Schatzkin, chief of the NCI's Nutritional Epidemiology Branch and lead investigator in this study. Unfortunately, the researchers did not investigate the protective effects of whole grains, which contain many beneficial phytochemicals besides fiber.

The second NCI study, the Wheat Bran Fiber Study, investigated possible benefits from taking a high-fiber supplement (13.5 grams daily) without any dietary restrictions. A group of 1,429 men and women, who had at least one colorectal adenoma removed within three months of beginning the trial, were enrolled in the three-year study. Again, the results of the study were disappointing in that participants given the supplement developed just as many new adenomas as those who were not supplemented. This study shows that isolating one component from foods and hoping it will protect against cancer doesn't necessarily work. Whole grains offer a family of protective phytonutrients, not just fiber.

When results such as these are reported, they create a stir within the scientific community because they seem to contradict what has previously been demonstrated by numerous other studies. Why have scientists focused on fiber as a means to prevent colorectal cancer? Fiber increases fecal bulk and exercises colonic muscles to expel waste material more efficiently. This reduces the opportunity for toxic by-products to alter normal metabolism in cells lining the colon. And while fiber is very important, other compounds in whole grains, including phenolic acids, phytic acid, phytosterols, and saponins, play a significant role in maintaining healthy colon function. The best advice for health-conscious people is to consume several servings of *whole* grains daily in addition to several servings of fruits and vegetables. Other studies that were based on these dietary goals showed a protective benefit against colorectal cancer. Let's move on now to other health benefits that might accrue from eating whole grains.

Breast Cancer

Researchers in Besançon, France, who studied the effect of diet on primary breast cancer, found a significant reduction in risk among those eating the greatest amount of grains, garlic, and onions. Among postmenopausal women in the study, there was an added advantage if they consumed a diet low in saturated fats and increased their intake of unsaturated fats.

Despite the pitfalls in U.S. studies, nutrition experts continue to stress the importance of increasing your intake of whole grains, fruits, and vegetables. There is clear evidence that by doing so, you may alter, delay, or even prevent several chronic diseases. If you are diligent about choosing those foods that are your colors, you can increase the effect. The evidence is overwhelmingly in favor of replacing white flour, white sugar, and processed cereals with their whole-grain counterparts.

The scientific community continues to be intrigued by the prospect of identifying exactly which phytochemicals protect against a particular disease.

Effects of Fiber Intake on Appetite and Food Choice

Let's start with breakfast because most people have at least one grain serving for breakfast. How does your choice of which cereal to eat affect your appetite during the rest of the morning? Swedish scientists have found that eating a high-fiber breakfast is best. That's because it cuts down on snacking between meals and reduces appetite at the next meal, presumably lunch. Carbohydrate release and breakdown into sugars are the reason why whole-grain cereals more effectively reduce appetite. Whole-grain cereals are low on the glycemic index—an indicator of how quickly a carbohydrate-rich food will raise blood sugar levels and trigger the release of insulin. I will discuss more on the topic of the glycemic index a little later in this chapter.

Australian researchers wanted to know if you added fat to your breakfast, say regular cream cheese on your bagel, would that affect your satiety level and choice of foods at lunch? They gave test subjects either a fat-rich breakfast, a high-fiber breakfast, or a low-fiber meal. All of the meals contained the same number of calories. Apparently the people who got the high-fiber meal complained about their food not being tasty, while the high-fat people enjoyed the creamy texture of their meal. However, the people in the latter group paid the price at lunch. They were hungrier and picked more high-fat foods to eat than their high-fiber-eating counterparts, who had smaller appetites and didn't choose fatty foods for lunch. The people in this study were also asked about their mental alertness throughout the morning. Those who ate the high-fiber breakfast reported the greatest amount of sustained alertness between breakfast and lunch. By the way, this was a crossover study in which each person got to try both diets. Thus, they served as their own control.

How Quickly Will Dietary Change Work?

A research team in Los Altos, California, conducted a small study of 12 women that suggested switching to a phytochemical-rich diet can be effective in as little as four weeks, even for those at risk for cardiovascular disease. The women, who were hyperlipidemic (high blood fats and cholesterol), were divided into two groups, one receiving a standard refined-food diet and the other a phytochemical-rich diet of whole grains, fruits, and vegetables. The caloric content of the diets was the same and the women switched diets after four weeks, so each served as her own control. The phytonutrient diet was low in saturated fats and high in fiber, vitamin E, vitamin C, and carotene.

The women had significant decreases in total cholesterol (13 percent) and LDL cholesterol (16 percent) at the end of the four-week phytochemical diet. Surprisingly, the levels of their cellular antioxidant protective enzymes were reduced by 69 and 35 percent, respectively. This meant that their antioxidant status had been boosted by the phytochemicals so that fewer of these protective enzymes were needed. The women also reported improved colon function.

Phenols and Antioxidant Protection

Whole grains have strong antioxidant protection. A team of Polish scientists tested the antioxidant power of wheat, barley, rye, oats, and buckwheat. The strongest antioxidant was buckwheat, followed by barley, oats, and wheat mixed with rye. When the cereals were processed to remove their hulls, the hierarchy changed slightly. Buckwheat still came out on top but oats switched places with barley. The antioxidant activity came from the phenolic acids in the cereals. The next question we might ask is, what happens to the phenolic acids when grains are processed?

It is common to treat plant-derived foods with alkali in order to recover proteins from grains and legumes, remove the peels from fruits and vegetables, and destroy microorganisms. This process drastically alters the functional and nutritional properties of whole foods and destroys some natural phenolic compounds. These compounds supply us with antioxidant, anticarcinogenic, and anti-microbial protection.

Phytic Acid

Phenolic compounds make a very important contribution to human health as antioxidants and cancer preventives. Although they are found in fruits and vegetables, they are concentrated in whole grains. Phytic acid is another important phytochemical in whole grains that has powerful anti-cancer properties. These and several others have been proposed by several research teams for being just as important, if not more so, than fiber. This highlights the importance of eating whole grains rather than depending solely on dietary supplements of fiber.

Phytosterols

Plant sterols (phytosterols) are found in some grains, nuts, seeds, soy, fresh and dried peas, split peas, and saw palmetto berries. Phytosterols are unique phytochemicals in that they have a structure similar to cholesterol. Because of this, phytosterols compete with cholesterol for absorption in the colon. This reduces the total cholesterol load in the body without the side effects of drugs commonly used to reduce serum cholesterol. Phytosterols are added to margarine (Benecol, Take Control), making this product a functional food with FDA-approved claims for lowering cholesterol. Daily phytosterol intake in the United States is estimated to be 180 mg, while in Japan it is around 400 mg. The Japanese eat large amounts of soy foods, one of the best sources of phytochemicals.

The interest in phytosterols and cholesterol lowering in humans can be traced back to a 1984 Johns Hopkins study of diets of Seventh-Day Adventists living in the greater Los Angeles area. Most Adventists eat either a lacto-ovo (includes eggs, dairy) or strict vegetarian (no animal products) diet. Both of these diets contain less cholesterol and more phytosterols than the standard American diet. The vegan diet would not contain any cholesterol, which is an animal product. The ratio of phytosterol to cholesterol (phyto:chol) in the participants' blood was used as an indicator of their primary risk factor for cardiovascular disease. In the opinion of the researchers, the amount of total cholesterol consumed may not be as great a risk factor for disease as its ratio to phytosterols. Therefore, the higher the ratio, the better. Not surprisingly, vegans had the highest ratio, 16:1. Lacto-ovo vegetarians came in next at 3.26:1, non-vegetarian Adventists had a ratio of 0.98:1, and non-Adventists eating a standard diet had the lowest ratio of 0.49:1. Since that time, numerous studies have been published showing the relationship between phytosterol intake and cholesterol metabolism.

A recent review of sixteen published clinical trials showed that phytosterols lowered total cholesterol by an average of 10 percent. They also lowered LDL cholesterol by an average of 13 percent. This is exciting news because most of the drugs used to lower cholesterol have side effects.

Some people are genetically prone to pump out more cholesterol from the liver than is needed. For these people, cholesterol stubbornly remains high, even when they modify their diets. Phytosterols appear to alter the way the liver handles cholesterol and may block its manufacture. The exact mechanisms by which phytosterols work and which ones are most effective have yet to be defined.

Below is a table listing the various phytosterols in selected grains:

Phytosterol Content of Some Grains

Grain, Nut or Legume	Avenasterol	Campesterol	Stigmasterols	Oryzanol	Beta sitosterol	Gamma sitosterol
Oats		✓	✓			
Barley		✓	✓			
Rice		✓	✓	✓	✓	✓
Wheat						
Almond					✓	
Cashew	✓			✓		
Filbert	✓	✓	✓		✓	
Pistachio		✓		✓		
Olives					✓	
Flaxseed		✓	✓		✓	
Sesame					✓	
Sunflower		✓	✓		✓	
Pumpkin	✓			✓		✓
Soy			✓		✓	
Green Pea, Split Peas		✓	✓			

Source: James Duke, *Handbook of Phytochemical Constituents.* Boca Raton, Fla.: CRC Press, 1992.

From the table, it is apparent that rice contains a greater variety of phytosterols than other tan foods. This illustrates why eating more rice, particularly brown rice, is an important part of your meal plan. Most Americans eat more wheat than any other grain, and most of it is refined. Rice is a grain to pay close attention to. Rice is extremely versatile, with a lower tendency to raise blood sugar levels than potatoes, and whole-grain rice is more nutritious than pasta. Many kinds of rice are available, so you have an endless variety to choose from. The following table gives you the various kinds, what they taste like, and how to use them.

Rice Varieties and Blends

Short Grain (almost round)	Medium Grain (2–3 times length vs. width)	Long Grain (4 times length vs. width)
Full-flavored grains that hold together well after cooking. Use in recipes where stickiness is preferred.	Tender and slightly cohesive after cooking. Great for casseroles and stuffings. Excellent bakery flour.	Fluffy, slender grains that remain separate after cooking. Well suited for pilafs and stir-fry dishes.

Rice Varieties and Blends

Aromatics
(4 times length vs. width)

Fragrant long grain rices. Exceptional in exotic recipes. California varieties similar to Indian basmati and Thai jasmine.

Sushi
(pearl-like rounds)

Delicate flavor. Moist and translucent after cooking. Superb in Asian recipes. A Japanese variety is Akitako-matchi.

Arborio
(2–3 times length vs. width)

Al dente yet creamy after cooking. Perfect for risotto and paella. A superfino Italian variety.

Wehani
(3–4 times length vs. width)

Naturally aromatic and flavor-ful. Plump, separate grains after cooking. A delicious, deep honey-red rice.

Wild Rice
(4 times length vs. width)

An exotic black long grain. Elongates during cooking. Hearty nutlike flavor. Add to gourmet entrées.

Quick Brown
(4 times length vs. width)

Long grain brown rice. Cooks in one-third the time of regular brown rice. Use when quick cooking time is important.

Sweet
(2–3 times length vs. width)

Very soft after cooking. Good for Asian recipes, crackers, mochi cakes, and sauces. Also known as sticky or glutinous rice.

Adapted with permission: Lundberg Family Farms, 5370 Church Street, Richvale, Calif.

Most brown rice requires forty-five to sixty minutes to steam, so it's a good idea to cook it ahead of time and store in the refrigerator for quick meal preparation. It'll keep, refrigerated, for three or four days. Rice is easy to take with you for lunch, especially if you eat it with some vegetables.

Red rice gets its color from the pigment anthocyanins. I discussed these compounds in chapter 6. Anthocyanins, regardless of the source, have several protective effects, including blocking tumor growth. A group of Japanese scientists compared the protective effects of feeding red or white rice to mice. They found that the mice who ate the red rice developed fewer and smaller tumors when injected with cancer cells (lymphoma). The mice who ate plain white rice or standard laboratory chow developed several tumors, and their survival time as compared to the mice fed red rice was much shorter. Several other phytochemicals found in grains are important. These include complex carbohydrates known as oligosaccharides and lignins.

Oligosaccharides

Oligosaccharides are complex sugars that occur in various forms. They are found with other sources of fiber and are important because they are small molecules, with different effects from the much larger cellulose. Yet they are often overlooked in analyses of dietary fiber. Two oligosaccharides, fructo-oligosaccharides (FOS) and arabinogalactans (ABG), are of particular importance in human nutrition. These oligosaccharides are known for their ability to enhance the growth of friendly intestinal flora and moderate immune response. I will discuss the role of friendly flora more extensively in chapter 9 when I talk about yogurt and other cultured dairy products.

FOS and ABG, termed pre-biotics, have profound effects on the health of the colon and its ability to sustain the health of the entire body. FOS and associated oligosaccharides inulin and fructans are found in many foods, although in most foods the amounts are small. Bananas, chicory root, oats, wheat, rye, globe artichoke, asparagus, leek, onion, garlic, salsify, dandelion, and Jerusalem artichoke all contain FOS. Of these food sources, Jerusalem artichoke and chicory are the richest sources of FOS. It is primarily used as a dietary supplement to enhance the growth of beneficial bacteria in the large intestine. Since FOS does not contain raffinose or stachyose, the offending gas-producing sugars found in beans, you can enjoy its beneficial effects without running the risk of increased flatulence.

ABG occurs in carrots, radishes, black beans, pears, corn, wheat, red wine, Italian ryegrass, tomatoes, sorghum, and coconut. Because these foods are not particularly high in ABG, it is derived from other sources such as trees of the larch species. This source provides ABG as a dietary supplement. ABG is an excellent source of dietary fiber and is important to healthy bowel function and regeneration of cells in the colon wall. In studies that compared the effectiveness of several kinds of fiber, ABG was the only one that was completely broken down by gut flora, suggesting it may be a better supplementary source of fiber than pectin, psyllium, or bran.

Both FOS and ABG can activate immune function when necessary or slow down the action of overzealous immune cells. These oligosaccharides are found in several herbs that modify immune function, including *Echinacea purpurea, Baptista tinctoria, Thuja occidentalis, Angelica acutiloba,* and *Curcuma longa.* The oligosaccharides contribute significantly to the effectiveness of these herbs as immune modulators.

Earlier in this chapter I talked about the importance of the glycemic index as it relates to whole grains. Let's focus now on how various cereals, bread, pasta, and grains affect blood sugar levels.

Glycemic Index

Glycemic index (GI) is a measure of how fast a food is digested into sugars that are absorbed into the blood. This information is important if you are trying to lose weight or if you have blood sugar problems such as hypoglycemia or diabetes. But it's also important when you're trying to improve your food choices and eliminate swings in energy and your ability to concentrate. Blood glucose (a kind of sugar) is transported into cells and used to supply energy-rich molecules for all metabolic processes. If it is released into the bloodstream faster than it can be utilized, insulin quickly shuttles it into storage and glucose blood levels drop as a result. A steady, consistent supply of blood glucose is essential for sustained brain function, and when glucose blood levels drop, so does cognitive function.

Low glycemic foods include legumes, pearled barley, lightly refined grains such as whole wheat or whole grain pumpernickel bread, and pasta, especially whole-grain pasta. Foods low on the glycemic index release sugar into the bloodstream slowly and don't trigger a dramatic insulin response. Eating low GI foods helps protect against developing diabetes and is a standard part of dietary treatment for blood sugar disorders. Low glycemic index foods also delay gastric emptying, thus increasing the feeling of fullness. Plus, they encourage friendly bacteria to produce short-chain fatty acids that are useful in fatty acid and nitrogen metabolism. Foods are rated according to how fast they raise blood glucose levels as compared to a standard food, either glucose or white bread. Following is a table listing the glycemic index of various foods. The standard used for this table is white bread, which has a GI of 138. The closer a food comes to 138, the higher its GI and the less desirable it is.

Glycemic Index of Selected Foods
(Standard = White Bread, GI = 138)

Food	GI	Food	GI
Breakfast Cereals		**Cereal Grains**	
All-Bran	60	Pearled barley	36
Cornflakes	119	Cracked barley	72
Muesli	80	Buckwheat	78
Oat Bran	78	Bulgur	68
Porridge Oats	87	Couscous	93
Puffed Rice	123	Cornmeal	98
Puffed Wheat	105	Sweet corn	78
Shredded Wheat	99	Millet	101
Bran Buds, Bran Chex, Cheerios,		Rice, white	81
Corn Bran, Corn Chex, Cream of Wheat,		Rice, brown	79

Crispix, Golden Grahams,
Grapenuts, Grapenuts Flakes, Life,
Pro Stars, Sustain, Team, Total   83 to 127
Bran Buds with Psyllium,
Red River, Special K   67 to 77

Breads
Barley, whole grain   49
Barley flour   95
Rye, whole grain   71
Rye flour   92
Whole-grain bread   99
Bagel, stuffing mix, hamburger bun, rolls,
melba toast   100

Baked Goods
Cakes   87
Cookies   90
Crackers, wheat   99
Muffins   88
Rice cakes   123

Pasta
Linguine   71
Macaroni   64
Macaroni, boxed   92
Spaghetti, white   59
Spaghetti, durum   78
Spaghetti, brown   53
Other pasta   59

Potatoes
Instant   118
Baked   121
New   81
White, boiled   80
White, mashed   100
French fries   107
Sweet potato   77
Yam   73

Rice, instant   128
Rice, parboiled (converted)   68
Specialty rice   78
Rye kernels   48
Tapioca   115
Wheat kernels   59

Legumes
Baked Beans   69
Black-eyed Peas   59
Butter Beans   44
Chickpeas   47
Canned chickpeas   59
Black (Haricot) beans   54
Kidney beans   42
Kidney beans, canned   74
Lentils   38
Lima beans   42
Peas, green   68
Pinto beans   61
Soy beans   23
Split peas   45

Fruit
Apple   52
Apple juice   58
Apricots, dried   44
Apricots, canned   91
Banana, ripe/overripe   51/82
Kiwi   75
Mango   80
Orange   62
Orange juice   74
Peach, canned   67
Pear   54
Cherries, fruit cocktail,
grapefruit, grapefruit juice,
grapes, plum, pineapple juice   54
Pineapple, raisins, melons   92

Source: Carbohydrates in Human Nutrition, Food and Agricultural Organization Food and Nutrition Paper, 1997.

As you can see from studying the table, many of the foods you may be eating have a high glycemic index. Even breads made from whole-grain flour have a higher GI than the cooked whole grains. If you have had low energy, can't sustain consistent mental function, and can't lose weight, it could be the carbohydrate foods you have been eating. Carbohydrates supply energy for all the metabolic processes in the body and the brain consumes the greatest amount of energy. By choosing foods with a quick release of sugar (high GI) you are sabotaging your efforts to maintain adequate energy levels and keep focused on your work. That's because as blood glucose levels rise, insulin quickly lowers them by shuttling glucose into cells for metabolism. If your cells can't metabolize glucose as quickly as it's released, it will be stored as fat. Now let's explore some of the scientific highlights of individual grains.

Properties of Buckwheat

Buckwheat is not a true grain but rather a member of the rhubarb family. Strictly speaking, what we eat is the seed of the fruit of the buckwheat plant, and in digestion buckwheat has the longest bowel transit time, thus greater satiety, of any cooked grain. It also has numerous health benefits of its own. It is distinguished from cereals in being gluten-free—a plus for those with celiac disease and possibly other bowel disorders. Buckwheat has the added value of being rich in the phytochemicals rutin and quercetin. Japanese soba noodles are made from buckwheat and wheat flours and are lower on the glycemic index than white noodles. They are excellent tossed with sautéed vegetables and sprinkled with sesame seeds. Researchers in Brazil compared the nutrient characteristics of wheat and buckwheat flours and found that buckwheat was higher in iron, copper, and magnesium. They also found that buckwheat was superior to wheat in lysine content. Grains are low in lysine, one of nine essential amino acids. Therefore, grains are considered an incomplete source of protein because they don't supply all the amino acids needed by the body. This means they must be combined with another food that contains sufficient levels of lysine, such as legumes. Grains contain methionine, another essential amino acid that's missing in legumes. Consequently, these two tan foods form complementary proteins: grains supplying methionine and legumes supplying lysine. Buckwheat will not produce light and fluffy breads, pancakes, and other foods because it lacks gluten, the protein that gives wheat and other grains their lightness and elasticity. You will need to keep this in mind when substituting buckwheat for wheat in recipes.

Legumes

Legumes, or pulses, make up one of the largest botanical families, including plants that produce edible pods or peas (beans, peas), ornamental plants (sweet pea, lupine), trees (carob), and shrubs. Some scientists extend the word *pulse* to include plants that are harvested with a reaper, such as grains and some seeds. However, most confine the term "pulse" to members of the legume or pea family.

When most of us refer to legumes, we mean dried beans, split peas, and lentils. The group also includes green and edible pods such as green peas, sugar snap peas, and pea pods. Carob and tamarind are also legumes, as are red clover and alfalfa. Vetch, a common clover crop, is another legume.

Legumes supply more protein than grains. The amount of protein in 100 grams (½ cup) of legumes is between 7 and 8 grams, or around 27 percent of total calories in beans. By comparison, one-half cup of grains contains 3 grams of protein or about 15 percent of the total calories in the grain. Legumes supply all the essential amino acids except methionine. Strict vegetarians who shun eggs and dairy products must consume grains in addition to legumes in order to supply the proper proportions of amino acids for bodily needs.

Legumes, particularly soy, have numerous disease-preventing properties. Most research on legumes has focused on isoflavones, which I discussed in chapter 6. The most important isoflavones are genistein, daidzein, and glycetin. However, there are other important phytochemicals in legumes, including saponins, phytates, and protease inhibitors that all protect against cancer, and lignins and phytosterols that protect against cardiovascular disease. Some of these effects will be detailed below.

Soy Foods and Disease Prevention

The interest in soybeans and disease prevention began when scientists started to question why people eating Asian and other traditional diets had lower rates of heart disease, several types of cancer, osteoporosis, and hormonal problems. Epidemiological evidence suggested that low fat consumption, coupled with high-fiber, legume-based diets, protected these people from the killer diseases westerners commonly suffer.

Today, enough evidence has accumulated from population-based studies around the world to support the theory that soy products and their constituents are largely responsible for the lower rates of chronic diseases seen in many areas. Researchers debate over which soy constituents are most responsible for the anticancer effects of this remarkable bean. Research teams from leading American universities have investigated soy's many constituents. Each study contributed a piece to the puzzle of how soy helps prevent disease. They all agree that several constituents are responsible for the diverse health benefits of soy.

Prostate Cancer

A Harvard University group studied the link between soy protein intake and prostate cancer. The effects of soy protein, casein (milk protein), and concentrated soy isoflavones (phytoestrogens) upon transplanted prostate cancer cells in mice were compared. While casein showed little inhibitory effect, soy protein reduced tumors by 11 percent, and soy isoflavones inhibited the tumors by 30 percent. The most benefit was seen with soy protein plus isoflavones concentrated at specific amounts, where tumor growth was cut by up to 40 percent.

Endometrial Cancer

Researchers at Wake Forest University in Winston-Salem, North Carolina, looked at another way soy protein reduces tumor growth, in this case breast and endometrial cancer. Soy protein, as mentioned above, is low in methionine. Rapidly growing tumors need this amino acid for their growth just as normal cells do. However, since healthy cells are growing at a much slower rate, low methionine doesn't limit their growth as quickly as it does tumor growth. According to the Wake Forest team, during periods of short methionine supply it is the breast and endometrial tumors that cannot reproduce, thus curtailing their growth.

Breast Cancer

A research team at Rockefeller University in New York studied how genistein, one of the soy isoflavones, exerts its anticancer effects. They used cultures of normal human breast tissue and induced cancer in the cells by exposing them to a well-known carcinogen. Half of the cells were pretreated with genistein and the others were left untreated. After exposure to the carcinogen, the treated cells showed a 65 percent reduction in cellular progression toward cancer. All of the untreated cells developed cancer.

At UCLA, Dr. Dave Heber and associates have investigated the effects of a low-fat diet enriched with soy foods in both normal and high breast cancer–risk women. Their research, besides the advantage that it was on humans, expands our understanding of soy's effects on hormones. Soy fiber, and a low-fat diet similar to that eaten by Asians, lowers estrogen levels and lengthens the menstrual cycle. The implications for this are that the less estrogen present, the less opportunity for hormone-dependent cancers to begin or progress.

Colon and Other Cancers

Phytic acid is a soy component that for many years was considered an anti-nutrient because it binds minerals, primarily calcium and iron. Yet, iron-binding may be one of the most effective ways soy protects against colon, breast, and perhaps other cancers. Cancer cells rely on iron for their growth, which is slowed if not enough iron is available. Too much iron can also promote cardiovascular disease. Iron can act as a free radical, attacking vascular tissue and oxidizing LDL cholesterol, and generally creating havoc in the circulatory system. Phytic acid is found in all legumes—not just soy—and all whole grains including wheat, rye, barley, oats, wild rice, and corn.

Cardiovascular Disease

Cardiovascular disease (CVD) is a progressive disease that begins, at least in part, when changes in blood lipids cause damage to the interior walls of blood vessels in the heart, brain, and extremities. A lesion develops on the arterial wall, usually caused by free radical and enzymatic damage, but it can also stem from an infection. A cascade of events follows that eventually blocks blood flow. The lesion that forms erodes the vessel's smooth lining, and inflammatory debris, blood fats, cholesterol, dead cells, fibrous proteins, calcium, and collagen collect within the lesion. The deposit-filled lesion (plaque) becomes rough and cracked on the surface as it "matures." Blood platelets snag on the rough surface and form clots that finally cut off (occlude) blood flow through the vessel.

Depending on which vessels are affected, a heart attack, stroke, or peripheral tissue damage results. For many years, heart experts thought heart attacks and strokes resulted primarily from the gradual buildup of plaque on artery walls. However, recent findings suggest a more likely cause is "unstable" plaque that ruptures and precipitates a blood clot. It has been estimated that 60 to 70 percent of heart attacks are caused by eruptions of unstable plaques. Large "soft" centers packed with fats, cholesterol, immune cells, and inflammatory mediators distinguish unstable plaques and make them extremely volatile. Thus, prevention and management of cardiovascular disease now center more than ever on diet. Consumption of saturated fats and cholesterol should be kept to a minimum, while more whole grains, legumes, and fresh fruits and vegetables with many different kinds of phytochemicals should be added to one's diet.

Soy Foods and Blood Lipids

Animal products contain cholesterol and most are also high in saturated fats, both known to promote cardiovascular disease. A diet high in meat, poultry, dairy products, and butter raises serum triglycerides and harmful forms of cholesterol: low-density (LDL) and very low density lipoproteins (VLDL). Increasing your intake of legumes, particularly soy protein (25 grams or more per day) lowers total blood lipids, specifically total cholesterol, LDL, VLDL, and triglycerides. Dr. Clare Hasler, director of the Functional Foods for Health Program, based at the University of Illinois at Urbana-Champaign, and an expert on soy foods and heart disease, emphasizes that soy protein is what lowers cholesterol, although soy isoflavones appear to have other benefits.

A comparative analysis of thirty-eight controlled clinical trials confirmed that consumption of diets rich in soy protein, as opposed to those high in animal protein, significantly decreased blood levels of total cholesterol, LDL cholesterol, and triglycerides without lowering helpful HDL cholesterol. Numerous investigations have been done to find out if soy protein will also lower cholesterol in those who do not have high cholesterol. Although some benefit has been found among groups of "normal" men and women, the greatest improvement has been seen among the high-cholesterol groups. For several years, it has been accepted that people who had high triglycerides experienced lower levels of these blood lipids when they ate soy protein–enriched diets. More recently, it has been shown that cholesterol and triglyceride levels could be further reduced by those eating a diet low in saturated fats and cholesterol, in addition to increasing the intake of soy protein.

Soy Isoflavones

Isoflavones are naturally contained in soy foods and are an important component that aids soy proteins in lowering cholesterol. Isoflavones are also excellent free radical scavengers and some researchers propose that this action protects vessels. Additionally, soy is rich in soluble fiber. Some studies have shown that soy fiber is also important in lowering LDL cholesterol and triglycerides.

Several mechanisms have been proposed for the way soy protein selectively lowers total cholesterol, LDL cholesterol, and triglycerides. Soy appears to aid in clearing excess cholesterol from the body—partly by increasing its elimination in the colon and partly by increasing cellular efficiency in picking up excess serum cholesterol. Soy also appears to increase the conversion of cholesterol into bile acids, a necessary step for its excretion. Furthermore, resorption of cholesterol in the colon appears to be blocked by soy fiber, its phytic acid and saponins. Soy foods have shown numerous beneficial effects on women's health because of their phytoestrogenic properties.

Soy Foods and Menopausal Symptoms

Hot flashes are the most commonly reported symptom of menopause. For some women the flashes are mild—a rather pleasant warm rush that radiates from the center of the body. Other women experience extreme rushes in body heat that cause excessive perspiration and interrupted sleep. Irritability, slowed cognitive response, lowered immune resistance, irregular periods or spotting, and fatigue may also mark the menopausal transition. After menopause, the protective benefits of estrogen disappear and women are more prone to cardiovascular disease and bone loss. Doctors most often recommend hormone replacement therapy to alleviate the symptoms of menopause and protect against bone loss and CVD. However, adding soy foods to your diet will reduce hot flashes, and these marvelous legumes will also protect your heart, reduce bone loss, and help prevent cancer.

Soy phytoestrogens are weak estrogens, meaning that they are stand-ins for estrogen, binding to the same cellular receptors and eliciting similar metabolic responses. Estrogen receptors are located all over the body—in the brain, bones, heart, and blood vessels—which explains why menopausal symptoms involve so many parts of the body. While phytoestrogens mimic the effects of estrogen they are weaker in action and consequently don't cause the same problems.

It appears soy isoflavones are dual action—substituting for estrogen when levels are low and crowding out surplus estrogen that causes hormone imbalances and even cancer. Consequently, soy foods benefit women both before and after menopause. As estrogen levels diminish during menopause, phytoestrogens partially compensate for low estrogen by giving cells important signals that keep bone tissue healthy and heart and blood vessels working smoothly. Phytoestrogens also orchestrate cellular resistance to progression of cancer by blocking the effects of high estrogen levels.

It doesn't take a lot of soy foods to raise phytoestrogen levels in blood serum. Scientists have determined that one cup of soy milk, 8 ounces of tofu, or one-third cup of roasted soy nuts is enough to elicit an estrogenic response. As for hot flashes, studies in the United States and Europe suggest that 60 grams of soy protein powder taken daily for ninety days significantly reduced hot flashes.

The cardiovascular benefits of soy foods have been documented above, however, a 1999 study is especially noteworthy for women. Women with high cholesterol were enrolled in the study in which they were given 60 grams of soy protein per day. The soy contained two different levels of isoflavones, delivering either 1.39 mg or 2.25 mg per gram of soy protein. After six months, both levels of isoflavones raised HDL (good) cholesterol. The number of LDL (bad) cholesterol receptors on white blood cells was also increased, which was a positive indicator that cholesterol was being eliminated, vital to improved cardiovascular health. Isoflavones are also efficient antioxidants and may reduce free radical attack on blood vessel walls—a precipitating event in atherosclerosis.

Soy Foods and Osteoporosis

The solid appearance of bones belies a bustling interior. Underneath lies a vast network of bone tissue in a constant flux of rebuilding and breakdown. Although the greatest bone density develops before the age of thirty, the process continues throughout life. Bone tissue turnover, or "remodeling," gets rid of old bone cells and lays down new ones. Many nutrients are needed to nurture this process, among them calcium, magnesium, potassium, manganese, boron, vitamins C, D, K, and omega-3 fatty acids.

Estrogen protects a woman's bone-building process during her childbearing years. Following menopause when estrogen levels drop, remodeling shifts from bone building to bone loss at an increased rate. During the first years following menopause, up to 10 percent of bone mass is lost per year. The loss tapers off after five years as other hormone adjustments occur. However, the bone loss is not easy to reverse and is one of the chief reasons hormone replacement therapy is advised by doctors for postmenopausal women.

Recent scientific evidence has shown that eating soy foods not only slows bone loss but even helps rebuild bone structure. Researchers at the University of Illinois found that postmenopausal women who ate daily servings of 60 grams of soy protein containing 2.25 mg of isoflavones per gram for six months were protected against spinal bone loss. Moreover, animal research has shown that isoflavones do not increase uterine activity and thus are a safer approach to reducing bone loss than hormone replacement therapy.

The research is so compelling that soy isoflavones have become the newest trendy bone savers and ones that are becoming more popular in functional foods. Experts advise you should have daily servings of 90 mg of isoflavones—the amount in 2 ounces of soy protein powder, one-third cup roasted soy nuts, or 8 ounces of tofu. Or, you can look for supplements of ipriflavone.

Ipriflavone is an isoflavone that has been found to halt bone loss and increase bone formation. It is very effective and has virtually no side effects. Ipriflavone may also be useful in treating bone loss from overuse of steroids, removal of the ovaries, and parathyroid gland disorders. Although you won't find it naturally occurring in soy foods, ipriflavone supplements may be helpful if you suffer from bone loss.

The Menstrual Cycle and Soy Foods

The menstrual cycle consists of two phases: the follicular phase occurs between menstruation and ovulation and the luteal phase from ovulation to menstruation. During the follicular phase of the cycle, which is approximately fourteen to seventeen days, estrogen levels gradually rise along with other hormones that ready the ovary to release an egg. During the luteal phase, which is fourteen days, these hormone levels drop and progesterone levels rise to prepare the uterus for implantation of a fertilized egg. If the egg isn't fertilized, progesterone levels drop and menstruation follows. The average cycle repeats every twenty-eight days, with both longer and shorter cycles considered normal.

Scientists have found that intake of 45 mg isoflavones from soy products lengthens the follicular phase and extends the entire cycle by a few days. This results in fewer yearly cycles and lower amounts of estrogen released. Over a lifetime, this reduces the amount of estrogen that is available to bind to receptors in breast tissue. This may be one reason why Asian women are less likely to get breast cancer, and a good one for including soy foods in your diet. Although this is not considered the primary mechanism by which isoflavones prevent breast cancer, the phytoestrogen effects of soy include lessening premenstrual syndrome (PMS). That's because isoflavones smooth out hormone imbalances among premenopausal women. It appears the earlier that girls and young women are exposed to phytoestrogens, the more protective benefits they can hope to enjoy.

Soy Foods in Early Life

The health benefits of soy foods are becoming well known, and it seems the sooner they are introduced into the diet, the better. This has led scientists to investigate the benefits soy foods might have on fetal hormone development. A mother eating soy foods may be passing multiple benefits on to her unborn child, and these benefits may continue during breast feeding. Researchers are also studying the possible protection against later development of osteoporosis among babies fed soy formula instead of the typical milk-based preparation.

For teens, eating soy foods may help develop bone density. Since peak bone density occurs before the age of thirty, early consumption of soy foods might be good insurance against later bone thinning.

Some Concerns about Isoflavone Supplements

Research teams from several medical research centers have expressed concern over the possibility that genistein, the primary isoflavone, might actually promote progression of breast cancer in women who already have it. Researchers had observed this happening in animal models when they were fed extremely high doses of genistein. To find out more about this, I interviewed several experts who could shed some light on this perplexing situation. Dr. Mindy Kurzer from the University of Minnesota summed up the current thinking within the scientific community in saying that the data both for and against genistein are "theoretical" in basis and lack good human clinical evidence. According to Dr. Kurzer and Dr. Bill Helferich from Michigan State University, both authors of some of the research, there is little to be concerned about in consuming soy foods. The benefits of eating soy far outweigh any risk to women with breast cancer. As Dr. Helferich put it, you can't eat enough soy to get to the levels it took to produce adverse effects in mice. All told, the safest bet if you are a cancer sufferer or survivor is to stick to soy foods and perhaps avoid the genistein supplements, unless your doctor recommends them.

So how much soy should you eat to protect against cancer? Soy expert Dr. Mark Messina offers some sensible guidelines: eat the foods you enjoy and learn to make easy substitutions with soy, and add supplements if and when you can't fit two to three daily servings of soy in your diet. All the researchers interviewed agree that soy as part of a diet high in fruits and vegetables and low in saturated fats offers the best protection against disease. The sooner in life you begin to eat this way, the better chance you have of cancer protection.

Now that we've discussed the many disease-preventive phytochemicals in tan foods and how they work, let's look at additional things you should know about tan foods. Then we will see which of these foods are your color.

Possible Side Effects of Tan Foods

Cereals, Grains, Pasta, and Breads—Allergies are the most common reason to avoid these foods. Corn and wheat are the most likely to provoke a response, no doubt because they are encountered in so many foods we eat. Two wheat proteins, gluten and gliaden, may cause sensitivities, so exclude use of foods that contain them. Gluten is found in wheat, rye, spelt, triticale, and oats. All other grains are gluten-free.

Lentils—These contain the amino acid tyrosine and the peptide tyramine. Neither of these substances can be metabolized when one is taking monoamine oxidase (MAO) inhibitors for depression. MAO inhibitors are a group of antidepressants that inhibit the enzyme required to metabolize tyrosine and tyramine. Other high-tyramine foods that you should not eat when taking MAOs include aged cheese, bananas, alcoholic beverages, chocolate, cultured dairy products, liver, nuts, pickled foods, pineapple, prunes, soy sauce, vanilla, yeast, and MSG.

Legumes—These also contain the same amino acids as lentils and should not be eaten while taking MAO inhibitors. Legumes are also apt to provoke allergic reactions. This is particularly true for peanuts, peas, and some beans. I have mentioned the problem with flatulence some people have from legumes and on page 168 you will learn how to lessen this effect. Legumes are very good sources of protein, and when you digest them protein by-products called purines are produced. People who have gout or gouty arthritis need to avoid high-purine foods because they are broken down into uric acid, a waste product that accumulates in the joints of those who have this condition.

Rice—This is one of the foods least likely to cause allergies. However, a few very sensitive individuals may react to traces of mold on rice, especially if it's been stored for considerable periods of time in a damp place.

Buying, Storing, and Cooking Tan Foods

Tan foods are staples. This means you can stock up on them so you have a variety to choose from. An exception, of course, is fresh bread. Cereals and crackers will have an expiration date stamped on the box and should be used before the time of expiration or very shortly thereafter.

Whole grains need special consideration. Years ago the bran and germ were routinely removed from grains to lengthen their shelf life. Consequently, if you buy whole grains and whole-grain flours, you will have to use them within a reasonable amount of time. The length of time will depend on where you live and where you store your grains. If you have a cool room or cellar to store them, they will keep longer. If they are stored in a kitchen cupboard for more than a few weeks, you may get bugs in them. They will also turn rancid and lose some nutrients if not used within a few months. Don't use grains or flours that don't smell fresh or have a slightly nutty odor. The safest way to store these foods is in the refrigerator or freezer. Look for expiration dates on whole-grain flours, and if you buy them from bulk bins, make sure the store turns over its inventory quickly.

Whole grains and pasta can be boiled, steamed, or added to soups and stews before cooking time is finished. Follow package directions and don't overcook these foods. Couscous is not cooked but added to boiling water, then left to stand until the water is absorbed, usually five to ten minutes. Bulgur, which is cracked whole wheat, can be steamed, soaked, or not cooked at all. It is eaten either warm or chilled as a salad.

Legumes are another matter—you can barely overcook dried beans and peas. They are done if soft when pricked with a fork. Cooking time varies from one to three hours, depending on the type of legume. Split peas and lentils take only an hour to cook, while garbanzo beans take three. Indian dhal can be cooked quickly if you buy the split kind, and it should be slightly firm when cooked.

Which of These Foods Is My Color?

Tan foods are complementary for all color types and make up a significant portion of daily meal plans. Although these foods may not be as colorful and exciting to eat as others, they contain numerous disease-fighting phytochemicals, as you have seen. Tan foods are so important that they form the base of the food pyramid.

Reds: Tan foods are very good for you. The ones to avoid are amaranth, buckwheat, corn, cornmeal, millet, quinoa, and rye. All the other grains, cereals, flours, pasta, rice, and breads, are a major part of your daily food plan.

Greens: You also do well with legumes except for soybeans, kidney beans, and brown lentils. You can enjoy soy foods, just not the whole beans. Tempeh is made with a culture of mold and you should avoid it as well. Grains, cereals, and breads are good for you, with the exception of whole wheat, which is too heavy, cooked oats, which are also heavy, and sweet rice varieties. It's best to rotate eating brown and white rice because brown rice can get a little heavy for you.

Yellows: You are more restricted in which tan foods are good for you. You can eat all the grains except buckwheat, corn, cornmeal, millet, and rye. You should also avoid cereals that are dry and crunchy, or dry toast and croutons. As for legumes, most are too apt to cause gas and you should avoid them. The only ones you should have little trouble with are aduki beans, mung beans, mung dhal, tofu, and urad dhal.

9

White Foods

Foods in this group make up the top third of your food pyramid and are restricted to a few times a week, except for oils and dairy for Yellow and Red types. The white group of foods supplies important dietary oils and proteins that supplement your primary colors and complementary tan foods. This group of foods will also supply the first group of *zoochemicals*—protective nutrients from animal sources.

Americans have become accustomed to planning the main meal of the day around some kind of meat, poultry, or fish, and this automatically accords these foods a higher nutritional priority than they should have. As you implement your *Eat Your Colors* meal plans, think of these foods as "white," which is the least intense color. I have chosen this color in order to reduce the importance of these foods—not that they're unimportant, it's just that they're not the most important foods in your plan. I have been emphasizing the need to plan meals around your primary colors—Red, Yellow, Green—and complementary tan foods. This further helps establish that these foods are the most important components of your food plan and also form the base of the food pyramid.

Oils are the most important white food from the standpoint of phytochemical content and health maintenance, so I will begin by discussing dietary oils and their fatty acid components.

Dietary Fats and Fatty Acids

In the past decade, high fat intake has been blamed for a host of chronic problems, including obesity, cardiovascular disease, and cancer. And while curbing your total fat intake is paramount to staying healthy, avoiding *all* fats brings its own set of problems. What we need to do is distinguish health-promoting fats from those that can cause problems.

When thinking of fat, we usually consider the visible fat under the skin of chicken, around cuts of beef, pork, or lamb, and spreads such as margarine or butter. We may also be aware that many of our favorite foods contain various kinds of fats, and we try to avoid them by choosing fat-free items. However, the latest government food and nutrition survey has shown that while intake of saturated fats, considered "bad" fats, has decreased, total fat intake hasn't changed in the past ten years.

As for oils, the same government survey showed that consumption of a particular group of fatty acids, called long-chain polyunsaturated fatty acids, was practically nonexistent. Although fats in this group pack the same number of calories as saturated fats, these fats are necessary for health maintenance and are considered to be "good fats."

Oils: The Good Fats

Oils and fats belong to a family known as lipids. Lipids range in firmness from being soft and runny to very stiff. Oils are generally liquid at room temperature and are more healthful. We refer to them as unsaturated, monounsaturated, and polyunsaturated because of their molecular characteristics. Monounsaturated oils are considered the best for cooking, baking, and use in dressings. Olive, canola, peanut, and almond are monounsaturated oils. Polyunsaturated oils are more apt to turn rancid and must be stored very carefully. These include flax, corn, hemp, safflower, sesame, and sunflower. Oils contain fatty acids that the body converts into the special forms needed for numerous body functions.

Saturated fats, on the other hand, are solid at room temperature and are less healthful. Our bodies break down saturated fats and either store them for later use or convert them into energy. Saturated fats are difficult for the body to process into necessary components, and are more likely to accumulate in arteries and promote several chronic diseases.

Most dietary oils come from seeds, such as those mentioned above, and from leafy greens and sea vegetables. All of these are "good oils," supplying essential fatty acids (EFAs) from three families: omega-3, omega-6, and omega-9 fatty acids. The first two, alpha-linolenic (omega-3) and cis-linoleic (omega-6), the human body cannot manufacture. Consequently, we must get them from our diet. Omega-9 can be synthesized within the body and has many health benefits, as we'll see.

Traditional and Modern Western Diets

Relative amounts of omega-3 and omega-6 that we get from our diet have shifted dramatically over the centuries. Originally, the human diet was higher in omega-3 and lower in omega-6 because it contained lots of fish, wild game, and various kinds of plant-based foods. As cultivation of crops such as grains and legumes began to increase, intake of omega-6 was increased and the ratio between the two families shifted. However, grazing animals, chickens, eggs, and dairy products still provided significant amounts of omega-3. In the past hundred years, animals have increasingly been fed grain and thus they no longer provide omega-3. According to nutrition experts such as Dr. Artemis Simopoulous, president of the Center for Genetics in Washington, D.C., and a former nutrition advisor to the president's office of consumer affairs, the shift has been most pronounced in the past forty or fifty years. Today we consume an excess of foods containing omega-6, too few rich in omega-3, and we are paying the health consequences.

Consequently, nutrition experts are urging us to eat more omega-3–rich foods so that the proper ratios between the two families of essential fatty acids are restored. The oils richest in omega-3 and the amount each contains are: flaxseed (57 percent), pumpkin seed (15 percent), canola (10 percent), soy (8 percent), and walnut (5 percent). You can see more detail on this in the table below, "Fatty Acid Profiles."

Ready-made omega-3, long-chain polyunsaturated fatty acids, or LCPs, come from fish that have already synthesized them from various food sources. Omega-3 LCPs from fish are zoochemicals because of their diverse protective activities. The advantage of consuming omega-3 LCPs directly rather than waiting for the conversion process is greater efficiency. Many factors, including saturated fats, interfere with the body's ability to synthesize adequate levels of LCPs. That's why experts suggest increasing fish consumption to between 12 and 16 ounces per week. And, if you don't like fish, you can get the same benefits by using fish oil supplements. In fact, research teams have used supplements when studying the health benefits of fish oils. The supplements provide higher levels of these essential LCPs. Algae also provide LCPs and are an increasingly popular source. Dark green leafy vegetables and sea vegetables such as nori, kombu, and wakame are also good sources of LCPs. The charts of fatty acid profiles on the following pages will guide you in the proper choice and use of oils. Choose those with a high percentage of monounsaturates, preferably those that contain omega-3s, such as canola and flaxseed. Low-heat oils are contained in dietary supplements. Flaxseed oil is found in some salad dressings.

Saturated Fats

Foods from animal sources, particularly beef, pork, and lamb, but not fish, contain saturated fats, those that are solid at room temperature and are stiff and unyielding. These fats do not slide into cell membranes and other body structures as easily as long-chain polyunsaturated fatty acids (LCPs). Instead, saturated fats wind up clogging arterial walls and impairing cellular function. Healthy oils can become saturated through a process called hydrogenation.

Fatty Acid Profiles for Culinary and Nutritional Oils

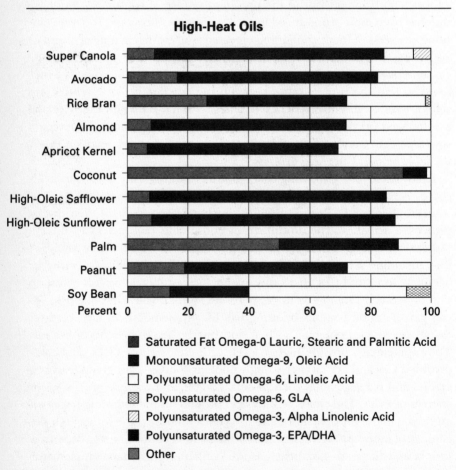

High-Heat Oils

Legend:
- ■ Saturated Fat Omega-0 Lauric, Stearic and Palmitic Acid
- ■ Monounsaturated Omega-9, Oleic Acid
- □ Polyunsaturated Omega-6, Linoleic Acid
- ▦ Polyunsaturated Omega-6, GLA
- ▨ Polyunsaturated Omega-3, Alpha Linolenic Acid
- ■ Polyunsaturated Omega-3, EPA/DHA
- ▤ Other

High-heat oils, 500° F—refined oils, neutral flavor
Use for: All purpose cooking—sear, brown, deep-fry, tempura, breaded fry, fry
Source: Spectrum Organic Products, Inc., Petaluma, Calif.

Medium-High-Heat Oils

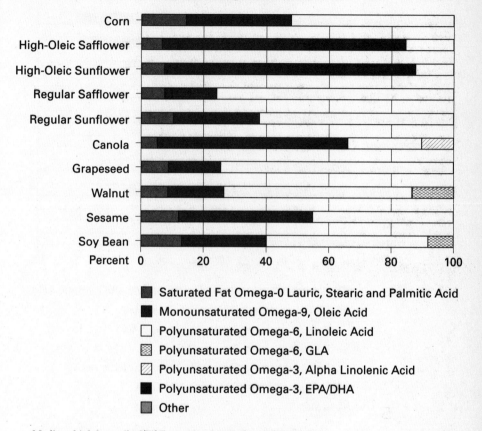

Legend:

- ■ Saturated Fat Omega-0 Lauric, Stearic and Palmitic Acid
- ■ Monounsaturated Omega-9, Oleic Acid
- □ Polyunsaturated Omega-6, Linoleic Acid
- ▨ Polyunsaturated Omega-6, GLA
- ▧ Polyunsaturated Omega-3, Alpha Linolenic Acid
- ■ Polyunsaturated Omega-3, EPA/DHA
- ▦ Other

Medium-high-heat oils, 375° F—semi-refined oils, mild flavor
Use for: Baking and sautéing—bake, crisp sauté, medium stir-fry, medium wok-fry, oven cooking
Source: Spectrum Organic Products, Inc., Petaluma, Calif.

Trans Fats

Unfortunately, hydrogenation causes chemical changes in oils that make them extremely unhealthful. The high temperatures and pressures under which oils are processed to make them saturated produce fat molecules that are completely foreign to the body. It is widely believed that trans fats are even more of a risk factor for chronic disease than saturated fats. Americans eat far more saturated and trans fats than healthy oils, leading health experts to recommend that we curb our total fat intake to 30 percent, with no more than 10 percent (about one teaspoon) of total daily calories as saturated fat. To do this, we need to avoid fatty meats, butter, margarine, commercial

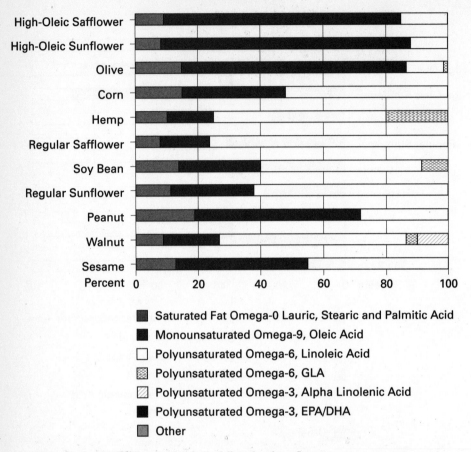

Medium-Heat Oils

Saturated Fat Omega-0 Lauric, Stearic and Palmitic Acid
Monounsaturated Omega-9, Oleic Acid
Polyunsaturated Omega-6, Linoleic Acid
Polyunsaturated Omega-6, GLA
Polyunsaturated Omega-3, Alpha Linolenic Acid
Polyunsaturated Omega-3, EPA/DHA
Other

Medium-heat oils, 320° F—unrefined oils, full seed and nut flavor
Use for: Light sautéing and sauces—sauce, low-heat bake, light sauté, pressure-cooking
Source: Spectrum Organic Products, Inc., Petaluma, Calif.

baked goods, deep-fried foods, snacks, and ice cream. Hopefully, labeling of trans fats will soon be made mandatory, making it easier to identify which foods contain them.

A growing body of evidence supports the idea that trans fatty acids found in margarine, shortening, fried foods, and snacks are major contributors to cardiovascular heart disease and that by eliminating them from the diet, we may lower the risk of this disease. Meanwhile, increasing consumption of fish and fish oils, and substituting flaxseed, canola and olive oils for butter and margarine may help avoid many chronic diseases we suffer.

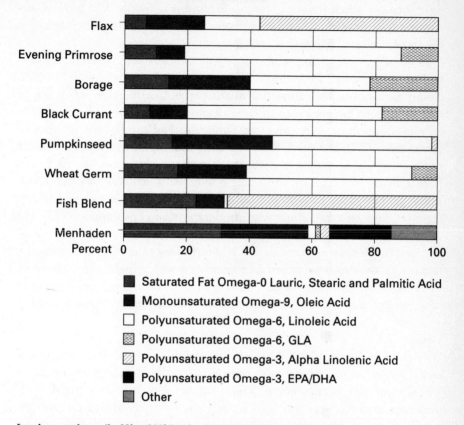

Low-Heat Oils

Low-heat, no-heat oils, 32° to 212° F—nutritional oils, full seed and nut flavor
Use for: Soups and salads—oils to be used as nutritional supplements, dips, dressings, and added to a dish after it has been removed from direct heat
Source: Spectrum Organic Products, Inc., Petaluma, Calif.

Fish, Fish Oils, and Disease Prevention

Cardiovascular Disease (CVD)

Data gathered between 1959 and 1996 have shown a strong connection between a diet rich in marine oils and reduced incidence of heart disease among Native American peoples. Research on the diets of Inuits (Eskimos) in particular has generated great interest because these people have extremely low rates of CVD and diabetes, despite a diet high in fat. Eating oily fish daily, especially those from deep cold waters, such as salmon, herring, tuna, anchovies, mackerel, lake trout, and menhaden, has been shown to raise HDL (good) cholesterol levels, lower total cholesterol, increase blood viscosity, and reduce platelet stickiness. These observations have been confirmed through autopsy reports on 104 Inuit natives by Greenland researchers, who found high tissue levels of omega-3 and selenium and low incidence of ischemic heart disease. Selenium is essential to antioxidant enzyme systems and may further protect the Inuits from other negative effects of eating a high-fat diet.

In another interesting study, populations from seven different world regions were studied for twenty-five years. Research teams identified which dietary factors besides eating fish might prevent or increase incidence of CVD. Northern Europeans from Finland and the Netherlands had the highest consumption of dairy products. Finns also had the highest number of deaths from CVD; 268 per 1,000, suggesting that high consumption of dairy products typical of people living in these areas may be a possible risk factor. People living in Crete, on the other hand, had the lowest; 24 per 1,000. These people, along with those from Italy, ate a diet rich in fish, vegetables, legumes, and olive oil, along with moderate wine consumption. This and other studies have given rise to the popular "Mediterranean diet." A food pyramid for the Mediterranean diet is shown. Low rates of CVD among the Japanese have also been noted and associated with a high consumption of soy, cereals, and fish. Meanwhile, high rates of CVD among Americans were most strongly associated with consumption of animal and processed foods.

Cancer

Diets high in meat with little or no intake of fish may pose a significant risk factor for breast cancer. Researchers compared the meat and fish intake of 740 women with occurrence of breast cancer. A significantly higher incidence of breast cancer was seen among premenopausal women who ate processed meats including cold cuts, hot dogs, and bacon at least once a week. The effects of eating processed meats weren't as conclusive for postmenopausal women. However, this group showed a reduced incidence of breast cancer when they ate fish at least once a week. The investigators concluded that among the women studied the kind of fat they ate was even more important in preventing breast cancer than their total fat intake. Studies done in twenty-four European countries confirm that eating fish or taking fish oil supplements may prevent breast and colorectal cancer.

Immune Response and Inflammation

Several animal studies have suggested that EPA-rich fish oils may boost immune function. (EPA is an LCP in the omega-3 family.) Human clinical trials have shown therapeutic effects from increased consumption of omega-3 oils in the treatment of acute and chronic inflammation and for autoimmune disorders, such as rheumatoid arthritis, that result from an inappropriately activated immune response. Omega-3 oils also appear to increase graft survival in plastic surgery patients.

The Traditional Healthy
Mediterranean Diet Pyramid

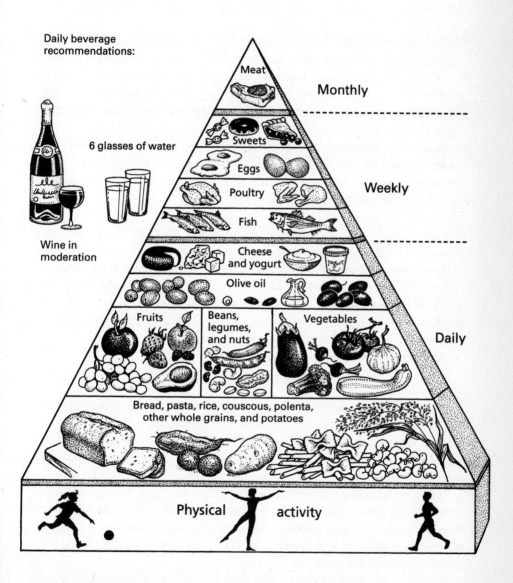

Daily beverage recommendations:

6 glasses of water

Wine in moderation

Meat — Monthly

Sweets

Eggs

Poultry — Weekly

Fish

Cheese and yogurt

Olive oil

Fruits | Beans, legumes, and nuts | Vegetables — Daily

Bread, pasta, rice, couscous, polenta, other whole grains, and potatoes

Physical activity

Rheumatoid Arthritis (RA)

Researchers reported that patients with rheumatoid arthritis receiving fish oil supplements showed significant improvement as compared to a control group of RA patients receiving corn oil capsules. The measures assessed included interleukin-1 levels (a measure of inflammation), morning stiffness, and joint pain. These patients had been taken off nonsteroidal anti-inflammatory drugs (NSAIDs) just prior to the study and essential fatty acids (EFAs) led to greater improvement than was experienced with the NSAIDs.

Multiple Sclerosis (MS)

Multiple sclerosis is an inflammatory condition in which the fatty myelin layers that protect the brain and nerves break down. The immune system is involved in the condition and although it's not known if immune dysfunction is the cause of the condition, moderating immune response with omega-3 fatty acids has shown favorable results. In a six-month trial, MS patients were given supplements of omega-3 capsules (3 grams daily) and several indicators of immune function were measured. Researchers determined that pro-inflammatory activity was reduced and this resulted in symptom relief, especially as the trial proceeded.

The importance of ensuring sufficient levels of omega-3 fatty acids cannot be overstressed. Adding flaxseed and canola oil to your diet and eating fish two or three times a week, while cutting down on saturated and animal fats, is a simple plan for ensuring health. In the case of most disorders, supplementation is usually needed to help correct long-standing imbalances. If you are using supplements to address specific problems, be sure to get your physician's advice before taking large amounts of fish oils.

Other Beneficial Oils

Rice bran oil has not attracted as much attention among researchers as fish oils have. However, leading scientists in Asia and India point out that rice bran oil lowers high cholesterol much better than other vegetable oils. Rice bran oil is also a unique source of gamma-oryzanol, tocopherols (vitamin E), and tocotrienols, the phytochemicals that may provide the benefits seen.

Tocopherols reduce the oxidative burden of the body and tocotrienols appear to act directly in the liver to reduce cholesterol synthesis. Rice bran oil is one of only five vegetable oils that contain alpha linolenic acid (2.2 percent), the essential omega-3 fatty acid. The other four are flaxseed, walnut, canola, and pumpkin seed.

Results of two trials in the United States confirmed results of the Asian studies, although American scientists expressed different opinions about what caused the lipid-lowering effects. A primate study done at the University of Massachusetts, Lowell, found that rice bran oil significantly lowered low-density serum cholesterol and total cholesterol without altering high-density cholesterol (the good kind). This research team suggested that the other phytochemicals in rice bran oil most likely caused the observed benefits.

Tocopherols and Tocotrienols

Rice bran, barley, palm, corn, olive, and soybean oils all contain the natural vitamin E complex including four tocopherols and four tocotrienols. In 2000, two new and potentially more potent tocotrienols were reported by Dr. Asaf Qureshi and colleagues from Advanced Medical Research in Madison, Wisconsin.

Corn, soybean, and olive oils primarily contain tocopherols, whereas rice bran, palm, and barley oils are the richest source of tocotrienols. Vitamin E compounds are the primary antioxidants in cellular membranes. (I discussed their antioxidant role and how they interact with carotenoids in chapter 5.) Not surprisingly, nature packages tocopherols and tocotrienols with oils to protect them and dietary oils supply us with these powerful antioxidants.

Cardiovascular protection is one of the major benefits of these phytochemicals. Dr. Lester Packer and colleagues from the University of California at Berkeley have shown that tocotrienols help prevent oxidation of LDL cholesterol, believed to be a precipitating event in atherosclerosis. Several other factors involved in progression of CVD were reduced by tocotrienols.

A research team from the Kenneth L. Jordan Research Group in Montclair, New Jersey, conducted an eighteen-month study with fifty patients who had carotid atherosclerosis. This disease involves blockage of the carotid arteries in the neck and results in significant reduction in cognitive function and increased risk of stroke. The amount of plaque in the carotid arteries was determined using ultrasound scans. Serum lipids, fatty acid oxidation, and platelet aggregation were assessed along with ultrasound after six, twelve, and eighteen months. During this period of time, half of the patients received tocotrienols daily. The other half received a placebo. All but two of the tocotrienol patients showed a significant regression in carotid narrowing while all of the placebo group and two of the tocotrienol group showed progression of their disease.

Tocotrienols are part of a family of protective antioxidants with anticarcinogenic properties. They are positioned within membranes and help combat mutagenic effects and the initiation and progression of tumor cell growth. Tocotrienols, tocopherols, and carotenoids affect intercellular signaling, an important event for cancer prevention. They prevent oxidative damage to DNA that could otherwise result in chromosome breaks—a first step in cellular aging and possible initiation of cancer.

Olive oil is associated with reduced incidence of colorectal cancer. Spanish researchers investigated the protective effect of olive and fish oils on development of colonic polyps in animals. The animals were fed one of three diets containing oils: safflower, olive oil, or fish. After being on these diets for twelve weeks, the animals were treated with a substance known to produce colon cancer. The researchers found that the animals receiving either the olive oil or fish diet had fewer colonic polyps and cancers than those who ate the safflower diet.

English researchers have found that olive oil appears to have a protective effect on the colonic membranes. While meat consumption inhibits an enzyme that helps colonic mucosal cells proliferate, thus leaving room for tumor formation, olive oil increases the enzyme's activity. Colonic mucosal cells, like those in other parts of the digestive tract, wear out and need replacing every few days. By protecting colonic cellular growth mechanisms, olive oil helps maintain the mucosa and prevent growth of tumors. Olive oil, particularly unprocessed dark green extra virgin oil, is monounsaturated and contains several carotenoids and xanthophylls. These powerful antioxidants may also contribute to the benefits of olive oil.

Another natural monounsaturated oil with health benefits is *avocado oil.* Several Mexican research teams have shown that avocado oil lowers cholesterol, LDL cholesterol, and triglycerides. One study was a short, one-week diet that included avocado oil or contained a combination of saturated and unsaturated fats, typical of a Western diet. Thirty-seven patients with high cholesterol and high triglycerides were studied along with thirty normal control subjects. Half of each group got the avocado diet and the other half ate the diet with the combination fat. All of the subjects who ate the avocado diet experienced lowered cholesterol levels, lower LDL cholesterol, and lower triglycerides. They also averaged raised HDL levels. The control subjects did not show any of these benefits. The results of this study have been corroborated by two other human studies, one that used avocado fruit and the other that used avocado oil along with a vegetarian diet.

Conjugated Linoleic Acid (CLA)

Eating beef has been justifiably maligned because it primarily contains saturated fat. In later chapters, you will find it's restricted in the meal plans to once a month. However, beef and milk from dairy cows contain another type of fat—one that has anticancer effects and may help you lose weight. The fatty acid in question is actually a group of fatty acid isomers (closely related structures of the same chemical) known as conjugated linoleic acid, or CLA. These fatty acid isomers may be an up-and-coming zoochemical. The presence of CLA in dairy products has been known for some time, since it was found by accident in raw hamburger in 1987. Subsequently it was discovered that CLA was better utilized by the body when beef was cooked. The research on CLA could possibly have an impact on future nutrition recommendations. With the information available to us at this time, however, it would not be wise to increase beef consumption. Fortunately, there are two ways you can add CLA to your diet without eating beef. The first is by utilizing CLA-enriched dairy products and the other is by using dietary supplements made from sunflower oil.

Farmers who supplement the diets of their dairy cows with sunflower oil see the CLA content of milk fat increase eight times over normal. This may be enough to have significant health benefits. Clement Ip and his colleagues from the Roswell Park Cancer Institute in Buffalo, New York, fed young rats CLA-rich butter in their chow. Another group of animals ate the same amount of regular butter that had not been fortified. After one month, the researchers injected all of the animals with a known carcinogen. Ninety-three percent of the animals on the regular butter diet developed cancer. However, only half of the animals eating CLA-enriched butter developed cancer.

Dr. Ip has also found in other studies that CLA reduces the formation of terminal end buds in breast tissue. These structures are where cancer develops. It appears one of the CLA isomers, called cis-9, trans-11, is the most effective in preventing cancer. Another CLA isomer, known as trans-10, cis-12, is most effective in reducing body fat and increasing lean muscle mass. Delbert R. Dorscheid, M.D., Ph.D., reviewed the published scientific literature on CLA and found that CLA has demonstrated several remarkable disease-preventive effects, among them being anticancer, anti-diabetic, anti-inflammatory, and cholesterol and triglyceride lowering. CLA may also be an effective agent for weight loss, by increasing your lean muscle to fat radio. Supplements are the best way to get this fatty acid because foods that contain it aren't healthful.

The Health Benefits of Dairy Products

Egg yolks are a good source of the yellow carotenoid lutein which gives yolks their color. Not surprisingly, yolks are good for Yellows.

However, studies have shown that eating egg yolks daily can have a significant effect on raising LDL levels. Taking lutein supplements (6 mg daily) may be a better option for protecting the macula of your eye. For more detail on this, please refer back to chapter 5. Also, absorption of fat-soluble vitamins is enhanced by intake of some fat, but don't start adding fat to your diet if you are using supplements. Just take these fat-soluble supplements with a meal containing some fat.

DHA, or docosahexaenoic acid, is the most important long-chain fatty acid (LCP) for the brain, eyes, and heart. In the brain, DHA is bound to membrane lipids and is intimately involved with signaling and neurotransmitter activity. In the eyes, DHA is bound to rods in the visual centers of the retina and affects visual adaptation to darkness and other visual functions. In the heart, DHA is found in the nerve centers that control heartbeat. These functions make DHA one of the most important fatty acids for maintaining health. We don't get much DHA from our diet, but it is possible to increase your DHA intake by eating egg yolks produced from chickens who are fed DHA-rich algae. The average DHA-enriched egg contains 150 mg of this valuable LCP and 20 percent of your vitamin E requirement for the day. This is about the amount you should get daily to ensure optimum intake. However, egg yolks should not be your only way to get this LCP because of the cholesterol problem. You can also get DHA from fish, fish oils, and marine algae supplements.

Cultured dairy products including yogurt, cottage cheese, and kefir, and some kinds of buttermilk provide various species of lactobacilli and bifidobacteria that enhance total body health. In addition to their high nutritional value, cultured dairy products have been reported to possess considerable therapeutic value. Early in the twentieth century observations by medical researchers led to the conclusion that the longevity of some European populations was due to the consumption of cultured dairy products. Today you can enjoy the multiple benefits of consuming cultured dairy products, but it is important to purchase only those products that contain live cultures, which will be indicated on the container's label. Depending on the species of bacteria used, yogurt products will have different flavors. You may have to try several brands before you find one that suits your taste buds. It's best to buy nonfat or low-fat products and those that have no artificial flavors or coloring agents. All color types can use these products, though Greens will have to restrict the amount used. It is also wise to consider a program for improving your colon health. In chapter 8 I discussed pro-biotics and how these polysaccharides enhance the growth of friendly flora in the colon and why that's important. Now I will explain how pro-biotics such as lactobacilli work, and why you should use foods cultured by these friendly bacteria and consider taking a pro-biotic supplement.

Pro-biotics are cultures of various bacteria that have a favorable impact on colonic metabolism. Included are several species of lactobacilli: acidophilus, casei, bulgaricus, thermophilus, and sporogenes. Lactobacillus cultures may reduce digestive complaints for travelers (tourista), ease diarrhea, aid those with lactose intolerance, reduce yeast infections, and resist the side effects of antibiotic use. Lactobacillus cultures should be part of any immune building program. It still amazes me that so few physicians recommend yogurt or acidophilus capsules for patients being treated with antibiotics. The job of antibiotics is to kill all bacteria, regardless of whether they are good or bad. Friendly intestinal flora are killed along with the pathogenic bacteria, and the environment in the colon is drastically altered as a result. Yeast, which normally live in the colon, no longer have the friendly bacteria to keep them in check and proliferate, generating several toxic by-products that can enter the system. Yeast can cause all kinds of other problems, including acute and chronic yeast infections. Another side effect of antibiotic use is reduced immune competence because intestinal flora aren't providing the necessary products that help regulate the immune response. A weakened immune system will likely again fall prey to opportunistic organisms and antibiotics will again be needed. And so the cycle is repeated. Today we know that strains of bacteria resistant to antibiotics are increasing. Using pro-biotic foods and supplements is one way of helping your body resist infection and increase its ability to overcome the effects of adverse environmental factors. It is also important to include pro-biotics to ensure that the friendly bacteria thrive in your body.

Yogurt cheese is a delicious low-fat or fat-free cheese made by placing a quart of low or nonfat yogurt in a cheesecloth bag and letting it hang until all of the whey—the watery part—has drained off. (Be sure to save the whey to add to beverages.) You will get a soft, creamy cheese similar to farmer's cheese, and you can make different flavors by adding herbs, spicy pepper mixes, pesto, garlic, horseradish, or onion. Use it to spread on crackers or bread. I like a spicy variety as a topping on steamed salmon and garnish it with several colors of chopped bell peppers.

Possible Adverse Effects of White Foods

Oils—Nut oils, such as almond, walnut, and peanut, can cause allergic reactions. Olive, canola, and flaxseed oils are the best to use. However, you can't use flaxseed oil for cooking because it will break down. And oils need to be restricted in your daily plan. Even healthy oils pack twice the number of calories as carbohydrates and fats.

Fish—Some people have allergies to fish, particularly shellfish, and should avoid them. Fish oil capsules usually don't pose a problem, but if you are especially sensitive you can use algae-based supplements to meet eicosapentaenoic acid (EPA) and docosahexaenoic acid (DHA) requirements. Many states have issued warnings about consuming fish from local waters. These fish are apt to have parasites and may be contaminated with environmental waste. Women who are pregnant or lactating need to be especially careful because the contaminants can cross the placenta and get into breast milk.

Dairy products—Commercial dairy products may be a source of a bovine growth hormone (BGH). It's difficult to detect this hormone, which naturally occurs in lactating cows. However, many dairy farmers add this hormone to feed in order to increase milk production. The use of BGH is controversial and a full discussion is beyond the scope of this book. If you wish to avoid BGH, look for a "no BGH used" statement on the label of the milk container. Any organic milk will be free of BGH. As I have explained, cultured dairy products are much healthier to consume, and you should buy reduced-fat products whenever possible. You can reduce the amount of saturated fat in butter by mixing one cup of flaxseed oil in a pound of softened butter. Eggs, a good source of lutein, can also be a good source of DHA and vitamin E, if you buy eggs that come from chickens who are fed proper diets.

Poultry—Many stores offer free-range poultry, which may be a little leaner. Avoid chicken that has a lot of fat on it, and remove the skin before cooking if you can. Otherwise remove it before eating. Whether you choose dark or light meat will depend on your color and this will be discussed below.

Meat—Beef is high in saturated fat and although it contains the beneficial oil CLA (conjugated linoleic acid), you should restrict your beef intake to a few times per month. Reserve pork for occasional use, if at all. It is the least desirable meat from a health perspective. Pork is also likely to cause allergies in sensitive people. Lamb is good occasionally, but it contains a lot of fat. Game meats, buffalo, ostrich, and emu are all good meats and you can eat them a couple of times per month if your color's eating plan allows them.

Grilling meat can result in a blackened coating that contains heterocyclic amines (HCAs) that appear to increase risk of colon cancer. There are several ways you can reduce the formation of HCAs or reduce their toxicity. Cynthia Salmon and colleagues from the Lawrence Livermore National Laboratory in Livermore, California, compared cooking methods on hamburger patties that raised the meat temperature high enough to kill pathogenic bacteria and still prevent formation of HCAs. The meat had been inoculated ahead of time with *Escherichia coli,* the deadly bacteria in tainted meat. They found that turning the patties once a minute cooked them faster and reduced the formation of HCAs. Hamburgers that were turned every five minutes took longer to cook and had higher levels of HCAs. Research presented in chapter 6 described protective effects against HCAs when meats are marinated with phenolic compounds including red wine, cherries, and herbs such as rosemary, thyme, and pepper. Curcumin, the active pigment in turmeric and a component of most curries, has also been reported to be protective against development of colon cancer. So you may be able to enjoy grilled foods and, by taking some simple precautions, reduce your exposure to HCAs.

Buying, Storing, and Cooking White Foods

Oils turn rancid quickly, especially the more highly unsaturated ones such as flaxseed, hemp, pumpkin, and wheat germ. It is best to store them in a dark container to protect them from light and refrigerate them. For monounsaturated oils such as canola and olive, you can keep small amounts in a cool cupboard for quick use and store the bulk of the bottle contents in the refrigerator. Olive oil is rich in carotenoids, and the best brands come in a dark glass container. Be sure to check the fatty acid profile table for which oils are monounsaturated and which are polyunsaturated.

Meat, fish, and poultry should be bought the day they are cut. Don't risk contamination by buying bargain meats that were cut several days ago. Find a reliable source for poultry and fish because they spoil even faster than meat. Fish should not have a "fishy" smell. Poultry should have a nice clear white skin, although some poultry growers feed their chickens carotenes which may give the skin an unusual yellow color. Chicken fat should be a pale creamy color. Refrigerate all of these foods as quickly as possible and eat them within a day or two of purchase. Don't rely on the date on the label, if there is one. Whatever you can't use that day should be carefully repackaged and frozen. Plan on using frozen meat within a month, unless you purchase professionally wrapped and frozen meats and keep them in a non-defrosting freezer.

Dairy and eggs will have a date on the carton. Be sure to check dates when you purchase these items and use them before the date expires. Again, you want to get them into the refrigerator as soon as possible after purchase.

Which White Foods Are My Color?

White foods are complementary for all color types and are less important than the other color foods I have discussed. All of these foods should be considered supplementary to your meal plans.

Yellow Types

You can eat nearly all of the foods in this group, although some are better for you than others.

Oils: almond, apricot, avocado, canola, coconut, evening primrose, fish, flaxseed, mustard or hot pepper, olive, peanut, safflower, sesame, sunflower, walnut, and wheat germ

Avoid: corn, soy, margarine

Dairy: butter, buttermilk, yogurt cheese (panir), cottage cheese, cream, hard cheese, ghee, kefir, milk, sour cream, yogurt
Avoid: ice cream
Fish: all fresh and saltwater fish, tuna
Avoid: shellfish
Meat: beef, buffalo, emu, ostrich, and venison
Avoid: lamb, pork
Poultry and eggs: chicken and turkey, duck, eggs and egg yolks
Avoid: eating only white meat from poultry; dark meat is preferable

Red Types

You are more restricted in white foods. Meats are too heavy and hot for you and saltwater fish and shellfish are more likely to cause allergies in your type than others. Some oils will work well for you, but others will not. You will do well with most dairy products; in fact, you are the only type who can tolerate a little ice cream occasionally.

Oils: avocado, black currant, coconut, evening primrose, fish oils, hemp, margarine, olive, soy, sunflower, walnut, and wheat germ
Avoid: almond, apricot, canola, corn, flaxseed, mustard or hot pepper, peanut, safflower, and sesame
Dairy: butter, yogurt cheese (panir), cottage cheese, cream, ghee, ice cream, milk, and yogurt
Avoid: buttermilk, hard cheese, kefir and sour cream
Fish: freshwater fish
Avoid: saltwater fish, shellfish, and salty pickled fish
Meat: Avoid all meats.
Poultry and eggs: chicken and turkey, especially white meat, egg whites
Avoid: egg yolks, dark meat, duck

Green Types

You will be the most restricted in which white foods you can eat. Most oils and dairy products won't agree with you. Freshwater fish, shellfish, and poultry are your best choices among flesh foods. Many Green types have trouble with fish and shellfish because of allergies. Once you get your body in balance, you may find your tolerance for these foods increases. However, you should use only small amounts of poultry or fish two or three times a week. Egg yolks contain too much cholesterol for you but egg whites are a good source of protein.

Oils: black currant, borage, canola, corn, evening primrose, fish, flaxseed, mustard or hot pepper

Avoid: almond, avocado, coconut, hemp, margarine, olive, peanut, safflower, sesame, walnut, and wheat germ

Dairy: cultured dairy products only on occasion

Avoid: all other dairy products, all cheese

Fish: freshwater fish and shellfish

Avoid: ocean fish, salty pickled fish

Meat: lamb

Avoid: beef, pork, venison

Poultry and eggs: egg whites, chicken, turkey, goose, and game birds

Avoid: egg yolks, duck

10

Herbs, Spices, Condiments, and Beverages

This subject brings me back to my earliest days in the kitchen when I began experimenting with spices. As a teenager, I was frequently left in charge of my two younger brothers, who were my unwilling guinea pigs. I added too much Tabasco sauce to the salad dressing one evening and my poor unsuspecting brothers each took a huge mouthful before I did. This taught me one of the first rules of cooking—taste everything before you serve it to someone else. Although it was a while before my brothers trusted me again, I continued to perfect my skills in working with culinary spices and herbs. Soon I was growing my own kitchen herbs, never thinking I would one day be exploring them as medicinal agents.

Technically speaking, herbs are the leaves and flowers of plants and spices can be seeds, roots, bark, or the fruit of a plant or tree. Any of the plant parts can be used as seasoning, teas, or medicines. Here, I will primarily use the word *spice* when referring to seasonings and *herb* when talking about teas and medicinals.

Why Use Spices and Herbs?

The obvious reason for adding herbs and spices to food today is to increase palatability. However, the ultimate reason spices have been used for centuries is to retard food spoilage and kill organisms that might otherwise cause disease. My own love and appreciation for culinary herbs and spices has grown over the years, especially since I have learned how important they are in combatting potential disease processes.

Herbs and spices can

- increase the palatability of food and reduce the need for salt
- help moderate food intake, increase its absorbability, and improve bowel function
- aid in weight reduction
- moderate recirculation of cholesterol from the colon
- provide antioxidant protection, phytoestrogens, and phytoprogestins
- prevent nausea
- retard food spoilage and kill disease causing organisms

Let's review some of the research that has revealed these beneficial properties of herbs and spices.

A British team of researchers tested the free radical damage to human tissues before and after being treated with a blend of spices commonly used in the Provence region of France. The blend included rosemary, thyme, French tarragon, basil, savory, fennel, lavender, and marjoram. The scientists found that the spices reduced free radical damage by 50 percent. In a human study of the antioxidant power of herbs and spices, Indian researchers gave ten patients with coronary artery disease and ten healthy people two cups of milk containing a pinch of saffron (50 mg) each day for six weeks. At the end of the trial, the blood cells from both groups of people showed a significant reduction in free radical scavenging ability. However, those with coronary artery disease derived the most benefit. This study shows that even for those who are sick, impressive benefits can be gained by increasing use of herbs and spices. Studies such as these are intriguing in that they suggest adding herbs and spices to foods might not only retard spoilage, but also help prevent free radical damage in your body.

Holy basil (*Ocimum sanctum* and *Ocimum album*) is considered one of the most revered plants in Indian medicine, having been used to treat Yellow and Green type conditions of the digestive, respiratory and nervous systems. Recent work at the University of Michigan has revealed two new phytochemicals in basil (*isothymusin* and *isothymonin*). These are among six phenolic phytochemicals identified by the scientists as powerful antioxidants and anti-inflammatory agents. The Michigan team reported that basil was as effective as ibuprofen, naproxen and aspirin in reducing inflammation and relieving pain. Researchers in India also found that holy basil is an effective agent for reducing blood sugar, and their research suggests this herb may be useful complementary therapy along with dietary change in the management of moderate non-insulin dependent diabetes.

Garlic and cloves are effective anti-microbial agents and a recent study showed that both were effective killing agents against strains of *Staphylococcus* and *Salmonella*. Garlic was 93 percent effective in killing the strain of *Salmonella* that causes typhoid fever in laboratory cultures. Garlic has also shown killing ability against antibiotic-resistant bacteria and the yeast *Candida albicans*, more effective even than the drug nystatin, commonly prescribed for this condition. Several other herbs have shown important effects. Both saffron and rosemary appear to effectively deter cancer cell growth by modifying DNA synthesis, and adding cayenne pepper to meals helps increase metabolism and aid weight loss. Oregano added to tomato sauce increases taste and appetite appeal, something Italian cooks discovered a long time ago. Oregano is a powerful antioxidant, anti-bacterial, and anti-viral agent, making it useful for countering the effects of sore throats and colds.

Increasing digestive efficiency and improving bowel transit time are important goals in any health enhancing program. Black pepper has been used as a digestive enhancer in India for centuries and is known by the Sanskrit name *pippali*. Modern scientific investigation has shown that the primary phytochemical in pepper, called piperine, increases assimilation and utilization of foods and dietary supplements. Of special importance, pepper seems to strengthen the intestinal wall and increase its absorptive function. Leaky gut syndrome is a term that doctors use to describe a weak intestinal wall that allows undigested food particles to pass into the bloodstream, inviting attack by marauding immune cells. This condition is considered by many allergists as a chief cause of chronic food allergies. Black pepper, but not cayenne pepper, appears to be effective in reducing leaky gut syndrome. Many of the most important spices, including cayenne, ginger, and pepper, are innately hot and are classified in Ayurveda as warming. They are good for Yellow and Green types who are most likely to experience sluggish or impaired digestion and poor bowel function. However, these warm spices must be used with caution by Red types.

Garam masala, a traditional Indian spice mixture containing coriander, charnushka (kalonji), caraway, cloves, ginger, and nutmeg has been found effective in reducing bowel transit time and in elimination of waste material. In a recent study, 18 healthy people had improved gastric emptying and faster bowel transit time when they added garam masala to their meals. Fecal mass also increased, indicating better bowel function. Adding this spice to meals could be an easy way to aid weight loss in addition to relieving sluggish digestion.

Curcumin, the carotenoid in turmeric, is known to be an effective deterrent to inflammation, cancer, and thrombosis (abnormal blood clotting). The anti-clotting effects of curcumin have been well established in the scientific literature. Curcumin works in several ways, among them by selectively blocking enzymes that promote clotting. Aspirin is the most widely used remedy for preventing clots and it also works by blocking enzymes, but not selectively, so that stomach protective enzymes are also blocked. That's why taking aspirin irritates the stomachs of many people. Studies have shown that curcumin is more effective than aspirin, and it doesn't have the undesirable side effects. Curcumin, a constituent of curry, is one of the most effective cardiovascular protective agents known.

A research team from Aeron Biotechnology in San Leandro, California, tested 150 herbs and spices for phytoestrogen and phytoprogestin activity. The specific competitive ability against estradiol and progesterone for receptor binding in cultured human breast tissue was assessed. This study is of particular interest for women seeking natural forms of these hormones. The six highest phytoestrogen herbs were found to be soy, licorice, red clover, thyme, turmeric, hops, and verbena. The six highest phytoprogestin herbs were oregano, verbena, turmeric, thyme, red clover, and damiana. The feasibility of using these phytoestrogen and phytoprogestin herbs depends on how well they are absorbed into the system. Saliva testing of human volunteers verified there was a dramatic rise in blood levels of phytoestrogens and phytoprogestins, demonstrating the uptake of the herbal actives. Further testing of the herbal actives from the volunteers' saliva showed that they were biologically active, either enhancing or reducing the effects of estrogen and progesterone.

Together, spices can have a powerful impact on your health because of the phytochemicals they contain. You will find some of the most important phytochemicals listed in the table below. The names may sound strange because they are unique to the herb containing them. However, they are the same phytochemicals you have already read about—phenols, carotenoids, terpenes, flavonoids, saponins, and sulfur compounds. All of the spices are antioxidants, although I have listed this function for just a few of the outstanding ones.

Later, when you have complete color meal plans appropriate for your color, you will encounter foods that are not your color and may wonder what to do to balance them. You can reduce the effects of off-color foods by adding spices and condiment sauces to them. You can also enhance the disease-fighting action of phytochemicals in your food by adding spices containing the same or complementary phytochemicals. For example, you increase the phenolic content and its antioxidant power when you add spices such as rosemary, thyme, oregano, and basil. As you may recall, phenols are excellent at trapping rogue free radicals before they cause cellular damage. This is the same function phenols perform in plants when they keep free radicals from the environment at bay. Adding parsley along with these herbs supplies a phytochemical called apigenin which is an antihistamine, bactericide, and anti-inflammatory agent.

You will notice a few things when you study this table. Many of the spices are effective agents in supporting respiratory function. That's because they contain volatile oils and aromatic agents that naturally increase respiratory efficiency. Herbalists call this action diaphoretic. You will also notice that many are useful digestive aids and reduce flatulence. This means the spices improve digestive and absorptive function in all areas of the gastrointestinal (GI) tract.

If you are a Red type, you will quickly notice that there are few spices listed here that are your color. Reds don't need the stimulation of warm and aromatic spices because they generally have good digestion. As a very general rule, Red types will do best with leafy spices and should avoid red or hot spices. Since roots and tubers concentrate actives, they are usually too warm for Red types. Generally, the spices that are good for you are cooler and sweeter and many support the cardiovascular system, cholesterol metabolism, and bile production—all Red concerns.

Culinary Herbs and Spices—Actives and Actions

Seasoning (Your Color)	Phytochemicals	Useful For
Asafoetida or asafedida (Yellow, Green)	asaresinotannol, allyl propylsulfide, farnesferol, foetidin	Abdominal distension, gas, cramping, yeast infections, delayed or difficult menstruation, palpitations, nervousness
Basil, holy (Yellow, Green)	cirsilineol, cirsimaritin, isothymusin, isothymonin, apigenis, rosmarinic acid, eugenol	Pain relief, headache, diabetes, antioxidant
Basil (Yellow, Green)	aesculin, monterpenes, anethole, borneol, cadenine, estragole, phytosterols, tryptophan	Congestion, fever, stress
Bay leaves (Yellow, Green)	costanolide, sesquiterpenes	Digestive and respiratory stimulant, flatulence
Black pepper (Yellow, Green; Reds, don't overdo it)	piperine, carvacrol, carvone, chromium	Antioxidant, digestive stimulant, expectorant
Caraway (Yellow, Green)	carene, carveol, carvone, phytosterols, monoterpenes	Digestive aid, flatulence
Cardamom (All colors; Reds, don't overdo it)	phytosterols, phosphatides (choline, inositol, ethanolamine), monoterpenes	Stimulant, expectorant
Cayenne and paprika (Yellow, Green)	capsaicinoids, carotenoids	Flatulence, dyspepsia, poor digestion

Cinnamon (All colors; Reds, don't overdo it)	cinnamaldehyde, eugenol, trans-cinnamic acid, tannins, monoterpenes	Anorexia, bloating, nausea, flatulence, colic
Chamomile (All colors)	apigenin, chamazulene, farnesene, farnesol, pinene	Dyspepsia, nervousness, sleeplessness
Citrus zest (All colors)	limonene, naringin, hesperidin, neohesperidin, auranetin	Improves nutrient absorption, relieves congestion
Cloves (Yellow, Green)	eugeniin, ellagitannins, casuarictin	Aphrodisiac, expectorant, decongestant, flatulence, laryngitis, headache, toothache
Coriander and cilantro (All colors)	linalool, pinene, limonene, phytosterols	Stomach distension, stomach cramps
Cumin (All colors)	apigenin, monoterpenes, cumene, cuminic acid	Restores homeostasis, anti-stress, mild stimulant
Dandelion (Red, Green)	eudesmanolides, triterpenes, lutein, phytosterols	Liver and gall bladder problems, digestive and GI complaints
Dill (All colors)	anethole, apiole, carveol, carvacrol, carvone, esculetin	Leaves: expectorant; seed: anti-colic, stimulates lactation
Fennel (All colors; Greens, don't overdo it)	trans-anethole, fenchone, estragole, pinene, limonene, flavonoids	Stomach and bowel remedies
Fenugreek (Light use for Yellows, Greens)	galactomannins (mucilaginous fiber), lysine, tryptophan, alkaloids (trigonelline)	Cholesterol management, gastrointestinal complaints
Flaxseed (All colors; Reds, don't overdo it)	linolenic, linoleic, oleic, stearic, palmitic, myristic fatty acids, lignins, sterols	Demulcent, laxative, lowers blood lipids, lowers platelet aggregation
Garlic (Yellow, Green)	allyl, sulfides, ajoene, vinyl dithiins, phosphorus, prostaglandins, flavonoids, saponins, stigmasterol	Restores homeostasis, expectorant, stimulant
Ginger (All colors; Reds, don't overdo it)	oleoresins, gingerols, shogaols, gisbalone, gingiberene	Lessens travel nausea, stomach pain, nausea, vomiting, flatulence, promotes gastric secretion

Seasoning (Your Color)	Phytochemicals	Useful For
Horseradish (Greens, Yellows, don't overdo it)	glucosinolates, allyl isothiocyanates, coumarin, phenols, peroxidase enzymes	Respiratory and urinary infections, promotes gastric secretion
Juniper berries (Red, Green)	terpinen-4-ol, lignins, amentoflavone, desoxypodophyllotoxin	Indigestion, stimulates appetite, flatulence
Marjoram (Yellow, Green)	carvone, hydroquione, saponins	Stimulant, expectorant, aids digestion, promotes menstruation
Mustard seeds (Yellow, Green)	allyl isothiocyanates, sinapic acid	Relieves excess mucus, digestive stimulant
Nutmeg and mace (Yellow, Green)	p-cymene, malabaricone, phytosterols, sabianine	Good sedative, induces sleep, abdominal pain
Onion (raw, Green; cooked, Yellow, Red)	diallyl sulfides, alliospirosides, isothiocyanates, flavonoids, sitosterols	Diuretic, expectorant, combats colds, flu, antiseptic, reduces putrefaction in colon
Oregano (Yellow, Green)	caryophyllene, phenolic acids, vitexin	Upper respiratory and GI stimulant, anti-viral, analgesic
Parsley (Red, Green)	apigenin, apiole, bergapten, carveol	Diuretic, promotes menstruation, calms nerves
Peppermint (All colors; Yellows, go easy)	anethole, betaine, carvacrol, monoterpenes, menthacubanone, menthol	Relieves congestion, soothes stomach, flatulence
Rosemary (Yellow, Green)	carnosol, carnosic, rosmarinic, chlorogenic, and caffeic acids, rosmanol, rosmaridiphenol	Antioxidant, aids stomach upset, flatulence
Sage (Yellow, Green)	thujone, salviatannin, monoterpenes	Reduces sweat, night sweats
Tarragon (Yellow, Green)	artemetin, isocoumarin, estragole	Diuretic, promotes menses, flatulence, bloating
Thyme (Yellow, Green)	borneol, carvacrol, flavones, luteolin	Reduces spasms, cough remedy, anti-parasitic, antiseptic

Turmeric (All colors)	volatile oils, curcuminoids	Abdominal bloating, appetite loss, improves flow of bile, gastric and pancreatic juices
Watercress (All colors)	glucosinolates, gluconasturtiin, trace minerals	Respiratory congestion, cholesterol management; mouth, throat, and lung cancer preventive

Sources: David Frawley and Vasant Lad, *Yoga of Herbs;* Swami Sada Tirtha, *The Ayurveda Encyclopedia;* James Duke, *Handbook of Biologically Active Phytochemicals* and *Handbook of Phytochemical Constituents of GRAS Herbs.*

This list is not meant to be all inclusive or even to identify exactly which phytochemicals may be responsible for the observed effects. It will take years to unravel all of the phytochemical secrets herbs and spices hold. In the meantime, you can enjoy the flavor spices and herbs add to your food, correct imbalances in your type, and benefit from the added medicinal benefits of using them.

Sauces and Condiments

I will give you recipes for sauces appropriate for your color in Part Three. These sauces, along with the spices listed in your food plan, will help you balance your metabolism and tolerate foods that are off-color. For example, Yellows have a hard time digesting green cabbage. Adding plum sauce, vinegar, or ketchup to steamed cabbage helps offset the tendency for this food to cause gas. Yellows can enhance digestibility of vegetables and legumes by adding caraway or fennel seeds during cooking. Sweet and sour cabbage is much better for Yellows, and Reds can enjoy this food also, particularly if red cabbage is used instead of green. Green types do well with any kind of cabbage. However, sweet and sour dishes don't agree with Greens because they don't tolerate either vinegar or sugar.

The following table lists popular condiments and which type can use them. The taste category of the condiment is also given as an indication of what makes it suitable or unsuitable for a particular type.

Condiments for Your Type

Condiment, Sauce	Yellow Type	Red Type	Green Type
Mayonnaise	yes—sweet	yes—sweet	no—too oily
Mustard	no—too pungent	no—too hot, spicy	yes—increases metabolism
Ketchup	yes—sour	no—too hot, spicy	no—too sour
Chutney	no—too pungent	no—too hot, spicy	yes—increases metabolism
Worcestershire	yes—sour, salty	no—too sour, salty	no—too sour, salty

Condiment, Sauce	Yellow Type	Red Type	Green Type
Tartar Sauce	yes—sweet	yes—sweet	no—too sweet
Plum Sauce	yes—sour	no—too sour	yes—not too sour
Mint Sauce	no—too pungent	no—too sour	yes—pungent
Steak Sauce	yes—sour, salty	no—too salty	no—too salty
Vinegar; cider, malt, wine, rice, balsamic, umeboshi	yes—sour	yes—rice or balsamic in moderation, umeboshi occasionally	no—too sour

From a nutritional standpoint, condiments offer little benefit and are meant to be used on occasion. It's much better to use spices and herbs to flavor food instead of adding condiments. Most of those listed in the table contain additives, sugars, and other ingredients that make them unsuitable for daily use. As for ketchup, choose brands that aren't sweetened and contain a minimal amount of salt. In purchasing mayonnaise, look for brands that are made from canola oil; some brands are also egg free and low in salt. Both of these condiments are available in brands made from organic ingredients. Spectrum and Muir Glen are good brands to look for.

Beverages

Milk, tea, and fruit and vegetable juices, along with their medical benefits, have been presented in previous chapters. Coffee and tea are the two most frequently consumed beverages among adults worldwide. Not surprisingly, they have been widely studied for their health benefits and their adverse effects.

Coffee—Caffeinated beverages including coffee, tea, and colas are consumed primarily because they stimulate the autonomic nervous system, which controls the actions of the brain, glands, and organs. Among its effects are control of arterial pressure, heart rate, gastrointestinal motility and secretion, sweating, body temperature, and breathing rate. Anyone who drinks caffeinated beverages is familiar with these effects. The most striking effects of caffeine, however, are on the brain. Caffeine increases alertness and elevates mood. It gives us energy and helps us focus—at least until we drink too much of it. Then it can make us jittery, nervous, and delay the onset of sleep because of its effects on the central nervous system. The effects of caffeine from coffee and tea are much the same, except that tea is less likely to disrupt sleep, according to a study published recently by British researchers.

Caffeine constricts blood vessels and reduces blood flow to the brain and can result in headaches and reduced short-term memory. Somewhat paradoxically, coffee also relieves headaches and enhances the effect of pain remedies such as acetaminophen by up to 40 percent. These effects are most pronounced in the elderly, but are also common side effects in younger people. And, though caffeine is an addictive and mood-altering substance, withdrawal doesn't leave any lasting effects.

Coffee drinking can also have deleterious effects on blood lipids and blood pressure, both of which are risk factors for cardiovascular disease. A Dutch research team reported that consumption of one liter of coffee a day raised homocysteine blood levels by 10 percent among 64 healthy forty-year-old men and women. Homocysteine is considered a marker for increased risk of cardiovascular disease. This study used French pressed coffee, which is unfiltered. Does the way coffee is brewed make a difference? Yes, according to another group of researchers in Spain. It seems the constituents in coffee that cause these deleterious effects are concentrated in unfiltered coffee and less concentrated in coffee brewed using filters or coffee bags.

Elderly patients are most sensitive to the effects of regular coffee, particularly if they don't eat sufficient amounts of protein, according to researchers at Johns Hopkins University. Other scientists have found that though drinking more than two cups of coffee a day may not harm older individuals and may do some good, those with impaired liver enzymes may not be able to handle regular coffee but do well with decaffeinated coffee. Among the older population, coffee drinking can raise blood pressure in those with already elevated blood pressure, however, an Australian researcher found that drinking five cups of coffee during a single day actually lowered blood pressure among seventy-five-year-olds who didn't normally drink it and among coffee drinkers who weren't hypertensive.

For men, coffee drinking may be associated with development of prostate cancer. Canadian researchers assessed risk of developing prostate cancer among 3,400 men who participated in the Nutrition Canada Survey from 1970 to 1972. Tea drinking and cola drinking didn't appear to be risk factors for prostate cancer. However, coffee drinkers had a 40 percent increased risk of developing the disease. Rheumatoid arthritis is also connected with coffee consumption. In a study of 18,981 men and women, Finnish researchers found that drinking four or more cups of coffee daily increased the risk of developing rheumatoid arthritis. This risk was only associated with those cases that were positive for rheumatoid factor (RA). Among those individuals who developed negative RA factor rheumatoid, there was no connection, suggesting that coffee may contribute to the production of RA.

A rather unpleasant side effect of caffeine consumption appears to be weakening of the sphincter muscle (detrusor) that closes off the urinary bladder. Two studies found that the higher the caffeine intake, the more likely a woman would experience urinary incontinence. Although the problem increased with age, it was seen in younger women who drank between 100 mg and 400 mg of caffeine daily but not those who consumed less than this amount. Women who consumed more than 400 mg of caffeine daily reported the greatest incidence of detrusor instability.

Coffee also has a number of reported positive effects. Dr. Edward Giovannucci, from Harvard Medical School and Brigham and Women's Hospital in Boston, has been a prominent investigator in the field of phytochemical nutrition for some time. Dr. Giovannucci and his colleagues have found that coffee appears to reduce the formation of gallstones. The scientific team analyzed data from ten years of dietary and health information obtained from 46,008 men in the long-term Health Professionals Follow-Up Study. They found that men who drank two to three cups of coffee daily had a 40 percent lower risk of gallstones than those who didn't consume coffee regularly. Men who drank the most coffee, four or more cups per day, had 45 percent less risk of having gallstones than those who drank the least amount of coffee. Coffee stimulates release of cholescystokinin (a satiety hormone), increases gallbladder motility, and possibly enhances bowel motility. One of the phytochemicals in coffee, cafestol, may affect bile cholesterol concentration and reduce synthesis of bile salts, ultimately preventing formation of gallstones.

The fact that coffee increases bowel motility may help prevent colon cancer. Dr. Giovannucci also analyzed several studies from a number of European, North American, and Asian countries that reported coffee decreased the risk of colorectal cancer. The studies included some done in hospital settings but the majority were done in clinical settings. Although the analysis of all the studies showed a clear connection between coffee drinking and lowered risk of colorectal cancer, these findings are merely suggestive until the results of several ongoing studies are reported.

Several studies were reported in 2000 that showed coffee drinking may significantly reduce the incidence of Parkinson's disease. Researchers from Hawaii reported that data from a thirty-year follow-up of 8,000 men showed that those who drank at least twenty-eight ounces of coffee per day were protected from this disease. In November, researchers at the Mayo Clinic found that heavy coffee drinkers were less likely to develop Parkinson's than moderate coffee drinkers. The Mayo scientists were not convinced that caffeine prevented Parkinson's. They theorized that those with brain abnormalities that cause Parkinson's may be less likely to enjoy coffee.

A number of other positive benefits from drinking coffee have also been reported. These include a reduced buildup of uric acid, a factor in gout, and reduced iron absorption, a risk factor for cardiovascular disease among some people. Menstruating women who need iron, however, should consider that drinking coffee with meals can reduce the amount of iron and calcium absorbed from the meal.

All of this data may seem confusing and you should keep in mind that I am reporting what is the latest "news" on coffee. You will continue to read conflicting information about this beverage. Consequently, you should adhere to the following guidelines for drinking coffee according to your color:

- Regular coffee should be avoided if you're a Yellow or Red type.
- Moderate coffee drinking, up to two cups per day, is probably not harmful for Green types, especially if it's brewed using a filter.
- Decaffeinated coffee, preferably water processed, has less impact on the central nervous system and may be preferable for Yellow types.
- Coffee is acidic and may be irritating to the stomach, and therefore is not good for Reds.
- If you have a serious medical condition, such as high blood pressure, heart arrhythmia, kidney disease or diabetes, eliminate coffee drinking entirely.
- Avoid cream or sugar if you're a Green type.

Herbal teas have medicinal benefits that have not been discussed. Many of the most popular ones such as mint and chamomile were included in the above section on herbs and spices. A couple of studies done on peppermint, caraway, and chamomile are of interest. Peppermint has traditionally been recommended for various GI complaints including dyspepsia, irritable bowel, and cramping. Several studies reported favorable results in using peppermint oil for irritable bowel syndrome. German researchers studied 118 patients with gastric pain, some of whom had *Helicobacter pylori* infections. *H. pylori* is implicated in gastric ulcers and gastric cancer. Half of the patients were given medication (cisapride) for their symptoms and the other half received a peppermint and caraway oil preparation (enteroplant). Both groups of patients responded favorably to the treatments and the herbal oil was as effective in relieving symptoms as the drug. An English researcher also reported that peppermint oil was effective in relieving postoperative nausea.

Sweeteners

Sugar and natural sweeteners, including fruit juice concentrates, maple syrup, and molasses, are high on the glycemic index (as discussed in chapter 9) and should be used sparingly. Sucanat and Rapidura are two brands of natural sweeteners and are the best ones to use. Stevia is a natural noncaloric sweetener, although it is sold as a dietary supplement. It is intensely sweet and holds up well during cooking. Artificial sweeteners including aspartame

(NutraSweet, Equal), acesulfame potassium (Sunett), and sucralose (Splenda) all have side effects and should be avoided. Some of the effects are neurological and others are gastrointestinal.

Possible Adverse Effects of These Foods

Herbs and Spices—Some people are sensitive to certain groups of spices. If you are one of them, you should be careful in using other spices from the same family. Here are some families of spices that have been reported to cause allergic reactions:

Apiaceae—angelica, anise, caraway, carrot, celeriac, celery, chervil, cilantro, cumin, dill, fennel, lovage, parsley, parsley root, parsnip
Piperaceae—black, white, red, green pepper, long pepper
Solanaceae—cayenne, chili peppers, paprika, pimento, tomatillo
Compositae—chamomile, chicory, dandelion, sunflower, tarragon

A few cases of contact dermatitis (skin rash) have been reported among people who handle rosemary because of the strong volatile oils. However, normal kitchen and cosmetic use should not pose a problem.

Condiments—Be sure to avoid those that aren't your color. Otherwise just keep in mind that you should use condiments infrequently. Herbs and spices are better to use as flavorings. If you are used to adding condiments such as mayonnaise to vegetables, try a little fresh lemon juice instead. I have had great success getting children to eat their vegetables by squeezing lemon juice on the veggies. This works well for getting them to eat fish too.

Beverages—The problems with caffeine consumption are discussed above. Carbonated beverages pose different problems even if they don't contain caffeine. Many contain phosphates that interfere with calcium absorption and utilization. Additionally, they contain sweeteners. If you drink them at all, be sure to avoid those with artificial sweeteners. Carbonated mineral water is a good beverage to use and it makes easy work out of swallowing dietary supplement pills that tend to be large. I have found that people who have difficulty swallowing pills never fail to be successful if they take them with carbonated water.

Buying, Storing, and Cooking These Foods

The biggest mistake most of us make with herbs and spices is trying to keep them too long. The leafy green ones lose their flavor more quickly than the root and bark varieties. Whole spices will keep longer than those that are cut or powdered. Buy a mortar and pestle to grind your spices and grow the ones you use most frequently, if possible. If you buy fresh herbs at the market, treat them as you would a bouquet of flowers. Cut off the end of the stems and keep them in a container of water in a cool place. Do not refrigerate them. Leafy green herbs such as parsley and cilantro should be thoroughly washed when you first bring them home. Cut off most of the stem and dry them as much as possible before storing in a waxed sandwich bag in your vegetable bin. By taking a little extra time when you bring herbs home, you will find them very convenient to use. Be sure to replace bottled dried herbs in six months or less. You can find small plastic containers that hold ¼ cup or around one ounce of herbs that you don't use often.

As for herbal teas, the same storage conditions apply. Most teas come in packages that are easy to reseal; if not, put the tea in a container with a tight-fitting lid. Don't keep teas for more than six months. If you enjoy coffee, buy whole beans and grind them just before brewing. Use a filter and fresh spring water to brew both tea and coffee.

Which of These Foods Are My Color?

Spices and Herbs
> **Yellows**—You can eat almost any spice or herb except raw garlic.
> **Reds**—You can enjoy most green herbs except basil, bay leaf, marjoram, oregano, rosemary, sage, and thyme. You need to avoid those that are hot and spicy such as cayenne, paprika, and mustard.
> **Greens**—All herbs and spices are good for you. Avoid spice blends that have sugar or salt in them.

Condiments and Sweeteners
> **Yellows**—You can use all condiments and sweeteners. Avoid the artificial ones.
> **Reds**—Avoid condiments that contain salt, vinegar, and chili peppers. All sweeteners except artificial ones are good for you.
> **Greens**—Condiments are OK for you, except sour, salty, or fermented ones such as miso and soy sauce. Avoid sweeteners as much as possible.

Beverages

Yellows and Greens—The best herbal teas are ginger, cinnamon, clove, cardamom, orange peel, mint, chamomile, ginseng, and hibiscus.

Reds—The best herbal teas are alfalfa, blackberry, borage, chrysanthemum, dandelion, green tea, licorice, marshmallow, nettle, raspberry, red clover, rose flower, saffron, sarsaparilla, and strawberry.

Greens—The best teas in addition to those mentioned for Yellows and Greens are burdock, eucalyptus, fenugreek, and juniper berry. Coffee can be used in moderation and so can red wine.

part three

Foods for Your Color Meal Plans

❖

11

Eat Your Colors Nutrition Plans

We have now established the importance of choosing the right foods for your type and what those foods are. So it's time to develop the personalized eating strategy to put this information into a workable plan that can change your life. Although we live in an age when nutrition information is more available than ever before, this information can be very confusing. The information on what is best to eat keeps changing as new evidence unfolds.

Nutrition data on cardiovascular disease is one example of how our understanding of the disease process has affected dietary advice. For years we were told cholesterol was the chief culprit in narrowing of arteries and increased risk of heart disease. Accordingly we were advised to avoid high-cholesterol foods such as eggs and butter while embracing egg-white omelettes and margarine. Then scientists warned that cholesterol wasn't the only risky food ingredient and we should shun saturated fats in favor of polyunsaturated fats. Later, it was discovered that polyunsaturated fats quickly turned rancid in the body, creating harmful free radicals faster than our antioxidant systems could disarm them. So we switched to monounsaturated fats such as olive and canola oils. Next came the low-fat wave and advent of fat-free foods. Now we know that fat-free foods are high in sugars and that we need some fats in order to be healthy. The emphasis has once again shifted toward the kind of fats—primarily oils—we should consume. Which oils to choose for your color type was discussed in chapter 10. How have Americans responded to nutritional advice from the experts?

Making Nutrition Information Work for You

Some nutritional advice appears to have made an impact. According to results of the U.S. Department of Agriculture's 1994 to 1996 food survey, we have embraced some healthful practices such as reducing overall fat intake. However, the recommendation to increase fruit and vegetable consumption has largely fallen on deaf ears. We also have better food labeling information available today to aid us in making informed buying decisions. The Food and Drug Administration took a giant step forward in the process of nutrition education by mandating use of a standardized food label format. The standards that took effect in 1994 are specific about the way nutrition information is presented. This allows the consumer to make comparisons between products without having to guess what's in the product or make computations for serving sizes. Reliable information on serving size is one example of a major improvement the new labels give. What constitutes a serving size is clearly stated in grams (metric) and a more familiar measure such as tablespoons, cups, or pieces. Although this may seem like a minor detail, it is an important step in making it easier to compare the nutritional value of comparable foods.

The nutritional composition of a packaged food must also be detailed in grams of protein, carbohydrate, fats, and fiber. Grams of sugars and saturated fats will also be listed, and some labels list the breakdown of total fats into polyunsaturates, monounsaturates, and saturates, although this breakdown is not mandated. Hopefully the trans fat content will soon be required, since these fats, widely found in margarine and hydrogenated oils, have been strongly implicated in several diseases. Until it is required, you can figure it out if the label lists monounsaturated and polyunsaturated fats. Just add the grams of these two, plus saturated fats. If the sum of the three is less than the total grams of fat listed, the difference is the trans fat content. Finally, the percentage of total daily calories (% of daily value) supplied by each of the four classes of nutrients is also listed. Larger food labels will list the number of calories each gram of protein, carbohydrate, and fat contains—for those who enjoy doing their own math.

The percentages of daily value listed on the right side of the nutrition facts panel are based on a daily intake of 2,000 calories. This is the approximate amount of calories that should be consumed by an average sample of people. It includes most young women between the ages of eleven and thirty who are not pregnant or nursing. It also provides the correct number of calories for men who weigh around 150 pounds, are between the ages of thirty and fifty, and aren't particularly active. You will be given the specifics of serving sizes for your type in the next three chapters.

Other important information listed on the label includes the amount of cholesterol and sodium (salt) contained in the product. The label also lists the amount of vitamins A and C and the minerals calcium and iron contained in the food. Label sizes and format can vary, depending on the size of the package. Small items such as snack bars usually list the nutrition information in paragraph format while larger packages will display the familiar nutrition facts box. You should make use of this information whenever you buy packaged products because it can help you decide which item offers the best nutritional value for your money. You will also be surprised how much of your daily intake of sugar, fats, and salt is contained in some of your favorite foods. You cannot afford to squander your health and shopping dollars on products that are high in calories but offer little nutritional value.

As we have seen, the way nutrition information is dispensed to the public has improved considerably in the last few years. With easy access to the World Wide Web, we can download reliable information from the USDA and other government sites, making it easier to make informed choices. However, for most people, there is still a long way to go in making nutrition information accessible and meaningful. Good nutrition is much more than what we can learn from studying dietary guidelines. And there is little to motivate us to change the way we feed ourselves until we get sick. We tire of hearing the same mantra, "Eat more fruits and vegetables," regardless of how true it might be. Unfortunately, current nutrition information makes no provision for individual tastes or needs. The one big fault with modern nutrition is that it lacks a provision for teaching us how to access our body's innate wisdom in choosing foods that are good for us.

The goal of this book is to teach you how to listen to your body and provide a customized eating plan for your type. The preceding sections helped you understand that food truly is medicine and that everything you put into your mouth has an impact on your health. This book provides you with a time-tested, exciting, and personalized way to apply what you have learned. All of us need a system that is easy to follow and will guide us in our food-buying decisions.

Now let's get into what the *Eat Your Colors* nutrition plans will offer you. I'm going to provide some additional details about the nature of foods you will find in your plan and why they are good for you. Since this information applies to all *Eat Your Colors* plans, I'm presenting it for all types. I'm going to present the properties of foods and then discuss the digestive process and why it's the basis of good health. We'll start with food tastes and explain which are most nourishing for your color, which you should avoid, and why.

Eat According to Taste
with an Eye for Food Quality

Several chapters back, I explained how the Ayurvedic system classifies foods according to their properties. The system includes the sensation a food provokes on the taste buds, the food's properties (hot/cold, soft/hard, oily/dry, etc.), and the post-digestive composition of foods. Food is broken down during digestion as it is acted on by digestive enzymes. According to the Ayurvedic model, digestion modifies some food properties. For example, salty foods become sweet while astringent and bitter foods become pungent. These changes in food tastes are believed to influence the food's effect on the individual. This has been considered in making food selections for each type. For our purposes, the taste we perceive as we chew a food is the most important in determining which foods are best. Later in this chapter you'll learn why this is so important for proper secretion of digestive juices.

Food quality is also important in judging healing potential. We westerners think of freshness and appearance when considering quality. These attributes are also important to the Ayurvedic practitioner. However, the conditions under which a plant grew or an animal was raised are equally important. In the mind of the Eastern practitioner, quality begins with the seed. Only high-quality seeds are capable of producing healing foods. The less processing a food has undergone, the better for us it will be. Genetically modified foods have become an issue in several European countries and have begun to raise safety concerns among Americans. Bio-engineered foods are not acceptable to many health-conscious consumers and raise questions about the quality of foods that contain them.

Food quality extends to food preparation as well. The Ayurvedic cook possesses great skill in combining foods to enhance nutritional value. The liberal use of spices and herbs improves digestion and absorption. In designing food plans, Ayurvedic cooks consider the nutritional composition of foods—whether they are rich in minerals (alkali foods), or high in proteins, fats, or carbohydrates. Food plans are carefully balanced to provide good nutrition.

The Importance of Food Plans

Food plans provide a road map to improved health and are a necessary part of overcoming our Western "grab and feed" mentality. Ayurvedic food plans provide a model for *Eat Your Colors* food plans. The Ayurvedic plans are based on a variety of fresh mineral (and phytochemical)–rich fruits and vegetables. Of equal importance are complex foods that contain carbohydrates, proteins, and vitamins. (We now know these provide other important disease-fighting phytochemicals). Oils are important in food preparation with specific ones advocated for each body type. Animal products, including dairy, eggs, meat, fish, and poultry, assume minor roles in the overall plan. A vegetarian diet is strongly encouraged, especially for Red and Green types. The Ayurvedic plans completely avoid any foods that are heavily processed and those that are nearly devoid of nutrition. Ayurvedic nutrition has always been based on the physiological, psychological, and spiritual beliefs that are rooted in a culture thousands of years old. The system is highly complex, takes years to master, and includes more information than most of us can apply. Though the Ayurvedic model is one to which some of us might aspire, permit me to spare many of the finer details in order to provide a westernized presentation in the *Eat Your Colors* plans. Here, my comments will be to the tastes and quality of foods matched to your type. If you are suffering from a serious illness, I suggest you visit a skilled Ayurvedic healer.

> ❖ There has been a tradition of regarding food merely as 'fuel' for the body, not to be particularly enjoyed but to be got out of the way as quickly as possible so that everyone can get on with something more important . . . The idea that you should eat more of or avoid certain foodstuffs according to your individual constitution is a relatively recent idea among Western dietitians.
>
> —Dr. Shantha Godagama, 1997

In chapter 2, I introduced the concept of tasting food to determine its suitability for your type. Most of us aren't too skilled in doing this and seldom think about what we are tasting. That's an unfortunate side effect of our fast-food culture.

However, those who like to cook appreciate the tongue's ability to judge taste and use this ability to properly season what is being prepared. Cooks around the world have traditionally planned meals to optimize taste sensations, and we have all used taste to choose which foods we prefer. Ayurveda takes us one step further by using taste to determine the suitability of a food for our type. Let's review the six tastes and how they are perceived by our taste buds.

The Six Tastes

Sweet Taste

Foods with a sweet taste are considered the most nourishing. That's not to say eating "sweets" is a good thing, because these items are energetically "cold" and create nutritional deficits. They pull valuable vitamins and minerals from the body that are needed to assimilate the sugars. By sweet foods in Ayurveda we mean complex carbohydrates, such as whole-grain cereals, breads, pasta, and rice. These foods contain or are enriched with the essential vitamins and minerals needed for use in your body. These foods form the basis of the food pyramid in Ayurveda just as they do in Western nutrition. (The food pyramid can be found on page 115.) Most fruits are also sweet and many vegetables are as well. Dairy products, seeds, nuts, freshwater fish, poultry, and beef are also sweet. Sweet is the taste with which we are most familiar. It's no accident that most snack items are sweet. Eating something sweet satisfies our immediate hunger, increases our energy (at least temporarily), and raises levels of calming chemicals in the brain. *Eat Your Colors* recognizes the need for snacks, especially in some color types, and provides plenty of complex sweet foods instead of sugary snacks. Yellow and Red types benefit from the sweet taste while excessive use of sweet foods unbalances the Green type and leads to such disorders as obesity and diabetes.

Sour Taste

Lemons and grapefruit certainly taste sour. Oranges are sweeter but can also be very sour, depending on how ripe they are.

Some other foods with a sour taste are cultured dairy products, including buttermilk, sour cream, yogurt, and cottage cheese. Sour foods are good for Yellows, and small amounts of sour fruits are good for Greens as well, though dairy products are extremely limited for Green types. Reds should avoid eating anything with a sour taste. Foods with a sour taste improve the appetite and increase the flow of saliva and digestive juices. You're no doubt familiar with the "pucker" and mouth-watering sensation you get when something sour hits your tongue.

Salty Taste

This is another taste with which most of us are very familiar. Naturally salty foods such as kelp have been used for decades to cleanse the body and tone the adrenal glands, kidneys, prostate, and thyroid gland. Kelp also contains potassium, iodine, and other minerals that help balance sodium. Naturally salty foods represent a stark departure from our concept of salt, a highly purified substance devoid of its natural balancing elements. Green types who normally shun salt can eat kelp, nori, wakame, arame, and other sea vegetables.

Salty foods have traditionally provided a boost in digestive capacity and are popular additions to many Asian dishes. The Japanese have made good use of the digestive properties of seaweed by combining it with rice, vegetables, and a little fish to make sushi. They also use umeboshi, a small salty black plum, as a digestive condiment with heavy meals. Asian cooks also use shoyu, tamari, or soy sauce to flavor food and increase its digestibility. These sauces are made from fermented soybeans. Natural sea salt is also used as a condiment and unlike its highly refined counterpart contains other minerals.

Together sodium and potassium fuel cellular membrane "pumps" that control the flow of nerve impulses and other molecular traffic across membranes. One might think of these minerals as stop and go signals for cellular traffic—sodium being red and potassium green. Both minerals need to be in balance for the smooth flow of metabolic processes. When we overeat salty tastes, we keep the traffic light red and halt signaling between cells. One of the effects of this is increased retention of fluids. The kidneys cannot properly process fluids and they back up in tissues. This puts pressure on the blood vessels and all organ systems. The body cannot rid itself of toxins, becomes sluggish, and we become sick. From both a Western and Eastern perspective, overeating salted foods is bad for you. However, addition of naturally salty foods to the meal plans for Yellow types helps retain moisture in tissues that tend to be dry and aids sluggish digestion. For Greens who tend to retain fluids (the water element) salty tastes are a minor dietary constituent. Reds should avoid use of salty foods and condiments because they are too warming for their fire element.

Pungent Taste

Most people have an aversion to this taste. It's the acrid, somewhat unpleasant sensation you'd get by biting into a raw artichoke leaf, raw asparagus, or cauliflower, brussels sprouts, or horseradish. It's also the sensation you get from ginger, mustard, curry powder, chili powder, fenugreek, basil, or rosemary. Pungent foods are extremely healing and we temper their taste by cooking them. Many of the spices we enjoy are pungent, and you will learn to use them to balance your color when it's "off."

Pungent foods contain the powerful phytochemicals that were discussed in the preceding chapters. Included are organosulfur compounds (green foods) and carotenoids (yellow foods). As you might expect, pungent foods are excellent for Greens and to a lesser degree for Yellows, and the phytochemicals in these foods are what gives them their taste. Pungent spices are generally too hot for Reds and some pungent foods such as beets, garlic, and eggplant also disagree with Red types.

Pungent foods have the opposite effect from salty foods and reduce the fluid content of tissues. Consequently, they are the primary taste for Greens, the water type. They are therapeutic for clearing congestion in the head and upper respiratory tract. The typical brain fogginess that accompanies a cold or allergy attack can be relieved by pungent foods and spices. Yellows must use pungent foods with care because though they supply the warming energy this type needs, they can be too drying. The herb goldenseal is an example of how this works. Goldenseal is extremely pungent and drying. It is suitable for clearing congestion, which is a Green condition. Yellows who have congestion can use goldenseal but must exercise care, using it for only a day or two to clear congestion. Otherwise, it dries them out so much that they get nervous and can't sleep.

The most pungent green foods—brussels sprouts, cauliflower, and cabbage—have a similar effect on Yellows. Many people who are a Yellow type have a natural aversion to these vegetables.

Bitter Taste

This taste is closely associated with the Red type although Greens also do well with bitter foods and herbs. Bitter foods tend to deplete Yellows, who can become agitated and fearful if they consume too many foods with this taste. Bitter is the sensation you get when you eat deep-green leafy vegetables such as arugula, collards, endive, kale, or spinach, especially if they're raw. Bitter spices include cumin, coriander, dill seeds, and tarragon. Unsweetened chocolate, coffee, black and green tea are also bitter. We naturally gravitate toward these foods after a big meal. However, only Greens can drink coffee at all and should do so sparingly. Tea is better tolerated by both Reds and Greens. Spiced tea or chai is best for Yellows. Bitter beverages should be drunk after meals because they aid digestion. Bitter herbs have traditionally been used to increase digestive capacity. A bitter tonic typically includes herbs such as gentian, fenugreek, and peppermint—all bitter herbs—as key ingredients. Reds do especially well with "bitters" after meals.

Astringent Taste

When we taste a sour food, we pucker up and the juices start to flow. With astringency, the opposite happens since astringent foods and spices reduce the flow of fluids including saliva. The astringent taste is a sensation we don't particularly relish and it definitely gets us to sit up and take notice. Green sprouts of alfalfa, broccoli, and red clover are astringent. We enjoy the "bite" they provide when sprinkled on salads or sandwiches. Celery, cucumbers, eggplant, lettuce, mushrooms, and soy are astringent foods. Many fruits, including apples, avocados, berries, cranberries, grapes, pears, peaches, persimmons, and pomegranates are astringent. Imagine how your tongue would respond if you bit into a persimmon. That's a good example of the sensation of astringency. Astringent spices and herbs include dill, marjoram, and oregano. Several important medicinal herbs are astringent, such as frankincense (*Boswellia*), grape seed and pine bark extracts, resveratrol, and aloes. These herbs are anti-inflammatory and each has other benefits as well.

In chapter 6 on Red foods you may have identified the foods mentioned

here as being good for Reds. They are, because the astringent taste has traditionally been used to cleanse body fluids—blood, lymph, and sweat. It also
prevents capillary leakage and bruising and helps heal skin and mucus membranes. The phytochemicals in astringent foods and spices are *polyphenolic
antioxidants,* which protect the cardiovascular system, improve circulation,
boost immune response, and prevent some types of cancer.

Astringent foods are also beneficial to Greens because they reduce moisture and increase physical mobility. They are excellent expectorants, antihistamines, and diuretics. As you might expect, these are properties that can
give Yellows trouble if they are consumed in excess.

Heating and Cooling Effects of Food

Foods have specific properties from the molecules they contain and this
determines their effect on the body. The heating and cooling characteristics
of foods are strongly linked with the phytochemical content of the food. For
example, cayenne is heating, due to the red phytochemical carotenoids
unique to this food. On the other hand, turmeric, which contains yellow
carotenoids, is cooling. You have probably experienced the effects of
cayenne on the body, but you may be less familiar with the effect of turmeric.

Our innate wisdom guides us in selecting foods and spices that are best for
our type, once we become attuned to what our body is telling us. However,
that takes a lot of practice! In the meantime, you'll need to know what to
choose for your type. In the lists I'll provide later you'll notice I refer to the
heating and cooling properties of the foods selected.

Eat with Your Eyes

In Part Two of *Eat Your Colors,* you were introduced to the concept of choosing foods that match your color. When planning your meals, it is important
to design as colorful a plate as possible. Imagine your plate is sectioned. One-
third to one-half of your plate, depending on your type, will be filled with
vegetables and fruits that are your primary colors. Another third to half will
contain your tan "earth" foods, and the remaining space will be filled with
white foods—dairy, oils, seeds, nuts, and a little fish or poultry. The proportions that are right for each type will be given in chapters 12, 13, and 14.

Now that you understand your constitutional strengths and weaknesses,
you can better nurture yourself by choosing appropriate foods. The best
thing about the *Eat Your Colors* plan is that it will help you to overcome the
tendency to grab what's most convenient and instead to stop and consider
the impact a particular food will have on you. As you study the detailed Yel-

low, Red, and Green food plans in the next three chapters, you will see that you will be shopping and preparing meals with your eyes, rather than just grabbing something to satisfy your immediate hunger. And remember—don't shop when you're hungry! That's when you'll be most tempted to buy processed foods with little nutritional value.

As for the nutrition plans, you will naturally study the one for your type. However, keep in mind that you are a blend of all three colors. You will need to familiarize yourself with all three nutritional plans so that you will know what to choose when you are out of balance. Part Four of *Eat Your Colors* will highlight weaknesses peculiar to each type. This will help you recognize the color that's off.

Now, on to the *Eat Your Colors* nutritional plans!

12

Nutrition Plan for Yellow Types

The Yellow body type is most associated with *movement*, the action of air that is your element. All bodily movement is governed by the Yellow constitution according to Ayurveda. This includes:

- Breathing: movement of air in and out of respiratory organs
- Heart activity: rhythm and movement of blood
- Speech: process of verbal communication
- Peristalsis: movement of food along the alimentary canal
- Secretion of digestive enzymes
- Elimination of waste
- Menstruation
- Labor and delivery
- Circulation
- Body locomotion: movement of muscles, tendons, joints, bones
- Nervous system activity: brain, nerves, eyes, ears, tactile sensations
- Mental clarity: acquiring new information, processing it, memory, and output

When you are healthy and in balance, all of these functions happen uneventfully. According to Ayurveda, the Yellow element is charged with maintaining homeostasis and the body's adaptive response. The Yellow air element—present in Reds and Greens as well as Yellow types—maintains the balance between the body and the external environment. Because of this, it is considered the principal color.

Yellows who are out of balance experience symptoms in at least one of the areas listed above. In this chapter, we will address digestion and nutrition plans for Yellow types because this is the basis for maintaining health and overcoming problems. In Part Four of *Eat Your Colors*, we will address each of these areas and what else you can do to reduce symptoms.

Digestion and Elimination

Digestion for Yellows is a challenge. If you are this type, you have a creative mind and are very responsive to sensory stimulation—noises, smells, bright lights, and tactile sensations. You are also very changeable, prone to get intensely involved in what you're doing and forget about taking care of yourself. Good digestion relies heavily on sensory stimulation, which is one of your strengths, once you recognize it. You need to slow down, take a break from what you're doing and enjoy meals. You will do best with small, frequent meals. You get very scattered when too much time has passed since you last ate and you'll find your work productivity decreases accordingly. Consequently, Ayurvedic physicians recommend that you eat every three or four hours. Your digestive process is fast and your bowel transit time is probably closer to one rather than two days. However, constipation is always a problem, and this can lengthen the time from eating to evacuation.

Planning Meals

Yellow types benefit most from simple meals, well prepared with appropriate spices and seasonings. By simple, I mean food that is served without heavy sauces or dressings. Oil and vinegar with some black pepper is the best dressing for salads and eliminates the need to keep a variety of dressings in your refrigerator. However, I do recommend that you combine vegetables for color. Instead of serving just one color, combine them so that all your colors are represented in a single serving. Do the same thing with fruit. Mix yellows, oranges, reds, blues, and greens. This is one of the best ways to cope with preparing meals for people who are different color types. Mixing colors helps overcome irritation from eating too much of an offending food. The best meals for Yellows are soups and casseroles where the ingredients have cooked together and blended the properties of the individual components.

You should avoid overeating and choose brightly colored fruits and vegetables that delight your eyes as well as your palate. Fortunately, the brightest foods are the best colors for Yellows, and you have lots to choose from. Another plus for you is the love for adventure—you will try new things and will easily adapt to a new way of eating. Being a naturally creative person, you will find new ways to combine the tastes of foods that are good for you and will be easiest for you to digest. Your appetite is apt to vary from day to day and you will have to avoid skipping meals or eating on the run. Plan to eat at regular times each day and make up your shopping list from foods for Yellow types that are listed in tables at the end of this chapter.

As a Yellow, you have likely been bothered by frequent gas and wondered what foods were responsible. Since your digestive problems occur several hours after eating, it's been hard to pin down exactly what's causing the problem. You may have wondered about nuts, cornmeal products, wheat products, sweets, dairy or rye bread. Your instincts were probably correct, some of these foods are difficult for Yellow types to digest. Others work for you at some times but not others. And then there's constipation, which is always a continuing problem when you eat the wrong foods.

Food Tastes

Sweet: Yellow types do best with foods that are sweet, salty, and sour. Sweet foods are considered the most nourishing. Yellows can eat nearly all sweet foods with the emphasis on the two bottom levels of the food pyramid, which include all the yellow and orange fruits and vegetables and most red and green ones, plus whole grains, cereals, and breads.

Salty: Yellows are the only ones who tolerate salty foods and these include ocean (saltwater) fish, sea vegetables, table salt, and most condiments. Unfortunately, we find that salty foods make up the majority of food choices most people make. Though you do better with the salty taste than either Reds or Greens, the kind of salty food you have been eating may not agree with you. Salty foods are at the top of the food pyramid for Yellows and should be eaten no more than two or three times a week.

Sour: Include soured dairy products (cottage cheese, yogurt, kefir) in your daily nutrition plan. Vinegar, citrus fruit, fermented foods, pickles, and pickled foods are other sour foods you can enjoy frequently. These foods increase your digestive capacity. You will find food choices from this group in your daily nutrition plan at the end of this chapter.

Tastes to Avoid

Bitter or Astringent: Avoid foods that are bitter and astringent and choose carefully among those that are pungent. Eating an excess of these foods increases gas and flatulence and may disturb your sleep, increase stress, nervousness, and anxiety or cause headaches. You will likely have difficulty sleeping and may find you're worrying too much over the little stuff.

Foods that are bitter or astringent include arugula, collards, dandelion, eggplant, greens, endive, spinach, sprouts, barley, and most legumes. Some of these will be on the foods to avoid list in your food plans. Others will be listed on the limited use list, meaning that you can eat them on occasion or for balance when you are ill. You will find that nearly all fruits are good for Yellows because none are bitter or astringent. Overuse of astringent foods increases dryness in your body and invites abdominal distension and constipation. Bitter foods increase intestinal gas and cause headaches and joint stiffness.

Pungent: Pungent foods are strong-tasting and you may not like them much. Included are brussels sprouts, cabbage, cauliflower, green peas, kale, raw garlic, and onions. Like most things in life, you may be able to eat these foods occasionally, especially if they are well cooked. On the other hand, cruciferous and sulfur-rich vegetables that are less pungent like artichokes, asparagus, bok choy, broccoli, horseradish, and watercress are good for your type.

Pungent spices and herbs can help balance Yellow types, although these need to be used in small amounts. For example, adding turmeric to food helps you digest it, even though turmeric is a bitter and pungent spice. In chapter 16 several medicinal herbs that are pungent are suggested for Yellows.

Food Texture

Those with a Yellow constitution are innately dry—dry skin, dry hair, dry eyes, and dry nails. Dry or crunchy foods aggravate a dry condition. Crackers, chips, popcorn, dry or toasted bread, dried fruit, and dry roasted nuts aren't good for Yellows. Even the dry brown skin on almonds is aggravating and should be removed. Dry cereals, croutons, or toasted soy nuts can all cause problems. Even some grains such as buckwheat, cornmeal, millet, and rye are a problem. Dry psyllium husks, oats and wheat bran can cause nausea, vomiting, and even constipation instead of aiding in its relief. These fiber bulking agents can be helpful but at first must be used in small amounts. Psyllium should be taken as a warm beverage, and use only cooked oats and wheat bran. Be sure to increase your intake of warm (not iced) water when eating these foods.

Moist, oily foods and oily fish are good for you because they increase moisture. Yellow types can eat more oils than other types but should avoid use of saturated fats, and of course go easy on the oils. More substantial grains such as whole grains, brown rice, bulgur, whole grain pasta, and whole-wheat bread are better for you than light quick (instant) cooking grains, white bread, and white rice. When considering your tan "earth" foods, always choose those that are less processed and more nourishing.

Food Temperature

Yellow types are cold by nature and need to cultivate a warmer internal temperature. Eating smaller frequent meals is one way to increase body temperature, since a frequent supply of energy and nutrient-rich foods will help you keep warm. Obviously, cold and iced foods should be avoided unless it's a hot day. You have no doubt already found out that you like your food served hotter than others and prefer hot drinks to cold ones. Another way to increase the temperature of food is to use warm, hot spices such as ginger, curry, and chili peppers. Liberal use of black pepper is also helpful. Instead of salting your food, add spices and pepper. For breakfast cereal, you can add cinnamon, cloves, and nutmeg and add pepper to foods you eat later in the day. If you fix yourself a fruit cup, be sure to add ginger.

Your Daily Schedule

Certain times of the day present a challenge to each body type. These periods occur twice daily (diurnal) and are part of our normal biorhythm cycles. We are most vulnerable to an imbalance during these times, when aggravation is most likely to occur. For Yellows the times are between 2 P.M. and 6 P.M. and between 2 A.M. and 6 A.M. You may have noticed that your sleep is more easily interrupted during the early morning hours and you may like to get up early, although this tendency increases for everyone as we age. You may also get sleepy between 2 P.M. and 6 P.M. If you can rest or nap sometime during these hours, you'll feel refreshed.

Midafternoon is a stressful time for Yellows and you should avoid scheduling important appointments during this time. It is usually more difficult to work efficiently, and projects that require a high level of concentration are best tackled at another time of day. If you work at home or can work your schedule to fit your needs, you should consider a rest time midafternoon.

Since energy levels vary in Yellows, you should plan to be in bed by 10 P.M. It is a good idea to listen to soft music or read something soothing before going to bed. If you have difficulty quieting your busy mind, a little warm spiced milk and a soft nonchocolate cookie, preferably homemade, may help lull you into a restful sleep. Never eat cold desserts such as ice cream before going to bed.

Plan to get up early and have breakfast around seven o'clock. Your day will go much more smoothly if you allow an extra fifteen or twenty minutes to have a good breakfast before heading out the door to work. You will also do better if you have some protein for breakfast. You can eat leftovers from the night before or mix yourself a smoothie with a high-quality protein powder and fresh fruit such as bananas or berries. Use fruit or vegetable juice, yogurt, soy milk, milk or kefir as the base and to supply fluid. If your protein powder is designed to mix in water, use warm water instead of cold.

Pack yourself a snack of trail mix, nuts, nut butter, flatbread, fruit, veggies, or yogurt. You can eat these midmorning and midafternoon. A cup of chai (spiced tea) midafternoon helps overcome fatigue and restores mental alertness. Plan to have a vegetable or fruit salad with greens for lunch. Have some sprouted lentils, a hard-boiled egg, a little tuna, chicken, or turkey on your salad, depending on how hungry you are.

If at all possible, eat dinner before or around six o'clock. Ideally, this meal is lighter than the other two. However, with most people's schedules this isn't possible. Plan as light a dinner as possible that includes all your colors of vegetables, a green salad, and complementary grains. You can add a little poultry or seafood and red meat three or four days a week. Eggs and cheese also supply extra protein if you are making a meatless casserole. If you don't eat animal foods, add a side dish of lentils or mung beans for protein. You can have some fruit, yogurt, or warm spiced milk before going to bed. Avoid eating heavy desserts after meals or during the evening because these tend to interrupt sleep. Midafternoon is the best time to enjoy an occasional dessert.

Your Seasonal Schedule

Seasons of the year have different effects on each type. For Yellows, the months from mid-August to mid-November are the most challenging time of year. As autumn leaves turn and the days get shorter, Yellows are prone to greater stress and anxiety. This is when you are more vulnerable to colds, allergies, digestive complaints, headaches, and other nervous conditions. Take extra care of yourself on windy days, especially if they are chilly. Stay indoors as much as you can and bundle up if you have to go outside. If you do get chilled, drink plenty of fresh ginger tea.

During this season of transition, it is important to adhere strictly to your nutrition plan and be careful to get sufficient rest. This is not the best time of year to make big decisions or plan major events in your life. It's an excellent time to go on a relaxing vacation. Plan to take extra care of yourself, get a sesame oil massage frequently, enjoy light exercise, and try to slow down.

Nutritional Composition of Your Plan

Imagine that all your food for the day was arranged on a large plate. What would your plate look like? One-third would be occupied by your primary food colors—yellow, orange, red, and green fruits and vegetables. The other two-thirds would be covered by your complementary colors, one-third by tan foods and one-third by white foods.

We can make it easier to decide at a moment's notice what you should eat. Keep in mind that every third food you eat should be one of your colors. The other two choices will be your complementary colors tan and white. Just keep

Daily Food Plan

Yellow Types

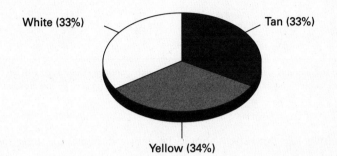

a mental tally or make a list of how you're doing as the day progresses and balance it out at the end of the day. At first you will probably find that you're running out of choices by dinnertime, but as you use this plan more, you will become more adept at choosing the ideal times to eat foods in your plan.

Now we need to design your daily meal plan, distributing your primary and complementary colors among the six food groups: grains, vegetables, fruits, dairy, meat, and oils. In designing your daily meal plan, we also need to maintain proper ratios between percentages of carbohydrates, proteins, and fats that make up your daily diet. These ratios differ among the three body types. For Yellows, the percentages are: carbohydrates, 50 percent; proteins, 20 percent; and oils, 30 percent.

The distribution of foods in the menu plan looks like this:

Daily Meal Plan for Yellow Types

Food Group ▶	Cereals, Grains, Breads, Starchy Vegetables	Fruit and Fruit Juice	Non-starchy Vegetables	Yogurt, Kefir, Soy milk, Grain Milk	Fish, Poultry, Meat, Skim Cheese, Eggs, Legumes, Nut Butter, Seeds	Oils and Fats, Parmesan Cheese
Serving Size ▶	½ cup	½ cup cut up or 1 small or ¾ cup juice	½ cup cooked, 1 cup raw, or ¾ cup vegetable juice	1 cup or ½ cup cottage or ricotta cheese	1 ounce fish, poultry, meat, or skim cheese or 1 egg or ½ cup legumes or 2 T. nut butter	1 teaspoon oils/fats or 2 T. Parmesan cheese

Daily Calories ▼	Number of Servings ►					
2,000	9	3¾	5	2½	6	3½
1,200	5½	2⅓	3	1½	3¾	2
1,500	6¾	3	4	2	4⅔	2¾
1,800	8¼	3½	4¾	2⅓	5½	3¼
2,200	10	4⅓	5¾	2¾	6¾	4
2,400	11	4¾	6¼	3	7⅓	4⅓

Note: To calculate the amount you should put onto your plate, multiply the number of servings by the serving size. For example, for a 2,000-calorie diet, 7 servings times ½ cup serving size equals 3½ cups.

The number of calories you should be eating depends on these factors:

- Body frame—light, medium or heavy
- Height and weight
- Activity level
- Age
- Body mass index (BMI)

Perhaps you know how many calories you should consume and can go directly to the table above. If you don't, you can get this information from my Web site, www.thenutritionsolution.com/quiz. Typically Yellow types have low BMIs and light body frames.

Activity Level and Age

You no doubt know your activity level and whether you are active or sedentary. We naturally slow down as we age and will need fewer calories. However, we don't need a special allowance for age as long as activity level is considered. (Some nutritionists calculate a decrease in daily calories for every ten years of age.) As long as we allow for increasing sedentary lifestyle, we automatically allow for advancing age. You will find this allowance for your activity level in "determine ideal daily calories" on my Web site.

Note that for calorie counts in the food plan, all starchy vegetables have the same nutritional composition as grains and are listed with them. When you are selecting which color vegetables to eat, you will be getting the phytochemicals that account for a particular color, regardless of how you account for its calories. If you move one of your vegetable choices into the grains column because it's starchy, just replace one grain serving with your starchy vegetable and add another non-starchy vegetable to your intake for the day.

Now that we have established how many servings of each food you will need to eat, let's see how you might plan your daily menus.

Daily Menus for Yellows

Yellow menu plans are designed to provide a good breakfast, which you will need in order to work efficiently during the morning. You have no doubt found that skipping breakfast doesn't work well for you. Others may get by with just a slice of toast and coffee, but if you do this you'll have difficulty concentrating and will find it hard to complete tasks. Before much of the morning has passed, you will be anxious, nervous, weak, and hunting for a snack. Yellows metabolize food quickly and need protein foods early in the day to anchor them. Leftovers will provide excellent breakfasts for you, and you might try rearranging your meals so that a portion of the dinner meal will be your breakfast. That way you'll have plenty of protein in the morning and will eat less before going to bed at night. Lunch is also important for Yellows, and ideally this would be your main meal.

As for sugary snacks, Yellow types have highly sensitized nervous systems that overreact either to too much sugar or skipped meals. If both breakfast and lunch are substantial meals, you can eat a lighter dinner of vegetables and grains or a hearty soup. As you have found out, Yellows tend to tire between 2 P.M. and 6 P.M. since this is the time of day your natural biorhythms are at low ebb. As I suggested above, plan your day for lighter work in the afternoon. A hearty lunch will help offset the afternoon fatigue you are likely experiencing.

An afternoon cup of coffee is not the answer for Yellows, except perhaps for an occasional latté. Coffee is bitter and diminishes digestive power in Yellows. Plus, it is a powerful central nervous system stimulant that makes it even harder for unfocused Yellow types to be productive. Yellows get a temporary mental and physical lift from caffeine, but soon find themselves fighting either to keep from bouncing off the walls or collapsing in a chair.

Day One

Breakfast
1 cup cooked oatmeal topped with ½ cup yogurt (2 grains, ½ dairy)
1 T. honey, ½ tsp. cinnamon, ½ cup of berries (1 fruit)
6 oz. fresh carrot juice (1 veggie)

Snacks and Lunch
Tuna sandwich: ¼ cup flaked tuna on two slices of whole-grain bread with mayonnaise and baby greens (4 meat, 2 grain, 1 fat, ½ veggie)

½ cup cucumber slices marinated in dill yogurt dressing, on a bed of greens (1½ veggie, ½ dairy)

½ cup grapes (1 fruit)

¼ cup nuts (1 fat, some protein, lots of fiber)

Westbrae Vanilla Royale lite malted soy beverage (2 dairy)

Dinner

1½ cups lean beef stew with carrots, turnips, potatoes, onions—no thickened gravy (4 meat, 2 grain from root veggies, 2 fat from meat)

2 plain biscuits with a little honey (2 grain, 1 fat)

Salad of 1 cup romaine lettuce, ½ cup jicama and ½ cup grapefruit topped with 1 T. ranch dressing diluted with a little orange juice (2 veggie, 1 fruit, 1 fat)

Water or beverage of your choice after dinner

Day Two

Breakfast

While I discourage eating on the run, busy women and men heading out the door can mix themselves a tropical juice smoothie:

1 cup papaya, passion fruit, or mango juice (2 fruit)

½ banana or ½ cup berries or ½ cup fresh pineapple (1 fruit)

½ cup low-fat yogurt (½ dairy)

1 scoop soy protein powder with isoflavones (1 meat)

This is a primary color smoothie for Yellows, loaded with phytonutrients. What a great way to start the day! If possible, the juices should not be ice cold and for heaven's sake, don't add ice! Since this is primarily a fruit beverage (carbohydrate, fiber) with protein added for balance, emphasis on the rest of the day's meals should be on vegetables and grains with additional protein and a little fat.

Lunch

Salad of 2 cups mixed greens, topped with a sliced hard-boiled egg, ½ cup mung bean sprouts, ½ cup radishes, and 2 T. dressing (2 veggie, 1 meat, 2 veggie, 2 fat)

4–6 wheat thin crackers (3 grain)

Soy malted beverage (2 dairy)

For convenience, this lunch can be assembled the night before and refrigerated.

Dinner

First selection:

> Pasta of your choice, 2 cups, topped with 1 cup of a meat, vegetable, and tomato sauce (4 grain, 2 veggie, 2 meat, 1 fat)
>
> Mixed green salad topped with 1 cup of steamed root veggies and an olive and balsamic vinegar dressing (1 veggie, 1 starchy veggie counted as a grain serving, 1 fat)
>
> 1 slice garlic bread with 1 T. grated Parmesan cheese (1 grain, 1 fat)

Second selection:

> Baked sea bass, 6 oz., topped with the Simple Dipping Sauce listed among the recipes below (6 fish, 1½ fat)
>
> Steamed couscous, 1 cup, with onions, bouquet garni, and bouillon in the water (1 grain)
>
> Steamed root veggies, 1 cup (1 grain)

Both of these dinner plans are quick and easy. They almost cook themselves while you mix up a salad and watch the evening news or catch up on the activities of other family members.

✑ Simple Dipping Sauce for Yellow Types

This sauce is a good source of phytochemicals, including apigenin and calcium. Use it for stir fries or marinating fish or poultry.

3 T. tamari sauce	1 tsp. roasted and lightly
3 T. dark sesame seed oil	crushed sesame seeds
½ tsp. raw honey	

Combine all ingredients. Mix again before serving, as the oil tends to rise to the top. Use the sauce for dipping vegetables, or in stir fries. Refrigerate any leftover sauce. Makes six 1 T. servings (1½ fat).

Balancing "Off" Colors

Another way to eat your colors is to mix them up into a soup or stew. You can add ingredients that aren't your colors and they will blend in so that the entire dish is nourishing and easy to digest. In this soup recipe, celery blends well with the other ingredients, and even though it is not your color in its raw and solitary state, it will work for you here.

Sample Recipe for Yellows

Creamy Golden Squash and Bacon Soup

2 cups of peeled and cut up golden winter squash (butternut, acorn, or delicata are nice)
2 slices of low-salt bacon
2 tsp. ghee or olive oil
1 cup of diced celery
½ cup chopped onion
1 cup of peeled and diced white or sweet potato
2 cups of peeled, seeded and diced golden apples
4 cups chicken stock
1 cup orange juice
1 cup fat-free sour cream or yogurt
1 tsp. salt
¼ tsp. black pepper
1–2 tsps. sweet curry blend; add according to your taste preference (turmeric, coriander, cumin, ginger, nutmeg, fennel, cinnamon, fenugreek, white pepper, cloves, cardamom, red pepper)

1. Steam the cut-up squash for about 20 minutes or put the seeded and cut halves upside down on a baking dish, add ½ inch water and bake at 350° F for 60 minutes.
2. Meantime, brown the bacon and drain well on a paper towel. In a 4-quart kettle, melt ghee or olive oil and cook the onions and celery until soft.
3. Add the potatoes, apples, steamed squash, and chicken stock; cover and simmer until the vegetables are tender, about 20 minutes.
4. Using a food processor, blend the soup until smooth, then return to pot.
5. Add orange juice, cream, salt, pepper, and curry powder.
6. Heat to serving temperature and serve with condiments.

Condiments:
1 cup of coarsely chopped hazelnuts
1 cup of freshly grated coconut
1 cup of golden raisins

Makes 12 servings

Nutrition information: Serving size: 1 cup; calories: 104; servings per food group: grains, ¼; fruit, ½; vegetables, ½; meat, ⅓; fat, ⅓; milk, ⅒

Yellow Food Selections

Now you'll need a personalized shopping list for foods, beverages, spices, and condiments. Your foods are listed by category, first by where they fit into your daily menu plan—grains, vegetables, fruits, dairy, meat or oils—and then by food color. Finally, comments about each food will guide you in shopping for and preparing them.

Eat Your Colors Vegetables: Yellow

Your food selections will include vegetables that are four colors—yellow, red, orange, and green. The comments column is a guide to how best to enjoy each of these foods. In general, Yellow types do best with cooked or warmed food. That's because cooking breaks down cellulose and other plant constituents that interfere with your absorption of nutrients. Be sure to add your color's spices and condiments to your shopping cart (see next to last table in this section) to enhance food digestibility and nutrient absorption.

Vegetable Color	Description	Comments
Yellow	bell peppers, yellow	raw or cooked
Yellow	chili peppers, yellow	cooked
Yellow	corn, fresh	cooked
Yellow	daikon	raw
Yellow	jicama	raw
Yellow	mushrooms, button	cooked
Yellow	onions, yellow	cooked
Yellow	parsnips	cooked
Yellow	potatoes, yellow	cooked
Yellow	rutabagas	cooked
Yellow	squash, yellow	cooked
Red, Blue, Purple	beets	cooked
Red, Blue, Purple	bell peppers, red	cooked, raw in moderation
Red, Blue, Purple	radishes	raw
Red, Blue, Purple	tomatoes	cooked only
Orange	bell peppers, orange	raw or cooked
Orange	carrots	cooked
Orange	chili peppers, orange	cooked
Orange	pumpkin	cooked
Orange	sweet potatoes	cooked
Orange	winter squash	cooked
Orange	yams	cooked
Green	aduki sprouts	in stir fries
Green	artichoke, globe	well cooked w/herbs
Green	artichoke, Jerusalem	cooked
Green	arugula	raw or cooked
Green	asparagus	cooked
Green	baby green mix (mesclun)	raw or cooked
Green	bok choy	cooked

Vegetable Color	Description	Comments
Green	broccoli sprouts	raw or cooked
Green	broccoli, broccoli rabe	cooked
Green	chili peppers, green	cooked
Green	chives	cooked
Green	cilantro	raw or cooked
Green	collards	cooked
Green	dandelion greens	cooked
Green	garlic	cooked
Green	grape leaves	cooked
Green	green beans	cooked
Green	horseradish	prepared
Green	iceberg lettuce	raw
Green	kale	cooked
Green	leafy green and red lettuces	raw
Green	leeks	cooked
Green	mustard greens	raw and cooked
Green	olives, green and black	prepared
Green	parsley	raw or cooked
Green	parsnips	cooked
Green	scallions	cooked
Green	spinach	cooked
Green	turnip greens	cooked
Green	watercress	raw or cooked
Green	zucchini	raw or cooked

Eat Your Colors Fruits

Yellow types can eat almost any fresh fruit. However, some will need to be peeled, and others should be cooked before eating. The comments describe how your fruit should be eaten. If you enjoy dried fruit, soak it first to soften it and improve digestion. You can also add slices of raw apple to a jar of dried fruit to soften and moisten it so it's better for snacking. Raisins, dried cranberries, or dried cherries make good additions to cooked cereals such as oatmeal, cream of wheat, or rice. If you have been experiencing digestive problems, eat fruit alone, between meals.

Fruit Color	Description	Comments
Yellow	apples, yellow	peeled; raw or cooked
Yellow	applesauce, baked apples	cooked
Yellow	avocados	raw
Yellow	bananas	ripe only
Yellow	bilberries	cooked in jam
Yellow	cherries, Rainier	raw
Yellow	coconut	fresh, shredded
Yellow	dates	dried

Yellow	figs, yellow Kadota	fresh or cooked
Yellow	gooseberries	cooked
Yellow	grapefruit, white	raw or juice
Yellow	grapes, yellow/green	raw
Yellow	guava	raw or juice
Yellow	juices, tropical fruit	fresh or bottled
Yellow	lemon	raw or cooked
Yellow	pears, yellow Anjou or Bartlett	very ripe and peeled
Yellow	pineapple	raw or canned
Yellow	plantain	ripe; raw or cooked
Red, Blue, Purple	bananas, red	ripe; raw or cooked
Red, Blue, Purple	blueberries	raw or cooked
Red, Blue, Purple	boysenberries	raw or cooked
Red, Blue, Purple	cherries, bing	raw or cooked
Red, Blue, Purple	cherries, sour	cooked
Red, Blue, Purple	chokecherries	cooked
Red, Blue, Purple	cranberries	raw or cooked
Red, Blue, Purple	currants, red fresh	raw
Red, Blue, Purple	figs, fresh Mission	raw or cooked
Red, Blue, Purple	grapefruit, red or pink	raw or juice
Red, Blue, Purple	grapes, red, purple	raw or juice
Red, Blue, Purple	juices, tomato-based	yes
Red, Blue, Purple	marion berries	raw or cooked
Red, Blue, Purple	oranges, blood	raw
Red, Blue, Purple	pears, red Bosc, Comice, etc.	peeled, cooked
Red, Blue, Purple	plums, red, purple	very sweet, raw
Red, Blue, Purple	pomegranate	raw or juice
Red, Blue, Purple	raisins	dried
Red, Blue, Purple	raspberries, red, black	raw or cooked
Red, Blue, Purple	rhubarb	cooked
Red, Blue, Purple	strawberries	raw or cooked
Orange	apricots, fresh	raw or cooked
Orange	juices, orange	yes
Orange	mangos	raw or cooked
Orange	melons: cantaloupe, casaba, etc.	raw
Orange	orange, mandarin	raw
Orange	orange, navel	raw
Orange	papaya	raw or juice
Orange	passion fruit	raw or juice
Orange	peaches, fresh	raw or cooked, juice
Orange	tangerines	raw
Green	grapes, green	raw
Green	kiwi	raw
Green	limes	raw or cooked
Green	melons, green	raw
Green	pears, green Seckel	peeled and cooked
Green	plums, green	very sweet, raw

Tan Foods: Cereals, Grains, Breads, and Legumes

You can enjoy a wide variety of grains and cereals. The ones to avoid are buckwheat and rye. Otherwise most are good for you as long as they're soft. Avoid anything that's dry and crunchy. If you want to enjoy dry cereals, add warmed milk and cinnamon to soften them before eating. Liberal use of cinnamon and ginger also helps warm tan foods to improve digestion. Some of the grains listed are eaten as cereals or steamed and served with vegetables and protein foods such as fish. Others such as wheat can be eaten as grains and are also ground into flour for baking. Yellow types are severely restricted in legume choices. That's because most legumes cause flatulence in Yellows. If you prepare them, make sure they are well cooked and add antiflatulent-herbs such as asafoetida, ajwan, or epizote as you're cooking them to break down the legume sugars that cause gas.

Food Type	Description	Comments
Breads	biscuits	warmed
Breads	bread, mixed grain	not toasted
Breads	bread, white or French, sour	warmed, not toasted
Breads	bread, white or French, sweet	warmed, not toasted
Breads	bread, whole wheat	not toasted
Breads	cookies	in moderation
Breads	muffin, English	warmed
Breads	pita or flat bread, white flour	warmed
Breads	pita or flat bread, whole wheat	warmed
Breads	stuffing, bread	softened
Breads	tortillas, white flour	warmed
Breads	tortillas, whole-wheat flour	warmed
Breads	waffles and pancakes, white flour	hot
Breads	waffles and pancakes, whole grain	hot
Cereals, Grains	amaranth	hot
Cereals, Grains	basmati rice, white or brown	hot
Cereals, Grains	brown rice, short or long grain	hot
Cereals, Grains	bulgur	hot
Cereals, Grains	corn grits	hot
Cereals, Grains	cornmeal	cooked, hot
Cereals, Grains	couscous	hot
Cereals, Grains	mochi	baked, warm
Cereals, Grains	oat bran	cooked, baked goods
Cereals, Grains	oats	cooked
Cereals, Grains	pasta, basil	hot
Cereals, Grains	pasta, red pepper	hot
Cereals, Grains	pasta, spinach	hot
Cereals, Grains	pasta, tomato	hot
Cereals, Grains	pasta, white	hot
Cereals, Grains	pasta, whole grain	hot
Cereals, Grains	quinoa	cooked, hot

Cereals, Grains	rice, sweet	hot or in sushi
Cereals, Grains	rice; white, arborio, jasmine, etc.	hot
Cereals, Grains	spelt	hot or baked goods
Cereals, Grains	triticale	hot or baked goods
Cereals, Grains	udon noodles	hot
Cereals, Grains	wheat bran	cooked, baked
Legumes (pulses)	aduki bean	cooked
Legumes (pulses)	baked beans (tomato based)	cooked
Legumes (pulses)	mung bean	cooked
Legumes (pulses)	urad dhal	cooked

White Foods: Oils, Fish, Poultry, Eggs, Meat, Nuts, and Seeds

Yellow types can enjoy more white foods than either Reds or Greens. Oils help lubricate dry skin and maintain the integrity of cells and all body tissues. Oils are anti-inflammatory and help stave off the effects of aging. Take care to buy only high-quality oils that have minimal processing. Stock your pantry with a variety of them and refer to the usage guides for oils on pages 110–13. You will find a list of which oils to choose in the table below; use them as directed.

Fish contains healthy oils and should be a regular part of your diet. The American Heart Association is now recommending at least two servings of fatty fish such as salmon, tuna, whitefish, trout, or herring, per week. You can steam, bake, grill, or sauté most varieties of fish. Avoid frying, especially deep frying, because this breaks down the healthy oils and adds too many of the wrong kind of oils to your food.

Choose poultry that is lean and preferably animals that are "free range." They are less apt to have been fed antibiotics and may have had a more varied diet. The same criteria apply to eggs. You can purchase eggs from chickens that have been fed only organic feed, are free range, or those that have been fed omega-3 fatty acid rich diets. As for dairy products, most markets now offer organic dairy products. These come from cattle that have been fed food free of pesticides, hormones, and antibiotics. Some markets also offer meat from animals fed an organic diet.

You can eat most nuts and seeds in small quantities. Almonds are the best and you should remove the skin from them by blanching them in hot water. Peanuts are legumes and not good for you. Raw nuts are preferred, but you can eat a small amount of roasted lightly salted nuts. Avoid the dry roasted varieties. Eat a few nuts at a time (no more than ¼ cup at a sitting) and chew them well. If you have problems digesting nuts, avoid them for a few days and then try again. Nuts and seeds are an excellent source of healthy oils, fiber, and trace amounts of protein. You may find that mixed nuts are a problem, but eating a single kind of nut is not. Sprinkle raw, shelled sunflower seeds on salads instead of croutons, which are too dry and crunchy.

Type of Food	Description	Comments
Dairy	buttermilk	warmed or chilled
Dairy	cheese, hard (Parmesan, etc.)	added to food
Dairy	cheese, soft, and panir	alone or added
Dairy	cottage cheese	chilled
Dairy	cow's milk	warmed is best
Dairy	cream, half and half	chilled
Dairy	eggs	not fried
Dairy	kefir	chilled
Dairy	sour cream	as topping
Dairy	yogurt	chilled
Meat, Poultry, Fish	anchovies	as topping
Meat, Poultry, Fish	bass, sea	baked
Meat, Poultry, Fish	beef	grilled, simmered
Meat, Poultry, Fish	catfish (farm-grown)	baked
Meat, Poultry, Fish	chicken	dark meat only
Meat, Poultry, Fish	cod	baked
Meat, Poultry, Fish	duck	baked
Meat, Poultry, Fish	haddock	baked, grilled
Meat, Poultry, Fish	halibut	baked, grilled
Meat, Poultry, Fish	herring	steamed, snack
Meat, Poultry, Fish	mackerel	steamed, grilled
Meat, Poultry, Fish	menhaden	steamed, grilled
Meat, Poultry, Fish	mussel	steamed
Meat, Poultry, Fish	oily fish; sable, eel	baked, grilled
Meat, Poultry, Fish	orange roughy	baked, steamed
Meat, Poultry, Fish	ostrich	grilled, baked
Meat, Poultry, Fish	oyster	steamed
Meat, Poultry, Fish	perch	baked, sautéed
Meat, Poultry, Fish	pike	baked, steamed
Meat, Poultry, Fish	pollack	baked, sautéed
Meat, Poultry, Fish	pompano	baked, sautéed
Meat, Poultry, Fish	rockfish	baked, sautéed
Meat, Poultry, Fish	salmon, chinook	steamed, baked
Meat, Poultry, Fish	sand dabs	grilled
Meat, Poultry, Fish	sardine	snack
Meat, Poultry, Fish	scrod	baked, sautéed
Meat, Poultry, Fish	snapper, red	baked, sautéed
Meat, Poultry, Fish	sole, English, and petrale sole	baked
Meat, Poultry, Fish	squid	stewed or baked
Meat, Poultry, Fish	trout	grilled or sautéed
Meat, Poultry, Fish	whitefish	baked, sautéed
Nuts	almonds and almond butter	skin removed
Nuts	brazil nuts	raw is best; roasted
Nuts	cashews and cashew butter	raw is best; roasted
Nuts	chestnuts	roasted
Nuts	coconut	grated, fresh

Nuts	filberts (hazelnuts)	raw or roasted
Nuts	macadamia	raw or roasted
Nuts	pecans	raw or roasted
Nuts	pine nuts	raw
Nuts	pistachios	raw
Nuts	walnuts	raw
Nuts	water chestnuts	cooked
Oils	almond	high-heat cooking
Oils	apricot kernel	high-heat cooking
Oils	avocado	high-heat cooking
Oils	black currant	do not heat
Oils	borage	do not heat
Oils	butter	cooking or spread
Oils	canola, regular	medium-heat cooking
Oils	canola, super	high-heat cooking
Oils	coconut, liquid	high-heat cooking
Oils	evening primrose oil	do not heat
Oils	fish blends, salmon, etc.	do not heat
Oils	flax, liquid or capsules	do not heat
Oils	ghee (clarified butter)	for cooking or spread
Oils	grape seed	medium-heat cooking
Oils	mustard	medium-heat cooking
Oils	olive	medium-heat cooking
Oils	peanut	high-heat cooking
Oils	pumpkin seed capsules	do not heat
Oils	rice bran	high-heat cooking
Oils	safflower, regular	medium-high heat
Oils	safflower, high oleic	high-heat cooking
Oils	sesame	medium-high heat
Oils	sunflower, high oleic	high-heat cooking
Oils	sunflower, regular	medium-heat cooking
Oils	walnut	medium-heat cooking
Oils	wheat germ	do not heat
Seeds	flax seeds	baking, added to food
Seeds	poppy seeds	baking, added to food
Seeds	psyllium seed	dietary supplement
Seeds	pumpkin seeds	raw, small amounts
Seeds	sesame seeds, butter, tahini	spread
Seeds	sunflower seeds, sunflower butter	snack, spread

Gold Foods: Beverages, Condiments, and Spices

I am designating these food items as "gold" because they are extremely valuable but are to be used sparingly. Yellows can enjoy all of the unusual beverages such as rice, nut and grain milks, aloe vera, and all kinds of fruit juices. Avoid carbonated beverages that encourage flatulence. Spring water is very good for you and so are the teas listed below. Coffee and caffeinated beverages will make you too nervous and forgetful. Even decaffeinated coffee is too bitter for you. If you drink these beverages first thing in the morning, you are setting yourself up for digestive problems throughout the day. If you enjoy coffee once in a while, that's not going to hurt you. Just don't make a daily habit of drinking it. Try substituting warm chai and milk as a morning beverage. Hot cocoa or a carob beverage is also a suitable morning drink.

You will not find alcoholic beverages listed on your table because they have a powerful negative impact on your nervous system. They can cause irregular heartbeats, insomnia, and muscular tension. They also interfere with your ability to concentrate and work to your optimum capacity the following day.

Yellow types can use almost any kind of spice. Spices enhance the appeal and digestibility of foods. Use them to "warm up" any food you are eating or to balance off colors, such as adding ajwan to legumes during cooking to reduce flatulence. Chili powder and curry powder are popular spice combinations that have been used for centuries to enhance food digestibility and absorption. These "hot" spices are invigorating to the system and improve circulation to the extremities. Ginger helps clear the respiratory tract and is an excellent tonic when you have congestion.

Type	Description	Comments
Beverages	almond milk	warmed or cool
Beverages	aloe vera	cool
Beverages	amasake	cool
Beverages	apricot juice	room temp or cool
Beverages	berry juice	room temp or cool
Beverages	carob drinks	warmed or cool
Beverages	carrot juice	cool
Beverages	cherry juice	room temp or cool
Beverages	chocolate drinks, hot chocolate	hot or cool
Beverages	coconut milk	in cooking
Beverages	cranberry juice	room temp or cool
Beverages	grape juice	room temp or cool
Beverages	grapefruit juice	room temp or cool
Beverages	hot chocolate	hot
Beverages	mango juice	room temp or cool
Beverages	mineral water	room temp or cool
Beverages	orange juice	room temp or cool
Beverages	papaya or pineapple juice	room temp or cool
Beverages	peach nectar	room temp or cool
Beverages	pomegranate juice	very small amounts
Beverages	soy milk	hot, warm or cool
Beverages	spring water	room temp or cool
Beverages	vegetable juices	room temp or cool
Condiments	bouillon	hot

Condiments	capers	room temp or warm
Condiments	carob	hot or cool
Condiments	jam and jelly	room temp or cool
Condiments	ketchup	room temp or cool
Condiments	lemon juice	room temp or cool
Condiments	mayonnaise	cool
Condiments	miso paste	warm or hot
Condiments	mustard	room temp or cool
Condiments	olives	room temp or cool
Condiments	pickles, sour	room temp or cool
Condiments	pickles, sweet	room temp or cool
Condiments	tamari, soy sauce	room temp
Condiments	tamarind paste	in sauce, gravies
Condiments	tomato sauce, paste	warmed
Condiments	umeboshi plums or paste	room temp or cool
Condiments	vinegar	room temp
Condiments	wasabi	room temp or cool
Herbal Teas	alfalfa	hot
Herbal Teas	bancha	hot
Herbal Teas	chamomile	hot
Herbal Teas	comfrey	hot, not for pregnancy
Herbal Teas	elder flowers	hot
Herbal Teas	fennel	hot
Herbal Teas	ginger, dried or fresh	hot
Herbal Teas	ginseng	hot, not for pregnancy
Herbal Teas	hops	hot
Herbal Teas	jasmine	hot
Herbal Teas	lemon balm (melissa)	hot
Herbal Teas	lemon grass	hot
Herbal Teas	licorice	hot
Herbal Teas	marshmallow	hot
Herbal Teas	nettles	hot
Herbal Teas	passionflower	hot
Herbal Teas	peppermint	hot or cool
Herbal Teas	raspberry leaf	hot
Herbal Teas	rose hips	hot
Herbal Teas	sarsaparilla	hot, not for pregnancy
Herbal Teas	sassafras	hot, not for pregnancy
Herbal Teas	spearmint	hot
Herbal Teas	wintergreen	hot
Seasonings	allspice	baking
Seasonings	almond extract*	baking
Seasonings	anise*	baking
Seasonings	asafoetida*	add to legumes
Seasonings	basil*	raw or in cooking
Seasonings	bay leaf*	cooking
Seasonings	black pepper*	added to food
Seasonings	caraway*	cooking, baking
Seasonings	cardamom*	cooking, baking
Seasonings	cayenne	cooking
Seasonings	chili powder*	cooking
Seasonings	cilantro	raw or cooking

Type	Description	Comments
Seasonings	cinnamon*	baking, at table
Seasonings	cloves*	baking
Seasonings	coriander*	baking, cooking
Seasonings	cumin*	cooking
Seasonings	curry powder*	cooking
Seasonings	dill weed and seed*	cooking, baking, at table
Seasonings	fennel*	cooking, baking, at table
Seasonings	fenugreek	cooking, tea
Seasonings	garam masala*	cooking
Seasonings	garlic	cooking
Seasonings	ginger	cooking
Seasonings	mint	cooking, at table
Seasonings	mustard seed*	cooking
Seasonings	nutmeg*	cooking, at table
Seasonings	oregano*	cooking
Seasonings	paprika*	cooking, at table
Seasonings	parsley	raw, cooking
Seasonings	peppermint*	raw, cooking
Seasonings	rosemary*	cooking
Seasonings	saffron*	cooking, baking
Seasonings	sage*	cooking, baking
Seasonings	savory*	cooking
Seasonings	spearmint*	cooking
Seasonings	tamarind*	cooking
Seasonings	tarragon*	raw, cooking
Seasonings	thyme*	raw, cooking
Seasonings	turmeric*	cooking
Seasonings	vanilla extract	baking, cooking
Sweeteners	barley malt, syrup or crystals	baking, at table
Sweeteners	brown rice syrup	baking, at table
Sweeteners	brown sugar	baking, at table
Sweeteners	cane sugar	baking, at table
Sweeteners	date sugar	baking, at table
Sweeteners	fructose	baking, at table
Sweeteners	fruit sugar or fruit juice	baking, at table
Sweeteners	honey, raw only	raw, at table
Sweeteners	maple syrup, sugar (real maple)	baking, at table
Sweeteners	molasses	baking
Sweeteners	raw sugar	baking, at table
Sweeteners	*Stevia*	baking, at table
Sweeteners	Sucanat	baking, at table
Sweeteners	turbinado sugar	baking, at table

*These seasonings are the most important for Yellow types.

Now that you have your personal list of foods to buy, mark your shopping list for what to buy at the market. Here is an example of what your list might look like.

Personal Shopping List for Yellow Types

Food Group	Food Color	Food
Vegetables	yellow	crookneck squash, fresh corn
Vegetables	red	beets, red bell pepper
Vegetables	orange	carrots
Vegetables	green	broccoli
Fruit	yellow	avocado, bananas, papaya
Fruit	red, blue, or purple	blueberries, grapes
Fruit	orange	mango, oranges
Fruit	green	kiwi
Grains	tan	brown rice, couscous
Breads	tan	whole wheat bread
Cereals	tan	rolled oats
Dairy	white	yogurt
Dairy	white	milk
Dairy	white	eggs
Oils	white	olive oil, butter
Fish	white	trout, salmon
Poultry	white	chicken thighs and legs
Meat	white	beef pot roast
Nuts, Seeds	white	almonds, sunflower seeds
Beverages	gold	herbal teas, spring water
Seasonings	gold	ginger, cinnamon, garlic, pepper

13

Nutrition Plan for Red Types

The Red body type is most associated with fire and, to a lesser degree, water. Fire (heat) is well known for its ability to transform substances into other forms. In our bodies, the fire element represents the enzymatic conversions that transform food into molecules we can assimilate, turning them into the functional and structural components of the body. The bodily attribute most associated with the fire element and hence with Red types is *function*. Following are the properties of the Red constitution—all major functions of the body.

- Digestion of food and digestive organ function; function of stomach, duodenum, intestines, pancreas, liver, and gallbladder
- Absorption of macro and micro nutrients, a function of the intestines
- Assimilation of food into tissues and cells
- All metabolic processes in cells, tissues, and organs
- Maintenance of body temperature
- All intellectual and emotional functions, memory
- Immune system function; formation of blood cells, thymus, and spleen function
- Vision and hearing
- Reproductive and respiratory function, including smell
- Skin function; primarily elimination of toxins, sweat, and heat

All these functions proceed smoothly when Red types are in balance. A disturbance in any of these bodily processes is considered a Red condition in Ayurveda. Red types are most prone to conditions that are a result of a dysfunction in any of these organs or tissues, such as gastric discomfort, anemia, cataracts, acne, and dermatitis. For any of the body types, the first sign of an imbalance will occur in the digestive system. In Red types, digestive disturbance occurs in the pyloric region of the stomach. This is the area where food enters the duodenum and in the duodenum itself. The duodenum is the first section of small intestine where digestive juices secreted from intestinal walls and neighboring organs break down food.

Digestion and Elimination

Digestive problems in Red types are felt in the area of the solar plexus and are often the result of mealtime conflicts. Reds are prone to carry over frustrations from the day's activities into mealtime and like to engage in lively conversation, which they tend to dominate. They may engage in heated debates over the dinner table and can become argumentative and combative.

If you are a Red type, it is important that you stick to fairly bland foods to keep from aggravating your digestive system. It is a good idea to take some time to disengage yourself from the day's activities before sitting down to lunch or dinner. Take time to appreciate the food in front of you and savor its aromas to get your digestive juices flowing. Enjoy soft music and a peaceful environment while eating. Although this is good advice for all types, it is especially important for Reds. Drinking alcoholic beverages before meals is sure to give you problems and you will do best if you avoid use of alcohol entirely or at least reserve it for drinking with meals on special occasions.

Planning Meals

Since Reds are intense in everything they do, this includes eating. Reds enjoy food and are apt to overeat and drink too much alcohol. Eat slowly and drink water or herbal tea with your meals. Take care not to overeat. Red types gain weight easily but can usually lose it. They often diet but dieting efforts do not yield long-term results. That's because you must change what you eat and your eating strategy. You must plan meals at regular times, because if a meal is late, you will be apt to snack, overeat and make poor food choices, relieving the fire that's burning inside you. Late meals also increase the likelihood that you will direct your digestive fire energy toward coworkers or family members. Think of yourself as having pent-up fire. If you don't quell the fire with food at the proper times, fire's intensity will escape in other ways.

Avoid the temptation to work late and finish a project, unless you take time out for dinner and then return to work. You will do best if you eat your heaviest meal at noon whenever possible. A light breakfast of cereal and fruit or a bagel with a little jam is best, and then make sure not to eat too large a meal at nighttime. Plan a snack of fruit and a cup of herbal tea around 4 P.M. if you need a break. Suggestions for these meals will be given later in this chapter. Be sure to use your personal shopping list at the end of this chapter to make sure you are getting the proper number of servings of your primary and complementary colors.

Red types have strong digestion and think they can eat anything. Your first clue that you have eaten too many of the wrong foods may be loose and frequent stools. If you consume too many hot and spicy foods, or large amounts of the wrong foods, your stools may also give a burning sensation as they leave your body. Reds do very well with raw and cold foods. The best herbs to add to your food are those from the aerial parts of the plant (fruit, leaves, and stems). The aroma from adding herbs to your food helps regulate your digestion. Avoid those that are roots or tubers such as ginger because they are generally too warming. You will find more on the best herbs to use along with nutrition plans for Reds later in this chapter.

You have no doubt experienced frequent gastric upset when eating the wrong foods or if you are upset about something. These symptoms usually occur within the first two hours after eating and are experienced as pressure in the solar plexus and abdominal bloating. You may even feel "itchy" on the surface of your skin in the solar plexus area. Reds are prone to gastric upset, nausea, and vomiting when eating the wrong foods.

You may have noticed that tomato products don't seem to agree with you, and if you eat them frequently your stomach feels acidic and stools are burning. Reds should not eat tomato products of any kind because they are too acidic. You may also have noticed that garlic and onions, especially if they are raw, give you problems. These foods will be listed in your foods to avoid. Deep-fried foods such as french fries are especially bad for you because the oils used to cook them are most likely to be broken down from repeated heating. Cellular function depends on having the proper fatty acids available, as you read in chapter 9. Fried foods interfere with your body's metabolism of essential fats. Reds do best on a vegetarian diet because eating concentrated proteins such as red meat increases the secretion of hydrochloric acid in your stomach—which you don't need.

Food Tastes

Most of us avoid bitter tastes. We carefully peel citrus fruits to avoid eating the bitter skin. Yet we enjoy sprouts on a sandwich or spicing up a salad with arugula—both of which are bitter greens. Many enjoy unsweetened grapefruit juice, too, so perhaps it's a matter of degree with bitterness. Other bitter vegetables are collards, eggplant, leafy greens, endive, and spinach. Mesclun, the popular salad mix, is composed mainly of bitter greens. Among grains and cereals, barley is the only bitter one. Bitter foods are the perfect tonic for Reds because they reduce excess acidity and help shed water weight.

Astringent tastes are those that cause our mouths to pucker and leave the tongue a little on edge. They help assuage drainage or leakage, especially from tiny capillaries near the skin surface. These foods are excellent for the cardiovascular system. Legumes, which are astringent, are prime foods for Reds. Considerable research has been done on the cardio-protective properties of legumes, especially soy, and this was discussed in chapters 6 and 8. Grapes, apples, and all kinds of berries are good for Reds and are also astringent. So are most cruciferous vegetables including broccoli, cabbage, and cauliflower.

Sweet tastes are good for you, but only those from whole foods. If you are a Red type, you may have noticed you love sweet foods, especially those that are sugary. Overconsumption of these foods typically results in digestive problems, weight gain, and an impatient, combative, angry disposition.

Tastes to Avoid

Sour and salty tastes are the worst ones for Reds. Tomatoes are sour, and although they are the first food we think of as "red" they do not agree with your type. Frequent consumption of tomato ketchup, juice, sauces, and fresh tomatoes can be a significant source of irritation for the Red type. Other sour foods that don't agree with Reds are pickles, olives, and vinegar. You can use lemon and lime juice provided you don't overdo it. Although these fruits are sour, they are energetically cold, making them suitable for Reds. Lemon or lime juice is an acceptable substitute for vinegar in making dressings. The result of eating sour foods will usually be a burning sensation in your mouth, stomach, or duodenum. Eating these foods may also cause skin eruptions, hives, or rashes. They can also cause ulcerations in the mouth or digestive tract. The presence of too much acidity in your system will sometimes reveal itself when your rings and other jewelry turn black while you're wearing them. Overuse of salty tastes increases inflammation, capillary leakage, and skin disorders. It also accelerates wrinkling and balding in Red types.

The strongest pungent tastes are found in members of the pepper family and in root and tuber spices. You should be wary of these tastes because pungent spices and foods increase burning sensations, fever, and thirst. Pungent vegetables include brussels sprouts, green peas, and kale. Cauliflower and cabbage have dual tastes and are pungent as well as astringent. This means you will have to judge how they affect you. If they don't seem to agree with you, avoid them.

Food Texture

Oily, greasy foods are a Red's worst enemy. Fats in foods that have been fried have had their molecules disarranged by heating and are energetically too hot for your system. Moist foods with a smooth texture are good for Reds. Crispy, crunchy raw vegetables are also good. Any vegetable that is cooked should be tender crisp so that it retains some of its texture. You can eat crackers, chips, or breads that are either soft or hard. However, you must avoid those that are salted.

Food Temperature

Reds are warm by nature and prone to perspire easily as the body attempts to cool itself. Consequently, you will do best with foods that are served cold or at least not really hot. You may have noticed that you get warm when you eat. If you eat hot and spicy foods, you will generate even more body heat. Since your digestive capacity is good and you don't need to add additional stimulation, avoid hot pungent spices such as cayenne, ginger, and garlic. Choosing the right foods, eating them on the cool side and not overeating are all ways you can reduce the heat your body generates during digestion. Eating foods such as red meat increases stomach fire and may cause gastric reflux, excess acidity, and stomach pain.

Your Daily Schedule

All body types have daily biorhythms. These are the times when various metabolic processes are at their peak. Hormone production, immune resistance, and even DNA synthesis follow a pattern of synchronism. The time of lowest circadian rhythm and most stress for Reds is between 10 A.M. and 2 P.M. You will find that though this is when you are fully awake and into the day, you are also most likely to get aggravated or impatient. Or, you may find that you "bottom out" on ideas and productivity. It is wise to plan activities that are less stressful during this time, if at all possible. Taking time for a substantial midday meal is paramount. Many Red types find midday a good time to take a break and go to the gym. However, if you do this, don't overexercise, drink plenty of fluids, and make sure to eat before going back to work.

The corresponding evening time that is most challenging for Reds is between 10 P.M. and 2 A.M. Reds often feel they get a second wind after ten o'clock and are likely to stay up until well past midnight. If you are one of these people, resist the temptation to do this on a regular basis. While you may enjoy the freedom from interruptions this time of night affords, staying up past midnight on a regular basis will have a negative impact on your health.

Start winding down in the evening by listening to music, reading, or watching nonviolent shows on TV. If you are hungry during the evening, you can snack on a little fruit. On rare occasions, you can enjoy a scoop of sorbet or good-quality ice cream. Red types generally sleep deeply when they are in balance and get along nicely on six or seven hours of sleep a night. Get up early the next morning and take time for a light breakfast before heading out the door. Best times to exercise are early evening (before 7 P.M.) or midday. Exercising late in the evening will get your adrenaline going too much and delay your desire for sleep.

Red types function best when following a schedule. Make to-do lists and check off completed items as you go through the day. Don't try to keep everything in mind. Although you have an excellent memory, stressful days will throw you off easily if you aren't following a schedule. Allow time for working with minimal distractions, and when you're tired or having trouble working through a problem, take a break. You'll come back to the task refreshed and able to accomplish your work more efficiently. Leave plenty of time to complete projects and don't try to leave everything for the last minute. The better organized you are, the easier your life will be. Delegate authority and don't try to control others or impose your work ethic on them.

Your Seasonal Schedule

Summer and early autumn months between mid-June and mid-October are the most difficult for Reds. That's because these are the warmest months of the year. It's a good time to take your vacation, and if you plan to travel during this time, choose cooler climates to visit. Since summer is traditionally vacation time, you are fortunate in that this coincides nicely with your seasonal rhythms.

If you must move your household during this time—the most popular time of year to do so—give yourself plenty of time for settling in. Don't try to rush back to work without first getting accustomed to your new surroundings. It is important that you take time to establish a comfortable, peaceful environment before resuming your regular hectic schedule. It's also the ideal time to throw out unsuitable foods and replace them with those that are your color. Think of it as a prime opportunity to begin your new healthier lifestyle!

Nutritional Composition of Your Plan

If you were to design your plate of food for the day, this is how it should look:

Daily Food Plan
Red Types

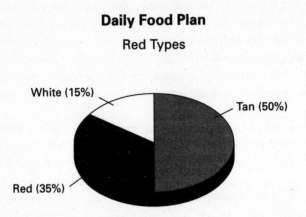

White (15%)   Tan (50%)   Red (35%)

Half of your plate should contain cereals, grains, legumes, and breads. Thirty-five percent would be Red fruits and vegetables, and the remaining 15 percent white foods.

Translated into nutritional composition, these proportions of colors you should eat yield 60 percent complex carbohydrates, 18 percent protein, and 23 percent oils. Each piece of the pie chart contains foods that are combinations of carbohydrates, proteins, and fats. Consequently, when we break these foods down by nutritional composition it may at first appear the percentages change. But remember that we are distributing your colors into more than six classes of foods (grains, vegetables, fruits, dairy, meat, and fats). We need the nutritional breakdown to design our daily meal plans.

Here is how your plan looks when spread over the various food groups in your daily meal plan.

Daily Meal Plan for Red Types

Food Group ▶	Cereals, Grains, Breads, Starchy Vegetables	Fruit and Fruit Juice	Non-starchy Vegetables	Yogurt, Kefir, Soy Milk, Grain Milk	Fish, Poultry, Meat, Skim Cheese, Eggs, Legumes, Nut Butter, Seeds	Oils and Fats, Parmesan Cheese

Serving Size ▶	½ cup	½ cup cut up or 1 small or ¾ cup juice	½ cup cooked, 1 cup raw or ¾ cup vegetable juice	1 cup or ½ cup cottage or ricotta cheese	1 ounce fish, poultry, meat, or skim cheese or 1 egg or ½ cup legumes or 2 T. nut butter	1 teaspoon oils/fats or 2 T. Parmesan cheese
Daily Calories ▼	**Number of Servings ▶**					
2,000	9½	7	5	2½	4½	2½
1,200	5⅔	4	3	1½	2⅔	1½
1,500	7	5	3¾	1¾	3⅓	1¾
1,800	8½	6¼	4½	2¼	4	2¼
2,200	10¼	7½	5½	2¾	4¾	2¾
2,400	11¼	8¼	6	3	5⅓	3

Note: To calculate the amount you should put onto your plate, multiply the number of servings by the serving size. For example, for a 2,000-calorie diet, 7 servings times ½ cup serving size equals 3½ cups.

The number of calories you should be eating depends on these factors:

- Body frame—light, medium, or heavy
- Height and weight
- Activity level
- Age
- Body mass index (BMI)

Perhaps you know how many calories you should consume; if you don't, you can get this information from my Web site, www.thenutritionsolution.com/quiz. Red types tend to fluctuate between ideal and overweight BMI. They also tend to have medium body frames that develop an "apple" shape when overweight.

Note that for calorie counts in the food plan, all starchy vegetables have the same nutritional composition as grains and are listed with them. When you are selecting which color vegetables to eat, you will be getting the phytochemicals that account for a particular color. Just replace one grain serving with your starchy vegetable and add another non-starchy vegetable to your intake for the day.

Now that we have established how many servings of each food you'll need to eat, let's see how you might plan your daily menus.

Daily Menus for the Red Type

Red menu plans provide a light breakfast and a substantial meal in the middle of the day between 10 A.M. and 2 P.M. Ideally, your main meal would be at lunchtime. The midday meal is important even if you can't make it the main meal of the day. It is important to take a break from work and retreat to someplace quiet to eat. Resist the temptation to eat at your desk. If your place of work doesn't have a lunch room, take your meal outside. Most offices have designated areas where you can take a break from the environment surrounding your desk. By taking this time for yourself, you will be less combative and able to work more efficiently in the afternoon. You may find that with this break you can work productively later in the evening. If you plan to do this, try to have a snack of fruit around 4 P.M. to keep your energy up.

The evening meal is less important and can be much lighter than lunch. Emphasize whole grains, legumes, and vegetables. One-dish meals with a green salad also make a good evening meal. Avoid heavy meats in the evening, especially red meat, which is difficult for you to digest. You can plan on fish or white poultry meat a couple of times per week, either at the midday or evening meal. Skip dessert but if you are hungry before retiring, have some berries, grapes, or an apple. Keep in mind that your chief foods are legumes, green vegetables, and red fruits. You will find your meal plans structured around these.

The best beverages for you are spring water and herbal teas. You don't do well with caffeinated beverages and sodas are too acidic. You can drink decaffeinated coffee, however. Alcohol is not good for you but an occasional glass of wine with dinner is all right, especially if your meal is composed of your colors only.

The following meal plans are for 2,000 calories. You can adjust the servings to match your desired calories as given above.

Day One
Lacto-ovo vegetarian version:

This meal plan offers dairy and legumes as the main sources of protein. It features pasta, vegetables, and fruit. Rice or other grains could easily be substituted for the pasta. Vegetables make a great topping and sauce for pasta or grains. Add a generous amount of fresh herbs—basil, parsley, oregano, and small amounts of freshly ground black pepper. A tablespoon of freshly grated Parmesan cheese may be added because you use very little oil to sauté the vegetables.

Breakfast
1 whole-grain bagel (2 grain)
4 oz. non-fat cream cheese (1 dairy)
4 oz. of orange, mango, or apricot juice (1 fruit)

Lunch

Cottage cheese, 1 cup on a bed of 2 cups mesclun salad mix (1 dairy, 1 vegetable)

Sliced pineapple, berries, kiwi, 1 cup (2 fruit)

Snack

1 small apple (1 fruit)

Dinner

Pasta, 1½ cups (1½ grain), tossed with

Sauteed mixed vegetables, 2 cups of all your colors, with 2 tsp. olive oil, plus 1 cup kidney or garbanzo beans (2 vegetable, 2 fat, 1 legume)

Mixed baby greens, 2 cups with herbs, ½ tsp. olive oil and lemon juice (1 vegetable, ½ fat)

Day Two

Baked fish or poultry option:

This menu plan offers a generous serving of fish or white chicken meat for dinner. If you are not eating fish, poultry or eggs every day, you can increase the amount you eat as long as you don't exceed the total number of servings per week. Or you can just substitute legumes for the meat servings to supply adequate protein.

Breakfast

2 cups of boxed whole-grain cereal (2 grain)

1 cup of milk or soy milk (1 dairy)

¾ cup of grapes or berries (1½ fruit)

Lunch

1½ cups of vegetable split pea soup (1½ legume, 1 vegetable)

4 small whole-wheat crackers (1 grain)

1 cup mixed green salad with 1 cup orange segments, 2 tsp. oil and lemon juice dressing (1 vegetable, 1 fruit, 2 oil)

1 cup of kefir (1 dairy)

Snack

½ cup of grapes (1 fruit)

Dinner

4½ ounces of baked trout (4½ fish)

1 cup of rice (1 grain)

1 cup of broccoli (2 vegetable)

1 cup mixed green salad with ½ cup sliced cucumbers, balsamic vinegar (1½ vegetable)

Day Three
Main dish option:
In this plan, grains, vegetables, and legumes (or fish or poultry) can be mixed into one dish and baked. All you need to complete the dinner is a green salad.

Breakfast
1 slice of whole-grain bread, toasted (1 grain), spread with
Sesame tahini or soy butter, 1 T. (1 fat)
1 cup of unsweetened yogurt (1 dairy)
½ cup of fruit or 4 oz. of fruit juice (1 fruit)

Lunch
Sandwich: 2 slices of whole-grain bread topped with ½ cup chopped egg mixed with 1 tablespoon mayonnaise, topped with arugula leaves (2 grain, 2 egg/meat, 1 fat)
Sliced jicama, apple, celery, and raisin salad, 1 cup, tossed with ½ cup non-fat yogurt, on 2 cups of greens. Add lime juice for added flavor (2 fruit, ½ dairy, 1 vegetable)

Snack
1 cup of kefir or soy milk (1 dairy)

Dinner
2½ cups of a mixed casserole; any recipe that uses a rice and legume (fish or chicken) mix, vegetables such as green peas, carrots, onions, celery, vegetable broth, and a green herb blend (1 grain, 2 vegetable, 4 legume, 1 fat)
Tossed salad, lettuce, cucumber, ¼ whole avocado, and ½ cup orange salad, balsamic or non-fat dressing 2 T. (1½ vegetable, 1 fruit, 2 fat)

These three options have endless variety. One of my favorite dinners is the pasta and vegetable combination which is made to order for busy people. Look for pasta that is interesting; basil, spinach, or even tomato—since it's not acidic in pasta form—would work for Red types. Mix up a sauté pan of all your colors—yellow, orange, red, and green vegetables—let them simmer together until just done and then toss with the cooked pasta. The vegetables will make their own juice, or you can add some vegetable bouillon to make enough moisture for the pasta. Top with some freshly grated cheese and you have a delightful and satisfying meal that is much better tasting than the tomato sauce–based pasta dishes most of us are used to fixing. You can reserve some of the pasta dish for lunch the next day. Legume or vegetable soups make good substitutes for the rice casserole suggested in the main dish menu plan. Soups make great lunches also.

Below is a wonderful sauce for Red body types—one that you can add to meals that may contain ingredients that aren't your color. It is so tasty you will want to have it on hand to use often.

❧ Mango-Orange Chutney for Red Types

This sauce is excellent to use instead of vinegar dressings that aren't good for Reds. It is also an excellent condiment for fish or poultry, and supplies vitamin C, bioflavonoids, alpha hydroxycitric acid, limonene, and terpenes.

1 mango, peeled and chopped	4 cardamom pods peeled and
1 orange, peeled and chopped	seeds crushed, or ½ tsp.
1 T. orange zest	ground cardamom
1 T. fresh dill leaves	1 tsp. tamarind paste

Toss all the ingredients into a food processor and process just until smooth.

Sample Recipe for Reds

The following soup recipe is especially good for Red types.

❧ Hearty Black Bean Soup

2 tsp. olive oil	1½ cups cooked and drained
1 large red onion, chopped	black beans
2 cloves garlic, minced	1½ cups low-sodium chicken
½ tsp. dried oregano, crumbled,	broth
or 2 T. fresh oregano leaves	4 T. sherry wine (optional)
¼ tsp. dried thyme, crumbled, or	4 tsp. chopped fresh cilantro or
1 T. fresh thyme leaves	parsley
½ to 1 tsp. ground cumin (adjust	
to your liking)	
⅛ tsp. cayenne pepper	

1. In a large heavy saucepan, heat the olive oil over moderate heat for 1 minute.

2. Add the onion and garlic and cook, uncovered, for 5 minutes or until the onion is soft.

3. Stir in the oregano, thyme, cumin, and cayenne and cook, stirring to release flavor for 1 minute longer.

4. Puree half of the black beans in a food processor and add to the onion and herbs.

5. Add remaining beans and the chicken broth to the pot.

6. Reduce heat and simmer for 15 minutes.

7. Add sherry, if desired, to soup, mix and ladle into serving bowls. Sprinkle cilantro or parsley over the top.

Makes 4 servings

Nutrition information: Serving size: 1 cup; calories per serving: 145; servings per food group: grains, 1¼; fruit, 0; vegetables, ¼; meat, ⅓; fat, ½; milk, 0

You can serve a marinated pasta and vegetable salad along with this soup. Warmed corn tortillas or bread make a good accompaniment.

Red Food Selections

Now you'll need a personalized shopping list for foods, beverages, spices, and condiments. Your foods are listed by category, first by where they fit into your daily menu plan—grains, vegetables, fruits, dairy, meat or fats—and then by food color. Finally, comments for preparing each food are listed.

Eat Your Colors Vegetables: Red

Red vegetables you can eat are pretty limited. Since tomatoes are too acidic and chili peppers, beets, and eggplant are too pungent and warming, the only red foods eligible are radicchio and red bell peppers. However, you can eat all the yellow, orange, and green vegetables with very few exceptions, and legumes will supply you with the most important phytochemicals for your type. Fruits make up the other important food group for Red body types.

Vegetable Color	Description	Comments
Red, Blue, Purple	radicchio	raw
Red, Blue, Purple	bell peppers, red	raw or cooked
Yellow	bell peppers, yellow	raw or steamed
Yellow	corn, fresh	steamed
Yellow	daikon	raw
Yellow	jicama	raw
Yellow	mushrooms, button	cooked, sautéed
Yellow	onions, yellow	same
Yellow	parsnips	steamed
Yellow	potatoes, yellow and russet	steamed, baked
Yellow	rutabagas	steamed
Yellow	squash, yellow summer	steamed
Orange	bell peppers, orange	steamed
Orange	carrots	steamed
Orange	pumpkin	cooked
Orange	sweet potatoes	baked
Orange	winter squash	baked or steamed
Orange	yams	baked or steamed
Green	cucumber	raw
Green	dandelion greens	raw or steamed
Green	edamame (green soybeans)	shelled, raw
Green	endive	raw or steamed
Green	escarole	same
Green	grape leaves	steamed, bottled
Green	green beans	steamed
Green	green juices	raw
Green	green lima beans	steamed
Green	green peas, pea pods	raw or steamed
Green	iceberg lettuce	raw
Green	kale	steamed
Green	kohlrabi	steamed
Green	leafy green and red lettuces	raw
Green	leeks	cooked
Green	mung bean sprouts	raw or stir-fried
Green	okra	sautéed
Green	parsley	raw or cooked
Green	parsnips	cooked
Green	sugar snap peas	raw
Green	turnip greens	raw or steamed
Green	watercress	raw
Green	zucchini	raw or steamed

Eat Your Colors Fruits: Red

Reds' primary fruits are red, blue, and black berries, cherries, plums, figs, grapes, pomegranates and melons. You can also enjoy any dried fruit—those that have not been sulfured are the best. Golden and orange tropical fruits, with the exception of bananas, peaches, and papaya, are also good for you, as are citrus fruits except for grapefruit. All fruits that are colored green, such as melons, grapes, green plums, and kiwi, are good for you.

Fruit Color	Description	Comments
Red, Blue, Purple	apples, red	unpeeled
Red, Blue, Purple	blueberries	raw or cooked
Red, Blue, Purple	boysenberries	sweet
Red, Blue, Purple	cherries, bing	ripe
Red, Blue, Purple	cranberries and juice	sweetened
Red, Blue, Purple	currants, dried	as is
Red, Blue, Purple	currants, red fresh	ripe
Red, Blue, Purple	figs, dried	as is
Red, Blue, Purple	figs, fresh Mission	ripe
Red, Blue, Purple	grapes; red, purple	ripe
Red, Blue, Purple	marion berries	sweet
Red, Blue, Purple	oranges, blood	sweet
Red, Blue, Purple	pears, red Bosc, Comice, etc.	ripe, cooked
Red, Blue, Purple	plums; red, purple	ripe, cooked
Red, Blue, Purple	pomegranate seeds and juice	ripe
Red, Blue, Purple	prunes, dried	as is or stewed
Red, Blue, Purple	prunes, fresh	ripe
Red, Blue, Purple	raisins	as is or cooked
Red, Blue, Purple	raspberries; red, black	very ripe
Red, Blue, Purple	strawberries	ripe, sweet
Red, Blue, Purple	watermelon	ripe
Yellow	apples, yellow	ripe
Yellow	applesauce, baked apples	add cinnamon
Yellow	avocados	ripe
Yellow	bilberries	ripe or in jam
Yellow	cherries, Rainier	ripe
Yellow	coconut	fresh shredded
Yellow	dates	as is
Yellow	figs, yellow Kadota	fresh or canned
Yellow	grapes, yellow/green	ripe
Yellow	juices, golden tropical	fresh or bottled
Yellow	lemon	juice
Yellow	pears, yellow Anjou or Bartlett	fresh
Yellow	pineapple	fresh or canned
Orange	apricots, dried	unsulfured
Orange	apricots, fresh	ripe
Orange	juices, orange	sweet
Orange	mangos	ripe
Orange	melons; cantaloupe, casaba, etc.	ripe
Orange	orange, mandarin	sweet
Orange	orange, navel	sweet
Orange	tangerines	sweet
Green	grapes, green	sweet
Green	kiwi	ripe
Green	limes	juice
Green	melons, green	ripe not sour

| Green | pears, green Seckel | ripe or cooked |
| Green | tamarind | as condiment |

Tan Foods: Cereals, Grains, Breads, and Legumes

Tan foods are most important for Red types. A well-balanced vegetarian plan including several kinds of legumes, whole grains, breads, and cereals in addition to red fruits and vegetables is the best for Reds. If you have been a big meat eater, now is the time to begin shifting to a lacto-ovo (dairy and eggs) vegetarian diet. Begin making the transition with several servings of fish and poultry weekly. As you find more vegetable, grain, and legume combinations you enjoy, you can gradually cut back on the flesh foods. You may find that you feel better if you keep them in your diet, and that's fine as long as your dietary emphasis is primarily vegetarian.

You can enjoy any grain except the yellow-colored ones: amaranth, corn, millet, and quinoa. Buckwheat and rye are too strong for you, and don't overdo it with white rice. There are many different kinds of rice and you should rotate the kind you eat. See pages 91–92 for the list of the varieties of rice and how to use them. You can also eat any legume except red lentils. Add cooked beans to your salads and stir them into vegetables. All it takes is a little awareness that these foods contain phytochemicals that prevent Red conditions and you'll find many ways to incorporate them into your meal plans.

Dry and cooked cereals work well for you and make a quick and nourishing breakfast. Fat-free whole-grain toast or a bagel are also good choices. Be sure to have at least one red fruit serving for breakfast and rely on fruit, vegetables, and seeds for snacks. Salt-free crackers and chips are also good for you. Look for rice chips, vegetable or seaweed chips, and high-fiber flat breads such as Wasa bread.

Type	Description	Comments
Breads, Crackers	bagels	warmed or toasted
Breads, Crackers	biscuits	baked
Breads, Crackers	bread, mixed grain	as is or toasted
Breads, Crackers	bread, white, or French, sweet	as is or toasted
Breads, Crackers	bread, whole wheat	as is or toasted
Breads, Crackers	chips	low salt
Breads, Crackers	crackers	low salt
Breads, Crackers	croutons	low salt
Breads, Crackers	muffin, English	plain or toasted
Breads, Crackers	pita or flat bread, white flour	plain or warmed
Breads, Crackers	pita or flat bread, whole wheat	plain or warmed
Breads, Crackers	stuffing, bread	low salt

Type	Description	Comments
Breads, Crackers	tortillas, white flour	plain or warmed
Breads, Crackers	tortillas, whole-wheat flour	plain or warmed
Breads, Crackers	waffles and pancakes, white flour	hot
Breads, Crackers	waffles and pancakes, whole grain	hot
Cereals, Grains	barley	as cereal or grain
Cereals, Grains	basmati rice, white or brown	cooked
Cereals, Grains	brown rice, short or long grain	cooked
Cereals, Grains	bulgur	cooked
Cereals, Grains	corn grits	cooked
Cereals, Grains	cornmeal	cooked
Cereals, Grains	couscous	cooked
Cereals, Grains	mochi	baked
Cereals, Grains	oat bran	cooked or baked
Cereals, Grains	oats	cooked
Cereals, Grains	pasta, basil	cooked
Cereals, Grains	pasta, spinach	cooked
Cereals, Grains	pasta, white	cooked
Cereals, Grains	pasta, whole grain	cooked
Cereals, Grains	puffed cereals	as is
Cereals, Grains	rice, sweet	cooked
Cereals, Grains	rice, wild	cooked
Cereals, Grains	rice; white, arborio, jasmine, etc.	cooked
Cereals, Grains	spelt	cooked or baked
Cereals, Grains	triticale	cooked or baked
Cereals, Grains	udon noodles	cooked
Cereals, Grains	wheat bran	cooked or baked
Legumes (pulses)	aduki bean	cooked or sprouted
Legumes (pulses)	black bean	cooked
Legumes (pulses)	black eyed peas	cooked, fresh or dried
Legumes (pulses)	black turtle bean	cooked
Legumes (pulses)	cannellini bean	cooked
Legumes (pulses)	chickpea	cooked
Legumes (pulses)	cranberry bean	cooked
Legumes (pulses)	fava beans	cooked
Legumes (pulses)	flageolet	cooked
Legumes (pulses)	green northern bean	cooked
Legumes (pulses)	kidney bean	cooked
Legumes (pulses)	lentils, brown	cooked
Legumes (pulses)	lima bean	cooked
Legumes (pulses)	mung bean	cooked or sprouted
Legumes (pulses)	navy bean	cooked
Legumes (pulses)	pinto bean	cooked
Legumes (pulses)	soybeans	cooked
Legumes (pulses)	split peas, green or yellow	cooked
Legumes (pulses)	tempeh	cooked
Legumes (pulses)	tofu	as is or cooked
Legumes (pulses)	urad dhal	cooked
Legumes (pulses)	white beans	cooked

White Foods: Oils, Fish, Poultry, Eggs, Meat, Nuts, and Seeds

Red types cannot use oils as freely as Yellows, but several are extremely important for healthy skin and maintaining cardiovascular health. Your largely grain- and legume-based diet will supply generous amounts of omega-6 fatty acids and oily fish will supply the equally important omega-3 family of fatty acids. At the same time that you are increasing your intake of these important oils, you will be eliminating the saturated fats and trans fats that interfere with your body's ability to process your dietary omega-3 and omega-6. Replace all hydrogenated fats (margarine, shortening, baked and fried goods), dairy fats, and fats from beef and pork with healthy oils and fish.

You can replace some fats without sacrificing flavor by using toasted sunflower, soy, and pumpkin seeds. These seeds make excellent snacks as well— they are high in fiber and protein as well as containing healthy oils. Poppy seeds and coconut make excellent toppings and provide that extra touch to dishes you prepare. And be sure to add water chestnuts to your stir fries.

Sweet dairy products, including milk, soft cheeses, butter, cream cheese, cream, and half-and-half are good for Reds. Select low-fat varieties and organic whenever possible. Reds can enjoy also cultured yogurt, especially with fruit. Yogurt is the only soured milk product that is good for Reds. That's because lactic bacteria "process" the milk rather than have a chemical process do it, and the end-product of bacterial action is healthful. Look for live culture yogurt, which supplies beneficial bacteria to aid your digestion. Use nonfat yogurt instead of sour cream to make delicious dressings and toppings.

Reds can get extra protein by using egg whites to make omelettes. You can also eat the whites of hard-boiled eggs. If you have a Yellow type in your family, they can eat the yolks or you can add them to baked dishes, hard-boiled and crumbled. If you do use egg yolks, you can modify any negative effects by adding turmeric. You'll find more information on why turmeric is one of your gold spices in the gold foods section of this chapter and in Part Four of *Eat Your Colors*.

Type	Description	Comments
Dairy	cheese, soft, and panir	choose low- or no-fat
Dairy	cottage cheese	choose low- or no-fat
Dairy	cow's milk	choose low- or no-fat
Dairy	sweet cream, half-and-half	use sparingly
Dairy	eggs	whites are best
Dairy	ice cream	on occasion
Dairy	yogurt	sweetened
Meat, Poultry, Fish	bass, sea	baked
Meat, Poultry, Fish	breaded fish	not fried
Meat, Poultry, Fish	chicken	white meat
Meat, Poultry, Fish	cod	baked or sautéed

Type	Description	Comments
Meat, Poultry, Fish	fish roe or caviar	as is
Meat, Poultry, Fish	haddock	baked, grilled
Meat, Poultry, Fish	halibut	baked, grilled
Meat, Poultry, Fish	orange roughy	baked, sautéed
Meat, Poultry, Fish	perch	baked, sautéed
Meat, Poultry, Fish	scrod	baked, sautéed
Meat, Poultry, Fish	sole, English and petrale	baked, sautéed
Meat, Poultry, Fish	squid	baked, sautéed
Meat, Poultry, Fish	swordfish	baked, grilled
Meat, Poultry, Fish	trout	baked, sautéed
Meat, Poultry, Fish	tuna	baked, grilled
Meat, Poultry, Fish	whitefish	baked, sautéed
Nuts	coconut	fresh, shredded
Nuts	soy nuts and soy butter	on salads, spreads
Nuts	water chestnuts	salads, stir fries
Oils	apricot kernel	high-heat cooking
Oils	avocado	high-heat cooking
Oils	black currant	no heat
Oils	borage	no heat
Oils	butter	cooking, spread
Oils	canola, regular	medium-heat cooking
Oils	canola, super	high-heat cooking
Oils	coconut	high-heat cooking
Oils	ghee (clarified butter)	cooking, spread
Oils	grape seed	medium-high heat
Oils	hemp	no heat
Oils	olive	medium-heat
Oils	pumpkin seed	no heat
Oils	rice bran	high heat
Oils	shortening, vegetable	high-heat baking
Oils	soy	medium heat
Oils	sunflower, high oleic	medium-high heat
Oils	sunflower, regular	medium heat
Oils	wheat germ	no heat
Seeds	poppy seeds	baking, on foods
Seeds	psyllium seed	dietary supplement
Seeds	pumpkin seeds, roasted	snacking, salads
Seeds	sunflower seeds, sunflower butter	roasted, as snacks

Gold Foods: Beverages, Condiments, and Spices

Reds can enjoy beverages that are naturally sweet such as apple and grape juice. Spring water is a better choice than distilled water because the latter pulls important minerals from your tissues. Herbal teas are extremely important because they can calm you down (chamomile, lemon balm) or enliven you (hibiscus, peppermint). Energizing teas such as ginger, ma huang, or Chinese or Korean Panax ginseng are too powerful for Red types and should be reserved for times when your green element is out of balance. There will be more on this in Part Four.

You will not see alcoholic drinks listed among beverages because they are too heating. Alcohol brings body heat to the surface, reducing digestive fire and increasing gastric acidity. In Red types alcohol has a powerful effect on the central nervous system and can result in increased anger, combativeness, and ultimately confusion and feelings of uncertainty. Alcohol also increases blood pressure and often causes heart arrhythmia.

Herbs such as cilantro, basil, dill, and mint are important for Red types who must avoid the use of salt. You will become skilled in the use of culinary herbs and spices as you concentrate on replacing salt in everything you prepare. Black pepper is an excellent digestive aid, but you'll have to exercise some restraint in its use. Too much pepper can overheat your system. Cayenne and other hot peppers are too intense and you should avoid using them. You can enjoy an occasional batch of chili beans if you use mild chili powder and enhance the flavor of the beans with cumin, cilantro, and parsley.

Another excellent spice for Red types is turmeric. Turmeric is a staple in curry powder and can be used liberally by itself in food preparation. Turmeric gets its yellow color from the carotenoids it contains. Turmeric overcomes the oxidation of fats, especially low-density cholesterol that is damaging to your cardiovascular system.

Type	Description	Comments
Beverages	almond milk	as dairy substitute
Beverages	aloe vera	juice
Beverages	amasake	rice drink
Beverages	apple juice	cool
Beverages	apricot juice	cool
Beverages	berry juice	cool
Beverages	carob drinks	cool
Beverages	coconut milk	in cooking
Beverages	grape juice	cool
Beverages	green drinks (spirulina, wheat)	cool
Beverages	mango juice	cool
Beverages	mineral water	cooled
Beverages	peach nectar	cool
Beverages	pear nectar	cool
Beverages	pomegranate juice	cool
Beverages	prune juice	cool
Beverages	soy milk	cool
Beverages	spring water	cool
Beverages	tea	warm or iced
Condiments	carob	cool
Condiments	lemon juice	sparingly

Type	Description	Comments
Herbal Teas	alfalfa	warm
Herbal Teas	burdock root	warm
Herbal Teas	catnip	warm
Herbal Teas	chamomile	warm
Herbal Teas	comfrey	warm, not for pregnancy
Herbal Teas	dandelion	warm
Herbal Teas	elder flowers	warm
Herbal Teas	fennel	warm
Herbal Teas	hops	warm
Herbal Teas	jasmine	warm
Herbal Teas	lemon balm (melissa)	warm
Herbal Teas	lemon grass	warm
Herbal Teas	marshmallow	warm
Herbal Teas	passionflower	warm
Herbal Teas	peppermint	warm or iced
Herbal Teas	raspberry leaf	warm
Herbal Teas	rose hips	warm
Herbal Teas	sarsaparilla	warm, not for pregnancy
Herbal Teas	spearmint	warm or iced
Herbal Teas	wintergreen	warm or iced
Seasonings	ajwan	stews
Seasonings	allspice	baking
Seasonings	almond extract	baking
Seasonings	basil	fresh or cooking
Seasonings	black pepper	cooking or table use
Seasonings	caraway	cooking or baking
Seasonings	cardamom	same
Seasonings	cilantro*	fresh or cooking
Seasonings	cinnamon	baking or at table
Seasonings	cloves	baking
Seasonings	coriander*	fresh or cooking
Seasonings	cumin*	cooking
Seasonings	curry powder	cooking
Seasonings	dill weed* and seed	fresh or cooking
Seasonings	fennel*	cooking or at table
Seasonings	garam masala	cooking
Seasonings	ginger	fresh or cooking
Seasonings	mace	baking
Seasonings	mint*	fresh or cooking
Seasonings	nutmeg	cooking, baking
Seasonings	orange peel	fresh or cooking
Seasonings	parsley	fresh or cooking
Seasonings	peppermint*	fresh or cooking
Seasonings	saffron*	cooking
Seasonings	spearmint*	fresh or cooking
Seasonings	turmeric*	cooking, curries
Seasonings	wintergreen*	fresh or cooking
Sweeteners	barley malt, syrup or crystals	baking or at table
Sweeteners	brown rice syrup	baking or at table

Sweeteners	cane sugar	baking or at table
Sweeteners	date sugar	baking or at table
Sweeteners	fructose	baking or at table
Sweeteners	fruit sugar or fruit juice sweetener	in juices and bars
Sweeteners	real maple syrup or sugar	at table, cooking
Sweeteners	raw sugar	at table, cooking
Sweeteners	*Stevia*	at table, cooking
Sweeteners	Sucanat	at table, cooking
Sweeteners	turbinado	at table, cooking

*These seasonings are the most important for Red types.

Now that you know the foods to buy, mark your shopping list for what to get at the market. Most staples from the tan foods category and spices for Reds can be stocked ahead of time. Add fresh produce items and white foods as you need them. Here is an example of what your completed list might look like:

Personal Shopping List for Red Types

Food Group	Color	Food
Vegetables	red	radicchio, red bell peppers
	yellow	daikon, jicama, mushrooms
	orange	carrots, pumpkin, squash
	green	leafy greens, artichoke, asparagus
Fruit	red, blue, or purple	apples, berries
	yellow	avocados, Rainier cherries, pineapple
	orange	apricots, orange, tangerines
	green	kiwi, sweet apples, grapes
Grains	tan	barley, bulgur, pasta
Legumes	tan	black beans, lentils, split peas
Breads	tan	whole-grain bagels, pita bread
Cereals	tan	Kashi, oat bran
Crackers, Chips	tan	rice chips, whole-wheat thins
Dairy	white	milk, soy milk
Dairy	white	yogurt, sweet cream, half-and-half
Dairy	white	eggs
Fish	white	trout, catfish, cod, haddock
Poultry	white	turkey or chicken breast
Oils	white	canola, flaxseed, olive
Nuts	white	coconut, water chestnuts
Sweeteners	gold	real maple syrup, raw sugar
Seasonings	gold	cilantro, cumin, coriander, dill, turmeric, peppermint, fennel

14

Nutrition Plan for Green Types

Water is the element associated with the Green body type and earth is the secondary element. All body *structures*, including the moistening and lubricating fluids, are governed by the Green constitution. In the previous chapters, you've seen how the three types complement one another. Bodily functions are Red properties, all molecular movement is due to Yellow, and body structures are maintained by Green. Let's see what structures Green maintains:

- Secretory and protective linings of the stomach
- Protective secretions of the esophagus
- Digestive juices containing enzymes
- Secretory and protective linings of the lungs (alveoli, bronchi) and heart (pericardium)
- Blood, lymph, and tissue fluids
- Linings and secretions of the mouth, tongue, and salivary glands
- Linings and fluids of the sinus cavities
- Linings of the brain and its fluids; spinal fluid
- Oily secretions of the skin; tears
- Mucus and protective secretions of the urinary and reproductive tracts
- Endocrine gland secretions (hormones)
- All bodily wastes

The maintenance and consistency of body fluids are supported by good nutrition. How much or how little of these fluids is secreted in a particular part of the body is highly dependent upon how the body is functioning. Consequently, Green is highly dependent upon Red for healthy balance. Green is also highly dependent upon signals it receives from the nervous system and is thus dependent upon Yellow. Imbalances in either Red or Yellow will affect Green by increasing the accumulation of fluids in the intestines and colon, and in the extremities or the respiratory tract. As the normal flow of fluids is impaired, toxins cannot be eliminated from the tissues and build up, causing disease.

Digestion and Elimination

Greens can be described as slow metabolizers. Greens are the folks who gain weight just by looking at food, and it takes very little food to satisfy them. Eating the wrong foods makes this type feel heavy, lethargic, and sleepy right after eating. All they want to do after a heavy meal is take a nap. Digestive problems in Green types occur right after eating. Often food doesn't appeal that much, and it may even be difficult to force it down. Consequently, this type is most prone to eating disorders such as anorexia, bulimia, and obesity.

Greens can fast with little difficulty and this can be an excellent way to rid the body of toxins and cut cravings for the wrong types of foods. When fasting, it's a good idea to use green drinks to help detoxify the body. Bowel elimination for Greens is very regular and should occur once a day. If you are constipated, you are eating the wrong foods and taking too little time to attend to your needs.

When Green types are healthy, they have a stable appetite, unlike Yellows, whose appetite varies from day to day, or Reds, who get grouchy when meals are late. Digestive function in Green types isn't as good as it is in Red types, so Greens must take greater care in how and what they eat. Green types also need a lot less food than either of the other types. One principal meal a day and a smaller meal are sufficient for Greens to maintain a consistent level of energy and good health. If you're this type and aren't hungry, skipping a meal won't hurt you. If you do decide to skip most of the meal and eat just a "little something," make sure you choose vegetables and skip the meat and potatoes. By all means, don't reward yourself for your restraint by having dessert! Since being overweight may plague you as a Green, let's address this problem now.

Weight Gain

Obesity is a Green condition. I will give more details on how to overcome this problem in Part Four of *Eat Your Colors*, but here we'll discuss eating strategy in weight management.

Green types can get along with very little food. It's always amazing how little you can eat and still retain or even gain weight. A poor sense of taste and smell is a big factor. The practice of grabbing whatever is handy to satisfy the need to put something into your mouth will also keep weight on.

You must learn to honor your body with what you eat. Before putting anything into your mouth, stop and ask yourself if what you're reaching for is really something your body needs. And if it isn't, then choose something you know is good for you. Good nutrition and effective weight management are a day-in, day-out practice of honoring the health you deserve. If you feel the urge to eat between meals, try drinking a glass of fresh spring water first. Your body could be needing water, but you misinterpreted its signal to mean food. If you truly need food, the water won't satisfy, and you can munch on some vegetables or some fresh or dried fruit. Baby carrots and sugar snap peas are excellent snack items. Drink at least one big glass of room temperature spring water before you sit down to eat. Eat only until you are satisfied, then push yourself away from the table. Lingering while food is still on the table and ready for the taking is poor strategy. When you put food on your plate, imagine you are preparing a child's plate.

When eating out, the portions you are served will likely be more than you need. Establish the practice of leaving at least half of what's served on your plate unless the portions are quite small. Most of us are tempted to eat as much as we possibly can because we paid for the meal and hate to leave any behind. This is especially true of Green types, who have a strong tendency to hoard money and possessions. However, the cost to your health isn't worth overeating—ever. Eating slowly helps trigger the satiety response and you will naturally eat less. Savor each bite and enjoy what you are eating. When you have finished, get up and move about. Best of all, go for a walk.

See how you feel in a little while. If you are still hungry at least an hour after finishing your meal, you can always fix yourself another small serving. Go to bed feeling a little lean and hungry and you'll lose weight, provided you haven't eaten too much earlier in the day. Adhere strictly to your daily food list. These practices are good mental exercises as well. Some of the most striking comments I have heard from people who are overweight involve issues of the mind: "I cannot remember ever feeling full when I finish a meal"; and "In my mind, I'm a fat person and always will be. Therefore, what I eat right now doesn't make a difference anyway." The mind also plays a powerful role in seeking gratification through eating.

Green types are prone to seek solace in food when stressed, bored, lonely, or unhappy. Not surprisingly, snacks, sweets, and highly processed foods are the likely food choices at these times. We develop a craving for them and they become our daily "comfort foods." These are the worst possible food items for Greens and eating them is a prescription for rapid weight gain. Snack foods are loaded with salt, sugar, and fat. As you will see a little later in this chapter, these are tastes you should avoid.

Instead, add hot and pungent spices to your food. You can use black pepper liberally but skip the salt because it increases fluid retention. Your primary foods are pungent green vegetables. You should avoid all heavy moist grains such as wheat, sweet rice, and oatmeal, sweet fruits and fruit juice, and starchy root vegetables. Stick to the leafy, aerial parts of plants and drying grains such as rye and buckwheat. Just keep thinking green when making food choices. Don't use heavy sauces or sweetened or fried foods.

Planning Meals

Greens need to plan an active life and overcome any tendency to eat whatever is handy. Most of the foods that are good for you will need to be purchased fresh from the market two or three times a week. When you go to do your shopping, begin in the produce section and plan all your meals around what vegetables you purchase. Remember that any vegetable you see— except white and sweet potatoes, tomatoes, and water chestnuts—is good for you. Skip the dairy, meat, deli, and processed food sections. You can add cereals, breads, beans, pasta, and grains to your shopping cart.

As for breakfast, a piece of toast with a little jam or a little unsweetened dry cereal will do nicely. If you like coffee or tea, you can have a cup in the morning to get going, but don't add sugar and cream. If you like to skip breakfast, that's fine—keep some mixed dried fruit at work for snacking. Lunch should consist of a salad or mixed vegetables along with a little rice, beans, millet, quinoa, or pasta. You have probably already discovered that having starches for lunch makes you sleepy and you need to switch to a high-protein lunch. You will find that you are sharper and more energetic in the afternoon. You may like to have leftovers from the night before for lunch and this is fine, especially if you can afford the luxury of resting after lunch. A mixed vegetable soup is also a good lunch when it's cold outside.

Dinner should be a light meal—soup, a vegetable stew or casserole, and salad make a great meal, especially when the weather is chilly. Avoid eating large amounts of starchy foods, including pasta, potatoes, or other root vegetables. Beef is heavy and hard to digest. You should eliminate it entirely if you can. However, if you are a beef lover, eat it at lunch or no later than mid to late afternoon.

Plan to eat dinner by six, leaving plenty of time for digesting your meal before going to bed. If you want something to eat before retiring for the night, have some fruit or a little nonfat yogurt (occasionally). You can also snack on roasted sunflower or pumpkin seeds. You should avoid sweet milk products except goats' milk and cheese but you can use soured dairy products such as nonfat yogurt and fat-free sour cream on occasion. Now, let's see which tastes you should go for.

Food Tastes

Pungent tastes are the best for Green types. All root, bulb, and tuber spices are pungent. So are aromatic spices like cinnamon, cloves, cayenne, pepper, rosemary, and thyme. Pungent herbs and spices are important for Greens to aid digestion and prevent weight gain. Greens are the only type who can eat raw garlic and onions. The pungent vegetables—brussels sprouts, cabbage, cauliflower, collards, and kale—are especially good for you as are the rest of the cruciferous vegetables discussed in chapter 7. Pungent tastes are light, dry, and heating—all properties that are good for you. Pungent tastes increase your desire to move about and seek out interesting people, situations that generally lend more excitement to your life.

Bitter tastes such as those in dark green leafy vegetables and sprouted seeds increase digestion. They are light and help overcome the heavy feeling you get as soon as you eat something. The best digestive bitter herb for a Green is fenugreek, and you will do well to drink it as a tea or add it to your food. Fenugreek is one of the primary ingredients in curry powder blends— often combined with turmeric, ginger, cumin, fennel, and coriander. Culti-vate a liking for curry powder, choosing blends that are hot and include red and black pepper. Curry powder combines bitter and pungent tastes, which are your two strongest tastes.

Astringent tastes are important for Green types. Most vegetables are astringent or pungent, which is the reason they are the primary foods for Greens. Astringent tastes complement pungency by promoting the normal flow of fluids within blood and lymph vessels. Astringent foods are known to strengthen the cardiovascular system. Red, blue, purple, and black berries, cherries, and the skins of apples and grapes contain powerful phytonutrients for preventing low density lipoprotein (LDL) oxidation and breakdown of arterial walls. Legumes such as soy, kudzu, and red clover contain isoflavones that have been shown to prevent cardiovascular disease. Kudzu is an excel-lent liver tonic herb and red clover is an effective blood cleanser. Many fruits are too sweet for Greens, and Greens depend less on cereals and grains than Yellows and Reds. Greens do not do well with dairy products or cold heavy foods such as ice cream.

Tastes to Avoid

Sweet taste is found in fruits such as avocados, bananas, coconuts, dates, figs, papayas, pineapples, and plums. Tropical fruit juice and carrot juice are too sweet for Greens, although orange juice is fine. Grains and root vegetables are also sweet, due to their high carbohydrate content. Consequently, Greens can't eat as many of these as Reds and Yellows. The grains that are drier in consistency, such as buckwheat, cornmeal, millet, oats, and oat bran, are the best ones for Green types. You should avoid wheat-based breads.

Artificial sweeteners of any kind, as well as white and brown sugar, are not good for Greens, but raw honey, barley malt, brown rice, natural maple syrups and fruit juice concentrates are fine as long as they are used in moderation. Amasake is a sweet rice milk beverage that can be used in place of other sweeteners or dairy products. Date sugar or any dried fruit can also be used for sweetness.

Sour and salty tastes occur in most condiments including coconut milk, miso (fermented soybean paste), olives, ketchup, tamari or soy sauce, vinegar, and soured milk products (yogurt, sour cream, kefir). These foods increase fluid retention, weight gain, and the tendency toward lethargy. Since this tendency is one to which Greens are prone, avoiding sour and salty foods helps diminish this characteristic.

Food Temperature

Green types have a warm exterior but a cool interior. Their skin is soft, supple, and warm to the touch and their body processes are slow and cool. Greens fall somewhere between Reds and Yellows, being neither as warm as Reds nor as cold as Yellows. Consequently, food temperature isn't as critical for Greens as it is for the other two types. As a Green type you can do well with either raw or cooked foods. Some Ayurvedic practitioners recommend that you don't eat raw and cooked foods at the same time. This is a good suggestion if your digestion hasn't been great or you're trying to lose weight. Eat salads and other raw foods at one meal and cooked ones at another. If this isn't possible, then eat cooked foods first and raw foods last because they will take longer for your digestive system to break down.

Cold dry cereals are preferable to hot cooked ones for you. You should toast your bread to cut down on moisture. Choose beverages that are warm or room temperature and have a glass of room temperature spring water before meals. You should never drink ice water with your meals and should wait until you have finished your meal before drinking anything. The exception to this is drinking wine with dinner. Wine is astringent, especially red wine, and Greens are the only type that can benefit from having a glass of wine with dinner.

Your Daily Schedule

Greens love to sleep and will languish in bed late into the morning whenever possible. It is important to get up and get going before 6 A.M. Your time of greatest challenge is between 6 A.M. and 10 A.M. That's one reason why you have always found it difficult to get moving in the morning. This is a good time to go to the gym or walk—whatever you can fit into your schedule. If you have to get up earlier to make it happen, do it. You will notice a tremendous boost in your mental outlook and energy levels. You can easily go directly from the gym to work and never miss eating breakfast. Greens have a tremendous capacity for exercise, are well-coordinated and natural athletes. However, this type is least likely to exercise regularly.

The other time of daily challenge is from 6 P.M. to 8 P.M. It's another good opportunity for exercise, and you should go for a short walk after dinner if you don't plan to exercise. You can plan an early bedtime but allow yourself no more than eight or nine hours of sleep each night.

Your Seasonal Schedule

The damp, cold weather of the late winter, changing into pollen season in the spring is the time of greatest challenge for you. Mid-March to mid-June is allergy season and the time of year when most change occurs. If you have allergies, you may feel least like exercising because you're bothered by respiratory congestion and a foggy mind. You will reduce these symptoms if you adhere strictly to your nutritional plan. Spring is the season of love and loving is one of your greatest attributes as a Green type. Make sure you direct love toward yourself and prepare your body for the months just ahead. Early spring cleansing is a good practice for you to have. Once winter has passed, you can cleanse your body, ridding it of the toxins that have accumulated during the holiday season.

Nutritional Composition of Your Plan

If you were to arrange all the food for a day on a plate it would look like the pie chart below. Your daily plate contains 50 percent vegetables and fruit. Forty percent should be tan foods—cereals, grains, and legumes—and the remaining 10 percent white foods.

Another way to think of your daily plan is that half of everything you eat should be green vegetables with limited amounts of green fruit. The other half of what you eat should be tan foods—grains, cereals, legumes, and, to a lesser extent, breads. The smallest portion of what you eat will be fish, poultry, seeds, and medium-heat oils.

Now we need to design your daily meal plan, distributing your primary and complementary colors among the six food groups: grains, vegetables, fruits, dairy, meat, and oils. In designing your daily meal plan, we also need to maintain proper ratios between percentages of carbohydrates, proteins, and fats. These ratios differ among the three body types. For Greens, the per-

Daily Food Plan
Green Types

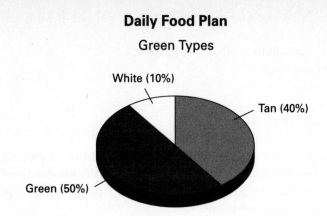

centages are: complex carbohydrates, 55 percent; proteins, 22 percent; and oils, 23 percent. When we distribute these calories among the six food groups, the meal plan will look like this.

Daily Meal Plan for Green Types

Food Group ▶	Cereals, Grains, Breads, Starchy Vegetables	Fruit and Fruit Juice	Non-starchy Vegetables	Yogurt, Kefir, Soy Milk, Grain Milk	Fish, Poultry, Meat, Skim Cheese, Eggs, Legumes, Nut Butter, Seeds	Oils and Fats, Parmesan Cheese
Serving Size ▶	½ cup	½ cup cut up or 1 small or ¾ cup juice	½ cup cooked, 1 cup raw or ¾ cup vegetable juice	1 cup or ½ cup cottage or ricotta cheese	1 ounce fish, poultry, meat, skim cheese or 1 egg or ½ cup legumes or 2 T. nut butter	1 teaspoon oils/fats or 2 T. Parmesan cheese

Daily Calories ▼	Number of Servings ▶					
2,000	7	5	11½	2	6	1
1,200	4½	3¼	7⅓	1⅓	3¾	1
1,500	5½	4	9	1⅔	4¾	1
1,800	6¾	4¾	11	2	5¾	1
2,200	8	5¾	13	2⅓	7	1¼
2,400	9	6⅓	14⅔	2½	7⅔	1⅓

Note: To calculate the amount you should put onto your plate, multiply the number of servings by the serving size. For example, for a 2,000-calorie diet, 7 servings times ½ cup serving size equals 3½ cups.

The number of calories you should be eating depends on these factors:

- Body frame—light, medium, or heavy
- Height and weight
- Activity level
- Age
- Body mass index (BMI)

Perhaps you know how many calories you should consume and can go directly to the table above. If you don't, you can get this information from my Web site, www.thenutritionsolution.com/quiz. Typically, Green types have high BMIs and large body frames.

You no doubt know your activity level and whether you are active or sedentary. Naturally we slow down as we age and will need fewer calories. However, we don't need a special allowance for age as long as activity level is considered. (Some nutritionists calculate a decrease in daily calories for every ten years of age.) As long as we allow for increasing sedentary lifestyle, we automatically allow for advancing age. You will find this allowance for your activity level in the determination "ideal daily calories" when you log on to my Web site.

Note that for calorie counts in the food plan, all starchy vegetables (which are restricted for Greens) have the same nutritional composition as grains and are listed with them. When you are selecting which color vegetables to eat, you will be getting the phytochemicals that account for a particular color, regardless of how you account for its calories. If you do move one of your vegetable choices into the grains column because it's starchy, just replace one grain serving with your starchy vegetable and add another non-starchy vegetable to your intake for the day.

Now that we have established how many servings of each food you'll need to eat, let's see how you might plan your daily menus.

Daily Menus for the Green Type

Green menu plans are designed for one main meal a day. You are the one type that can go without breakfast and still function well. You may like a piece of whole-grain toast—a cornmeal muffin is preferable—with a cup of coffee (no cream or sugar!) before leaving for work, and that's fine. Just be sure that you aren't tempted to snack on something sugary like doughnuts or cookies when you get to work. If you find that you get too hungry before lunch, just pack some vegetables to nibble on. You can also snack on roasted sunflower seeds, soy nuts, or pumpkin seeds. Vegetable, wasabi, or seaweed rice crackers are also good snack items for Green types.

If possible, plan a large meal for lunch and a lighter dinner. Since this isn't possible for most people, have a salad containing dark pungent greens such as arugula, mustard greens, endive, tatsoi, and sprouts for lunch. You can top your greens with raw broccoli, cauliflower, green peas, and carrots. Add some radishes or daikon to liven up the flavor and dress your salad with balsamic vinegar and croutons. Add lots of black pepper, no salt, and perhaps a salt-free salad spice blend.

In late afternoon, if you need a lift, you can enjoy a cup of Chinese or Korean ginseng, ginger tea, or black tea. Mineral or spring water is good for you but avoid sweetened carbonated beverages such as colas. If you can work out before dinner, this is a great time to do so. Otherwise, you can work out any time after 6 P.M. Your natural biorhythms are at low ebb between 6 P.M. and 10 P.M. and you probably want to fall into bed. A walk after dinner helps overcome the immediate fatigue you may feel after eating. You will find this tendency diminishes once you have been following your meal plan for a few days. Dinner should be mostly green vegetables, especially cruciferous vegetables, garlic, and onions. You can add a starchy vegetable and a whole grain serving to complete the meal. Avoid eating beef, pork, and lamb except on special occasions. On the days you don't eat any animal foods, be sure and add some legumes. A little fish or poultry two to three times a week is enough to keep you in good health. Limit yourself to no more than 6 ounces of protein foods each day (fish, poultry, eggs). You can eat large quantities of green vegetables and your meals should be planned around green.

Note: The following sample meal plans contain approximately the correct number of calories (2,000) for women. Green-type men follow the same plan, but should add approximately 20 percent more of each serving. Follow the daily servings guide listing how much of each food you should eat.

Basic Plan and Options

Breakfast
1 small cornmeal muffin or 1 slice of dry toast or ½ toasted bagel with 2 oz. nonfat cream cheese (1 grain, ½ dairy)
cup of black coffee
4 oz. fruit juice or ½ cup berries, cherries, or grapes (1 fruit)

Snack
¼ cup of roasted sunflower seeds (1 fat)

Lunch
2 cups of dark leafy green salad (2 vegetable)
1 cup of cruciferous vegetables, steamed or raw to go on salad (2 vegetable)

¼ cup of toasted croutons or soy nuts (½ grain or 1 legume)
Balsamic vinegar, black pepper and a salt-free salad mix

Lunch Option

Add 4 oz. of flaked water-packed tuna (4 fish) or a chopped egg (1 egg) to your salad

Mid-Afternoon

1 cup of herbal tea or iced tea and ½ cup of berries or grapes (1 fruit)

Dinner

2 cups mixed steamed vegetables (broccoli, carrots, cauliflower, peppers, onions, garlic), making this as colorful as possible and blending at least three different colors of vegetables; season with lemon pepper, basil, rosemary, coriander, parsley, oregano or paprika (4 vegetable)

Side dish of 1 cup black beans and 1 cup brown basmati rice flavored with hot curry powder (2 legume, 2 grain)

2 cups dark green leafy salad with ½ cup artichoke hearts and ½ cup sliced beets, top with oil free dressing, lemon juice, balsamic or brown rice vinegar, pepper, ¼ cup oil-free garlic-flavored croutons (1½ vegetable, 1 grain/root vegetable, ½ grain)

Dinner Option

If you don't have tuna, chicken or an egg on your lunch salad, you can have 6 oz. of fish or poultry with dinner. Eliminate the side dish of rice and legumes.

Another Dinner Option

A hearty vegetable soup can take the place of the vegetables and the grain/bean side dish in this dinner plan. Enjoy three cups of soup, the green salad, and add some crusty rye bread. If you want oil on your bread, don't use it on your salad. You'll find a recipe for vegetable soup below.

You may wonder about your calcium requirements since the Green plan does not use dairy. You can drink soy milk, which has the same amount of calcium as cow's milk. However, green vegetables are excellent sources of calcium, and if you are following your plan closely you are getting both calcium and magnesium (which dairy doesn't supply).

Add zest and variety to your meals by using the chutney sauce below. Be sure to have some of this on hand for dipping raw vegetables as well as dressing up cooked ones.

᥉ Peppermint and Cilantro Chutney for Green Types

I prefer this sauce for cruciferous vegetables like broccoli, cabbage, cauliflower, and brussels sprouts. It gives cauliflower character and overcomes the strong flavor of these vegetables. A good source of vitamin C, limonene, phenolic acids, allylic sulfides, and gingerols, this sauce is also a good alternative for salsa with tortilla chips, and it is excellent on poultry as well. It can also help overcome the heaviness of eggs, which are "off color" for Green types.

Juice of 3 lemons
1 tsp. lemon zest
2 cups washed peppermint and
   cilantro leaves
3 or 4 scallions, roughly
   chopped

1 T. peeled and chopped fresh
   ginger root
¼ tsp. sea salt (optional)

Toss all ingredients in a blender or food processor. Process until mixture reaches a smooth consistency.

Now for that vegetable soup recipe:

᥉ Hearty Vegetable Soup

2 small leeks (or 1 large), washed
   well; use white and light green
   parts, sliced thinly to yield about
   ¾ cup chopped leeks
2 medium carrots, peeled and cut
   into small dice to yield about ¾
   cup
2 small onions, peeled and diced to
   yield about ¾ cup
2 medium celery stalks, trimmed
   and cut into small pieces to yield
   about ¾ cup
1 medium russet potato, peeled
   and cut into small cubes to yield
   about 1¼ cups
1 medium zucchini, trimmed and
   cut into small cubes to yield
   about 1¼ cups

3 cups stemmed spinach leaves, cut
   into thin strips
1 large (28 oz.) can of whole tomatoes, drained and chopped into
   small pieces
1 15 oz.-can cannellini beans,
   drained and rinsed, about 1½
   cups
1 Parmesan cheese rind, about 5 ×
   2 inches
8 cups water
1 tsp. dried oregano, crushed, or 2
   T. fresh oregano, crushed
½ tsp. dried thyme, crushed, or
   1 T. fresh thyme leaves,
   crushed
Black pepper and sea salt or tamari
   to taste

1. Bring vegetables, tomatoes, water, herbs, and cheese rind to a boil.
2. Reduce heat to simmer, and cook uncovered until the vegetables are tender but still hold their shape, about one hour.
3. Add beans and cook just until heated through, about 5 minutes.
4. Remove and discard cheese rind.
5. Add Basil or Rosemary Pesto (see recipe below); add salt and pepper to taste.
6. Serve immediately.

Makes 8 servings

Nutrition information: Serving size: 1 cup; calories per serving: 102; servings per food group: grains, ¾; fruit, 0; vegetables, 1⅔; meat, 0; fat, 0; milk, 0

⌘ Basil or Rosemary Pesto

¼ cup prepared basil pesto sauce
—or—
1 T. crushed fresh rosemary

mixed with 1 tsp. minced fresh garlic and 1 T. extra virgin olive oil

Tomatoes are acidic and generally should be avoided by Green and Red types. However, when they are chopped and added to a hearty soup, the other vegetables and herb pesto improve their digestibility and neutralize their acidity. You won't have any problems with small amounts of tomatoes added to mixtures of herb and vegetable blends as long as you aren't eating other concentrated tomato products such as ketchup and tomato sauce.

Here is another excellent soup for Green types.

⌘ Purée of Broccoli Soup with Garlic and Red Pepper

1 T. olive oil
1 onion or leek, diced coarsely
2 carrots, peeled and diced
1 clove garlic, minced
6 cups chicken broth
1 bunch broccoli, trimmed and
    cut into ½-inch pieces or
    small florets

1 pound of potatoes (2 large or
    3 medium), peeled and cut
    into 1-inch diced pieces
¼ tsp. hot red pepper flakes
¼ tsp. tamarind paste
    (optional)
Sea salt or tamari and black
    pepper to taste

1. Heat oil in a large soup kettle. Add onion or leek and carrots. Sauté until vegetables soften, about 5 minutes.

2. Add garlic and sauté until fragrant, about 1 minute.

3. Add broth and simmer 1 to 2 minutes.

4. Add broccoli, potatoes, red pepper flakes, and salt or tamari and tamarind to taste.

5. Simmer until vegetables are tender, about 20 minutes.

6. Season with black pepper to taste.

7. Purée in batches in a food processor or blender. Return to the kettle, reheat and serve.

Makes 8 servings

Nutrition information: Serving size: 1 cup; calories per serving: 57; servings per food group: grains, ½; fruit, 0; vegetables, ⅔; meat, ¾; fat ¹⁄₁₀; milk, 0

Both of these soups can be made ahead of time and refrigerated. The flavor improves with storage. Extra amounts can be frozen for up to one month.

These soup recipes and the black bean soup in chapter 13 came from my late friend Kathy Barsotti, who with her family has been engaged in organic farming since 1974. Fresh organic produce from the Barsotti farm and those of their organic growers association are delivered weekly to our doorstep, here in Alameda. Kathy collected her family recipes in a small cookbook entitled *Farm Fresh to You—Savory Samplings of the Harvest.* You can obtain a copy from Farm Fresh to You, 23808 State Highway 16, Capay, CA 95607.

Green Food Selections

Now you'll need a personalized shopping list for foods, beverages, spices, and condiments. Your foods are listed by category, first by where they fit into your daily menu plan—grains, vegetables, fruits, dairy, meat or oils—and then by food color. Finally, comments about each food to guide you in shopping and preparing them are listed.

Your vegetable selections are easy. If it's green, it's good for you. Pungent foods that include all cruciferous vegetables, garlic, and onions are the best. However, less pungent ones like arugula, asparagus, endive, and spinach are also very good. Greens can eat any vegetable raw or cooked and use pungent spices liberally to speed up metabolism. Ginger, chili pepper, cayenne, fenugreek, and turmeric are all excellent additions to any meal. You should try new vegetables, blending them in among old favorites to vary your diet.

Eat Your Colors Vegetables: Green

Vegetable Color	Description	Comments
Green	aduki sprouts	you can sprout these at home
Green	alfalfa sprouts	you can sprout these at home
Green	artichoke, globe	look for compact, dark green
Green	artichoke, Jerusalem	firm, peel, eat raw, steamed
Green	arugula	raw or sautéed
Green	asparagus	steamed
Green	baby green mix (mesclun)	raw
Green	beet greens	steamed
Green	bell peppers, green	raw or cooked, stuffed
Green	bitter melon	chopped, added to stir fries
Green	bok choy	raw or steamed
Green	broccoli sprouts	raw
Green	broccoli, broccoli rabe	raw or steamed
Green	brussels sprouts	steamed
Green	cabbage	raw or steamed
Green	cauliflower	raw or steamed
Green	chicory	raw or steamed
Green	chili peppers, green	cooked
Green	chives	raw
Green	cilantro	raw
Green	collards	raw or steamed
Green	dandelion greens	raw or steamed
Green	edamame (green soybeans)	raw or steamed
Green	endive	raw
Green	escarole	raw
Green	garlic	raw and cooked
Green	grape leaves	bottled
Green	green beans	raw or steamed
Green	green juices	raw
Green	green lima beans	steamed
Green	green peas, pea pods	raw or cooked
Green	horseradish	prepared
Green	iceberg lettuce	raw
Green	kale	raw or steamed
Green	kohlrabi	steamed
Green	leafy green and red lettuces	raw
Green	leeks	sautéed or steamed
Green	mung bean sprouts	sprout at home, raw or cooked
Green	mustard greens	raw or cooked
Green	okra	sautéed
Green	olives, green and black	use sparingly, low salt
Green	parsley	raw or cooked
Green	parsnips	steamed
Green	scallions	raw or cooked
Green	spinach	raw or cooked
Green	sugar snap peas	raw or in stir fries
Green	Swiss chard	steamed, added to soup

Green	turnip greens	steamed, added to soup
Green	watercress	raw, added to salads
Green	zucchini	raw or cooked
Orange	bell peppers, orange	raw or cooked
Orange	chili peppers, orange	cooked
Red, Blue, Purple	beets	cooked, cold or hot
Red, Blue, Purple	bell peppers, red	raw or cooked
Red, Blue, Purple	eggplant	peeled, sautéed
Red, Blue, Purple	radicchio	raw
Red, Blue, Purple	radishes	raw
Red, Blue, Purple	tomatoes	raw in season, cooked in soup
Yellow	bell peppers, yellow	raw or cooked
Yellow	chili peppers, yellow	cooked
Yellow	corn, fresh	steamed or grilled
Yellow	daikon	raw
Yellow	jicama	raw
Yellow	mushrooms, button	sautéed
Yellow	onions, yellow	raw or cooked
Yellow	potatoes, yellow and russet	baked or steamed
Yellow	squash, yellow	raw or steamed

Eat Your Colors Fruits: Green

Greens are more limited in fruit selections than either Yellow or Red types. Sweet fruits are not on your list at all. Fruits that are listed are more pungent or bitter in taste. Your meal plan offers small amounts of fruit that should be eaten between meals, or, if you plan a fruit salad as part of a meal, eat it first. Fruit juice is not advised for Green types because it lacks the fiber that slows down the metabolism of fruit sugar. Better to drink green vegetable juices or choose pomegranate, berry, or cranberry in preference to citrus or tropical fruit juices. You can choose any of these fruits for snacks or serve them on a bed of dark leafy greens with daikon and radishes. You can also enjoy dried fruits as snacks. They are intensely sweet, so limit yourself to two or three halves.

Fruit Color	Description	Comments
Green	grapes, green	
Green	kiwi	
Green	plums, green	
Green	tamarind	paste added to stews, soups
Orange	apricots, dried	
Orange	apricots, fresh	
Orange	mangos	
Orange	orange, navel	
Orange	peaches, dried	
Orange	peaches, fresh	
Orange	persimmon	very ripe, slice in half, scoop out pulp
Orange	tangerines	

Fruit Color	Description	Comments
Red, Blue, Purple	apples, red	
Red, Blue, Purple	blueberries	
Red, Blue, Purple	boysenberries	
Red, Blue, Purple	cherries, sour	
Red, Blue, Purple	chokeberries	
Red, Blue, Purple	grapes; red, purple	
Red, Blue, Purple	marion berries	
Red, Blue, Purple	oranges, blood	
Red, Blue, Purple	pears, red Bosc, Comice, etc.	good baked
Red, Blue, Purple	pomegranate	seeds add to fruit combos
Red, Blue, Purple	raspberries; red, black	
Red, Blue, Purple	strawberries	
Yellow	apples, yellow	
Yellow	cherries, Rainier	
Yellow	grapes, yellow/green	
Yellow	lemon	
Yellow	pears, yellow Anjou or Bartlett	
Yellow	quince	baked or in jam

Tan Foods: Cereals, Grains, Breads, and Legumes

Sweet grains such as rice, especially brown rice, aren't good for Greens. However, plain white rice is good and so are brown and white basmati and jasmine rice. Both of these are aromatic and mildly pungent. Wheat is too dense and heavy for you, so you're limited in choosing products that contain wheat, including most pasta. The best grains for you are barley, buckwheat, corn, millet, and rye. Fortunately, corn pasta is available, as is Jerusalem artichoke pasta (De Boles brand), and Japanese udon and soba (buckwheat) noodles are good for you. You can eat most legumes, but avoid kidney beans, brown lentils, soybeans, and tempeh. Tofu (soybean curd) is good for you and is easy to add to dishes you prepare for extra protein. Tofu is also a good source of calcium. Since it takes on the flavor of anything it's mixed with, you can easily substitute tofu for meat or eggs in recipes.

Type	Description	Comments
Breads, Crackers	bagels	toasted
Breads, Crackers	biscuits	warmed
Breads, Crackers	bread, cornbread	warmed or cold
Breads, Crackers	bread, rye	plain or toasted
Breads, Crackers	bread, white, or French, sweet	plain or toasted
Breads, Crackers	chips	low salt
Breads, Crackers	crackers	low salt
Breads, Crackers	croutons	low salt
Breads, Crackers	muffin, English	toasted
Breads, Crackers	pita or flat bread, white flour	plain
Breads, Crackers	stuffing, bread	low-salt, fat-free

Breads, Crackers	tortillas, corn	plain or warmed
Breads, Crackers	tortillas, white flour	plain or warmed
Breads, Crackers	waffles and pancakes, buckwheat	well done
Breads, Crackers	waffles and pancakes, white flour	well done
Breads, Crackers	Wasa bread	as a snack or with salads
Cereals, Grains	amaranth	cold as cereal
Cereals, Grains	barley, grain or flour	cereal, steamed, added to soup, baking
Cereals, Grains	basmati rice, white or brown	steamed, eat hot or cold
Cereals, Grains	buckwheat, groats or flour	steamed or in baking
Cereals, Grains	corn, ground	cooked polenta or cornmeal, hot or cold
Cereals, Grains	corn grits	cooked, eat hot or cold
Cereals, Grains	cornmeal, corn flour	dip for sautéeing or in baking
Cereals, Grains	couscous	steamed
Cereals, Grains	millet, grain or flour	steamed or in baking
Cereals, Grains	mochi	baked, snack
Cereals, Grains	oat bran	in baking or sprinkle on food
Cereals, Grains	oats, oat flour	uncooked or in baking
Cereals, Grains	pasta, basil	boiled, serve with vegetables
Cereals, Grains	pasta, red pepper	boiled, serve with vegetables
Cereals, Grains	pasta, spinach	boiled, serve with vegetables
Cereals, Grains	pasta, white	very limited
Cereals, Grains	pasta, whole grain	very limited
Cereals, Grains	pasta, Jerusalem artichoke	boiled, serve with vegetables
Cereals, Grains	popcorn	no oil, salt, good snack
Cereals, Grains	puffed cereals	serve with soy milk
Cereals, Grains	quinoa	steamed, or in boxed cereals
Cereals, Grains	rice, wild	steamed
Cereals, Grains	rice: white, arborio, jasmine, etc.	steamed
Cereals, Grains	rye, grain or flour	steamed or in baking
Cereals, Grains	soba noodles	boiled, serve with vegetables
Cereals, Grains	udon noodles	boiled, serve with vegetables
Legumes (pulses)	aduki bean	sprout at home or cook dry beans
Legumes (pulses)	anasazi bean	cooked
Legumes (pulses)	black bean	cooked
Legumes (pulses)	black-eyed peas	fresh or cooked
Legumes (pulses)	black turtle bean	cooked
Legumes (pulses)	cannellini beans	cooked
Legumes (pulses)	chickpeas	cooked
Legumes (pulses)	cranberry beans	cooked
Legumes (pulses)	fava beans	cooked
Legumes (pulses)	flageolets	cooked
Legumes (pulses)	great northern beans	cooked
Legumes (pulses)	lentils, red	cooked, or sprout at home
Legumes (pulses)	lima beans	cooked
Legumes (pulses)	mung beans	sprout at home, eat raw or in stir fries
Legumes (pulses)	navy beans	cooked
Legumes (pulses)	pinto beans	cooked
Legumes (pulses)	split peas, green or yellow	cooked
Legumes (pulses)	tofu	add to dishes in place of meat
Legumes (pulses)	urad dhal	cooked
Legumes (pulses)	white beans	cooked

White Foods: Oils, Fish, Poultry, Eggs, Meat, Nuts, Seeds

Green types are severely restricted in dairy products. The only ones from cow's milk that work for you are low-fat cottage cheese, kefir (liquid yogurt), and low-fat or fat-free yogurt. If you like goat's cheese or goat's milk, you can enjoy these. Otherwise you should substitute soy milk, rice milk, or grain milk for cow's milk. Egg whites are a good source of protein for you, and egg white and vegetable omelettes make a good quick meal. You should enjoy red meat only on occasion and grilling it is best. Use the tips on marinating in chapter 6 to reduce formation of harmful HCHs. White chicken or turkey meat is good for you and you can enjoy several kinds of fish. You have good oils to choose from but use only very small amounts. Roasted sunflower and pumpkin seeds are good snacks, and you can eat peanuts but not tree nuts.

Type	Description	Comments
Dairy	cottage cheese	choose nonfat
Dairy	eggs	whites are best
Dairy	goat's cheese	good substitute for cow's cheese
Dairy	goat's milk	good substitute for cow's milk
Dairy	kefir	on occasion use instead of milk
Dairy	yogurt, live culture	on occasion
Meat, Poultry, Fish	bass, sea	baked, sautéed
Meat, Poultry, Fish	breaded fish	baked, not fried
Meat, Poultry, Fish	chicken	white meat
Meat, Poultry, Fish	clams	steamed
Meat, Poultry, Fish	cod	baked, sautéed
Meat, Poultry, Fish	crab	steamed
Meat, Poultry, Fish	fish roe or caviar	fresh or canned
Meat, Poultry, Fish	haddock	baked, grilled or sautéed
Meat, Poultry, Fish	halibut	baked, grilled or sautéed
Meat, Poultry, Fish	menhaden	baked, grilled or sautéed
Meat, Poultry, Fish	orange roughy	baked or sautéed
Meat, Poultry, Fish	prawn	steamed
Meat, Poultry, Fish	salmon, coho (farmed)	steamed, baked, or sautéed
Meat, Poultry, Fish	sand dabs	sautéed
Meat, Poultry, Fish	sardine	sautéed or canned
Meat, Poultry, Fish	scallops	baked, sautéed
Meat, Poultry, Fish	scrod	baked, sautéed
Meat, Poultry, Fish	sole, English or petrale	baked, sautéed
Meat, Poultry, Fish	squid	baked, sautéed
Meat, Poultry, Fish	trout	sautéed or grilled
Meat, Poultry, Fish	whitefish	baked, sautéed
Nuts	peanuts and peanut butter	unsalted, dry-roasted
Oils	black currant	no heat
Oils	borage	no heat
Oils	canola, regular	medium-high heat
Oils	canola, super	high heat
Oils	corn	medium-high heat
Oils	flax	no heat

Oils	ghee (clarified butter)	in cooking, as a spread
Oils	grape seed	medium-high heat
Oils	hemp	no heat
Oils	mustard	medium-high heat
Oils	pumpkin seed	no heat
Oils	rice bran	high heat
Oils	safflower, high oleic	high heat
Oils	safflower, regular	medium heat
Oils	soy	medium heat
Oils	sunflower, high oleic	high heat
Oils	sunflower, regular	medium-high heat
Seeds	flax seeds, meal	sprinkle on salads, add to beverages
Seeds	poppy seeds	sprinkle on food, baking
Seeds	psyllium seed	dietary supplement
Seeds	pumpkin seeds	roasted on salads, as a snack
Seeds	sunflower seeds, butter	roasted on salads, as a snack

Gold Foods: Beverages, Condiments, and Spices

Green types do well with warm and spicy beverages such as mulled apple cider and all pungent drinks including coffee and tea. Astringent juices—berry, cherry, cranberry, and pomegranate—are also good for Green types. Since most dairy products don't agree with Greens, soy milk is an excellent substitute. Nut milks—almond, coconut—do not work, however.

Most forms of sugar have not been listed on your plan, but natural sweeteners like raw honey, barley malt syrup, and real maple syrup will work for you. Greens can use several condiments, especially those that are hot and spicy like horseradish, mustard, and wasabi. All spices are good for you and so are most herbal teas.

Type	Description	Comments
Beverages	aloe vera	helps relieve congestion
Beverages	amasake	may be used instead of dairy
Beverages	apple juice	best juice for greens
Beverages	apricot juice	best Orange juice
Beverages	berry juice	astringent, excellent
Beverages	carob drinks	use instead of chocolate
Beverages	cherry juice	astringent, anti-inflammatory
Beverages	coffee	bitter, diuretic
Beverages	green drinks made from chorella, barley grass, or spirulina	excellent for detoxification
Beverages	lemonade	not too sweet
Beverages	mango juice	best Orange juice
Beverages	mineral water	helps digestion
Beverages	orange juice	rotate with other juices
Beverages	peach nectar	good for variety
Beverages	pear nectar	good for variety
Beverages	pomegranate juice	astringent, excellent

Type	Description	Comments
Beverages	prune juice	antioxidant and mild laxative
Beverages	soy milk	good substitute for dairy
Beverages	spring water	good, it's not fizzy
Beverages	tea	black, green, or herbal
Beverages	vegetable juices	not tomato-based
Beverages	wine and spirits	in moderation
Condiments	carob	use for baking instead of chocolate
Condiments	chutney	hot ones best; add to yogurt for a dressing
Condiments	lemon juice	sprinkle on vegetables to add zest
Condiments	mustard	best are dark, hot varieties such as Dijon
Condiments	pickles, sweet	these work, dills don't
Condiments	wasabi	improves digestion, eat with sushi, fish
Herbal Teas	alfalfa	hot, nutritive, phytoestrogens
Herbal Teas	bancha	cleanser and mild stimulant
Herbal Teas	burdock root	blood cleanser and mild stimulant
Herbal Teas	chamomile	calming
Herbal Teas	corn silk	diuretic
Herbal Teas	dandelion	thins congestion
Herbal Teas	fennel	digestive aid
Herbal Teas	ginger, dried or fresh	congestion, stuffy head, motion sickness
Herbal Teas	ginseng	energy boost, restores homeostasis
Herbal Teas	hops	sedative
Herbal Teas	jasmine	aromatic
Herbal Teas	lemon balm (melissa)	sedative
Herbal Teas	lemon grass	source of vitamin A
Herbal Teas	licorice	anti-inflammatory, anti-stress
Herbal Teas	marshmallow	stomach upset
Herbal Teas	Mormon tea or ma huang	stimulant
Herbal Teas	nettle	diuretic, anti-allergy
Herbal Teas	passionflower	sedative
Herbal Teas	peppermint	heartburn, nasal congestion
Herbal Teas	raspberry leaf	relieves nausea, uterine tonic
Herbal Teas	rose hips	astringent, rich in vitamin C
Herbal Teas	sarsaparilla	anti-rheumatic
Herbal Teas	sassafras	decongestant
Herbal Teas	spearmint	soothing to respiratory, GI tract
Herbal Teas	wintergreen	diuretic, cleansing agent
Seasonings	ajwan*	cooking
Seasonings	allspice*	baking
Seasonings	anise*	baking
Seasonings	asafoetida*	cooking
Seasonings	basil*	raw, cooking
Seasonings	bay leaf*	cooking

Seasonings	black pepper*	cooking, at table
Seasonings	caraway*	baking, cooking
Seasonings	cardamom*	baking, cooking, tea
Seasonings	cayenne*	cooking
Seasonings	chili powder	cooking
Seasonings	cilantro	raw and cooking
Seasonings	cinnamon*	baking and at table
Seasonings	cloves*	baking
Seasonings	coriander*	cooking and baking
Seasonings	cumin*	cooking, in dips
Seasonings	curry powder*	cooking
Seasonings	dill weed and seed*	fresh dill, marinades, cooking
Seasonings	fennel	cooking, at table
Seasonings	fenugreek*	cooking in curry powder
Seasonings	garam masala*	cooking
Seasonings	garlic*	cooking and sprinkle on food
Seasonings	ginger*	cooking, at table
Seasonings	horseradish*	prepared, use in sauces, at table
Seasonings	mace	baking
Seasonings	marjoram*	cooking
Seasonings	mint	fresh and cooking
Seasonings	mustard seed*	cooking
Seasonings	nutmeg*	baking, cooking, at table
Seasonings	onion*	raw
Seasonings	orange peel*	cooking
Seasonings	oregano*	cooking
Seasonings	paprika*	cooking, at table
Seasonings	parsley*	raw or in cooking
Seasonings	peppermint*	fresh or in cooking
Seasonings	rosemary*	cooking, marinades, sauces
Seasonings	saffron*	cooking, baking
Seasonings	sage*	cooking, baking
Seasonings	spearmint*	fresh, cooking
Seasonings	tamarind	paste in sauces, soups, stews
Seasonings	tarragon*	fresh and in cooking
Seasonings	thyme*	in cooking
Seasonings	turmeric*	in cooking
Seasonings	vanilla extract	baking, cooking
Sweeteners	barley malt, syrup, or crystals	beverages, baked goods
Sweeteners	brown rice syrup	beverages, baked goods
Sweeteners	date sugar	baking, at table
Sweeteners	fruit juice concentrate	beverages, baking, at table
Sweeteners	honey, raw only	at table
Sweeteners	real maple syrup or sugar	baking, at table
Sweeteners	*Stevia*	baking, at table

*These seasonings are the most important for Green types.

Now that you know the foods to buy, mark your shopping list for what to get at the grocery store.

Personal Shopping List for Green Types

Food Group	Color	Food
Vegetables	yellow	fresh corn, daikon, yellow squash, potatoes, onions
	red	beets, chili peppers
	orange	carrots
	green	cruciferous vegetables, peppers
Fruit (fresh, dried, juice)	yellow	yellow grapes, lemons, mango
	red	berries, pomegranate, apples
	orange	apricots, oranges
	green	guava, limes, kiwi
Grains	tan	barley, buckwheat pancake mix
Breads	tan	corn tortillas, rye bread
Cereals	tan	Kashi, corn flakes
Legumes	tan	red lentils, chickpeas, pinto beans
Dairy	white	cottage cheese
Dairy	white	eggs
Dairy	white	soy milk
Oils	white	canola, corn
Seeds	white	roasted sunflower, soy nuts
Fish	white	trout, white fish
Poultry	white	chicken breast, tuna, turkey meat
Seasonings	gold	ginger, chili, and curry powders
Beverages	gold	herbal teas, amasake

15

Nutrition Plan for Combination Types

Most people will be a combination of body types. If one type is clearly predominant with one or two other types present, you should follow the nutritional plan for your dominant type. If one type is dominant but a second has a significant influence, you may wish to make some of your nutritional selections from the second plan. If two of your types have equal scores, you will need to balance them with the third type.

In rare cases, you might be an equal combination of all three types. If you are a balanced combination type, follow the plan in this chapter. The combination plan offers foods that are good for all types. It is also the safest and best plan to follow when planning meals for several people who have different types. The drawback of using the combination plan all the time is that it is "neutral"—meaning it doesn't offer the therapeutic nutrition you get when you follow one of the *Eat Your Colors* nutrition plans.

Here is a summary of how to work in combining plans:

- Yellow > Red—follow Yellow plan, watch for (A) Green and (B) Red conditions
- Red > Yellow—follow Red plan, watch for (A) Green and (B) Yellow conditions
- Yellow > Green—follow Yellow plan, watch for (A) Red and (B) Green conditions
- Green > Yellow—follow Green plan, watch for (A) Red and (B) Yellow conditions
- Red > Green—follow Red plan, watch for (A) Yellow and (B) Green conditions

- Green > Red—follow Green plan, watch for (A) Yellow and (B) Red conditions
- Yellow = Red, low Green—follow Green plan
- Yellow = Green, low Red—follow Red plan
- Red = Green, low Yellow—follow Yellow plan
- Yellow = Red = Green—follow combination plan

(> means greater than, = means equal scores in two or more colors)

Although at first it may seem complicated, it's a question of balance. Since most people have a dominant color, carefully following the plan for your color will keep your dominant color from unbalancing the others. As you become more familiar with the symptoms associated with color imbalances, you will be able to switch to the plan for that color and restore your health.

You will find that even if you are a balanced type, your colors will be constantly changing. As Ayurvedic physician Dr. Robert Svoboda has said, the word *dosha* (which is your elemental constitution or body type color) means "things that go out of whack." In Part Four of *Eat Your Colors*, I will present therapeutic plans for balancing Yellow, Red, and Green conditions that can occur in anyone, regardless of body type.

For those individuals who are blessed with a balanced constitution, it will be important to study all three nutritional plans and the conditions that are peculiar to each color. When imbalances are detected, quickly adopting the menu plan for the color that is "out of whack" will restore the balance among all three colors. In cases where the condition is more deeply rooted, it will be necessary to add the therapeutic protocol in Part Four. Herbs make the subtle metabolic adjustments on the tissue level while nutrition corrects the visible signs of ill health.

Digestion and Elimination

Combination types generally have good digestion. However, digestive problems typical of the other types can occur. Difficulty swallowing, burping, belching, and a bloated feeling are typical of the Green type. Eating doesn't relieve this kind of indigestion but only makes it worse. Burning, stomach growling, and discomfort before eating are typical of Reds. Eating relieves this kind of indigestion. Gas and cramping are typical for Yellows and occur several hours after the offending food has been eaten. You may have eaten other foods before symptoms occur, making it difficult to pinpoint the cause. Depending on the kind of digestive problem you experience, adopting the appropriate nutrition plan with the correct spices will help remedy the situation.

Planning Meals and Your Daily Schedule

Find the daily plan that works best for you. Are you a person who gets out of bed fired up and ready to go? Is morning your most productive time of day? A yes answer to these questions indicates that you should eat a good hearty breakfast. Morning will be a good time for you to exercise, but do so moderately. Exercise will sharpen your mind and invigorate your body, but overdoing it will tire you out too much. You should follow with a light lunch and a hearty dinner.

If you are a person who gets going slowly in the morning, you may not need much breakfast but you should plan a hearty lunch and lighter dinner. If eating a high-carbohydrate lunch such as pasta or rice makes you sleepy in the afternoon, switch to a high-protein lunch with a vegetable soup or salad. Then you can save your carbohydrate-rich meal for evening.

Above all, be kind to yourself. Don't make adjustments too quickly and really think about what you're putting into your mouth. If you pay attention to the signals your body gives, you will find your ideal balance. And remember that if you make a soup or stew containing something not on your nutrition plan, its effects will be neutralized by the other ingredients cooked with it. Start making the changes suggested in this book and stick with it every day. The result will be increased energy, vitality, and freedom from disease.

Food Tastes

In the previous chapters, I discussed the six tastes—which are best for each type and which to avoid. For those who are balanced, choosing taste becomes a matter of which part of the body needs nourishing. Each of the six tastes supports an organ system and should be emphasized when strengthening that organ.

Sweet taste is the most nutritive of the tastes. It supports the digestive function of the pancreas. The pancreas has two important functions: digestive and hormonal. Several digestive enzymes are secreted by the pancreas that break down carbohydrates, proteins, and fats. When the pancreas is weakened, reduced amounts of these enzymes are secreted and foods are improperly digested. The partially digested food particles can make their way into the bloodstream and your "immune surveillance team" will move in to attack and destroy the foreign material. This causes a cascade of events that result in allergic symptoms.

Sweet foods are good for the pancreas, but only if they are from complex carbohydrates. Eating too many sugary sweet foods contributes to another pancreatic problem, and that's control of blood sugar. The pancreas also secretes the hormone insulin that regulates the transport of sugar from the bloodstream into cells where it's converted into energy. Too little or too much insulin released by the pancreas has disastrous results by upsetting the balance of sugar between blood and tissues. People who have a blood sugar imbalance, either too high or too low, must be very careful which foods they eat. They must choose only complex carbohydrates and avoid most fruit, fruit juices, and sweeteners. In short, they should follow a Green food plan. Not surprisingly, diabetes (high blood sugar) is classified in Ayurveda medicine as a Green condition.

Sour tastes are typified by acidic fruits such as citrus, vinegar, and pickled foods and support the liver, according to Ayurveda. The liver processes everything you eat, drink, and breathe, including nutrients of ingested toxins. Powerful detoxifying enzymes in the liver process toxic compounds so they can be eliminated safely from your body. Acidic foods high in vitamin C provide antioxidant protection for the liver and assist in its detoxifying processes. Vitamin C is also required for the conversion of cholesterol into bile acids.

The liver produces bile, an emulsifying agent that processes dietary fats so they can be broken down by lipases (fat-splitting enzymes). Bile acids also facilitate the absorption of fats into the lymphatic system. Bile is an extremely bitter, yellowish brown or yellowish green liquid that is concentrated in the gallbladder and released when fatty foods enter the duodenum.

Salty taste is, for most people, acquired through salt added to foods. Natural salts, however, which are really a combination of minerals and not just sodium, are found in all vegetables and fruits. The most highly concentrated natural sources of salt are sea vegetables (kelp, kombu, nori) and ocean fish. Minerals (salt) nourish the kidneys and maintain fluid balance in the body. We get an overabundance of sodium by oversalting food, shifting the balance between sodium and other essential minerals. Too much sodium impairs the kidneys' ability to maintain fluid balance. Hence, regular use of table salt is a major cause of fluid retention in susceptible individuals. It also weakens the kidneys and can lead to hypertension.

Use of foods that are high in minerals such as those mentioned above and replacing table salt with naturally salty condiments helps restore normal kidney function. Tamari, umeboshi plums, and low-sodium soy sauce are acceptable substitutes for salt. Sea salt contains trace amounts of other minerals and is a better choice than table salt for this reason, but sodium is its major mineral. If you have a tendency to retain fluids, avoid use of any salt including sea salt and watch your intake of condiments that have added salt such as olives, pickles, combination spices, and bouillon.

Pungent tastes support the lungs because they are aromatic and help move moisture from the respiratory tract into the air. Cruciferous vegetables, garlic, and pungent leafy greens are foods that nourish the lungs and clear congestion. Pungent spices include cinnamon, allspice, cloves, ginger, black pepper, anise, bay leaf, cayenne, nutmeg, oregano, parsley, rosemary, tarragon, turmeric, and thyme. All of these spices are warming to the body and many people like to add them to food when it's cold outside. Cold weather challenges your respiratory system and one way your body naturally responds is to increase your desire for pungent foods and spices. Satisfying this desire may help you avoid cold weather respiratory infections. Pungent foods and herbs are naturally drying and that's why they are less appealing in hot dry weather.

Bitter taste is one we don't encounter in most foods. Spring greens such as cilantro, dandelion, collards, endive, and sprouts are bitter. So are citrus peels which we discard because we don't like the bitter taste. Bitter herbs such as gentian have been traditionally used to reduce heartburn, cool the body, and reduce inflammation. They are popular tonics for aiding fat digestion and assimilation. In Ayurvedic medicine, bitter herbs are considered heart tonics. Since healthy heart and cardiovascular function depends on proper fat metabolism, there is a strong connection between the Western and Eastern therapeutic applications of the bitter taste. Bitter tastes commonly occur in foods along with either pungent or astringent tastes, thus forming a natural synergism.

Astringent taste is the opposite of sour. When you eat something sour, your lips pucker and your mouth waters. But if you eat something astringent, your lips will pucker but your saliva won't flow. You can most readily experience the astringent taste when eating spinach. It leaves a dry, almost gritty, feeling in your mouth due to the astringency of oxalic acid. Another astringent vegetable that may have gotten your attention is asparagus. Approximately half the population processes the astringent compound in asparagus, asparagusic acid, into an odoriferous substance eliminated in urine.

Ayurvedic medicine associates astringent tastes with the colon, where reabsorption of fluids is important. However, the drying effects of astringent foods and herbs can cause constipation, especially in Yellow types. On the other hand, for Reds, who are prone to loose stools, astringent foods help keep bowels in check.

We can now summarize which organ each of the six tastes is associated with and include the color type who benefits from each taste. This will give you a handy reference for which tastes to select when you need to balance one of your colors.

Taste	Organ	Color Type
sweet	pancreas	Yellow and Red
sour	liver	Yellow
salty	kidneys	Yellow*
pungent	lungs	Green*
bitter	heart	Red*
astringent	colon	Red and Green

*This indicates that the taste listed in the same row is most suitable for balancing that color.

Food Temperature and Texture

When you are in balance, you can eat food that's any temperature. But when one of your colors is off, you'll have to eat your food at the temperature that's best suited to that color. For example, if your Yellow is off, you'll eat mostly moist, hot foods. If Green is weak, eat warm and dry foods. And if Red is out of whack, eat cool and somewhat dry foods.

Your Daily Schedule

Rising and going to sleep—Most people do best if they get up by 6 A.M. and go to bed around 10 P.M. We generally need seven to eight hours of sleep a night for our body to restore proper organ function and relieve the day's stress. If you keep staying up past 10 P.M., you'll enter the Red Zone—that is the time when your Red color is most likely to be aggravated. Between 10 P.M. and 2 A.M. is the time of day you may get a second wind and want to work or study. However, repeated use of this time of night will eventually unbalance your Red element and increase gastric upset, combativeness, and indecisiveness.

If you work a nighttime shift, you will have to work around your natural biorhythms. One of your natural timing devices will be thrown off, and that's the hormone system that determines when you should go to sleep. Melatonin is a hormone secreted by the pineal gland in response to reduced amounts of light entering the retina of the eye. As it gets dark and less light hits the retina, a signal is sent to the pineal gland to release melatonin. This hormone makes us sleepy and signals release of several other hormones that restore our body systems as we sleep.

Exercise—Find your ideal time to exercise and make it a daily habit. If your stamina is low, use meditative exercises such as tai chi, yoga, or chi gong. Slow swimming or walking is also good for you. As your stamina increases, so can the kind of exercise you enjoy. High-impact aerobics should be reserved for those who have excellent stamina.

Alone time—Make sure that each day you leave time for yourself. Enjoy a warm herbal bath or spend time sitting under a shade tree. Read something inspirational, meditate, or just sit and pleasantly cogitate. Get a massage, enjoy a steam sauna, or stroll in a beautiful place. Whatever you enjoy doing, be sure and make it part of your daily routine.

Seasonal Schedule

When you are in balance, the season of the year has little effect on how you feel and function. You should be aware of the times of year that are challenging for each color. If you find a particular time of year is more of a challenge than the others, adopt the meal plan for the type whose season it is.

Your Yellow element will be most challenged during the late summer and early fall months. The times will vary depending on where you live, but as the leaves change color and dry winds blow Yellow tends to become unsettled. Your Red element will be most challenged during the hot summer months because Red embodies heat. Green is most challenged by the damp cold weather that occurs in late winter and the onset of pollen season in spring. You will read about the symptoms that indicate which of these elements is likely out of balance in Part Four of *Eat Your Colors*.

Nutritional Composition of Your Plan

If you were to arrange all your food for the day on a big plate, this is what it would look like:

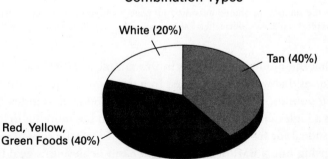

Daily Food Plan

Combination Types

White (20%)

Tan (40%)

Red, Yellow, Green Foods (40%)

Most of what you eat will be yellow, orange, red, green, and tan. The smallest portion of what you eat will be fish, poultry, seeds, nuts, and medium-heat oils.

Now we need to design your daily meal plan, distributing your primary and complementary colors among the six food groups: grains, vegetables, fruits, dairy, meat, and oils. In designing your daily meal plan, we also need to maintain proper ratios between percentages of carbohydrates, proteins, and fats that make up your plan. These ratios differ between combination types and the three individual types. I am also offering two plans here, one for women and one for men. That's because the percentages of carbohydrates, proteins, and fats are slightly different.

Daily Meal Plan for Combination-Type Men

Food Group ►	Cereals, Grains, Breads, Starchy Vegetables	Fruit and Fruit Juice	Non-starchy Vegetables	Yogurt, Kefir, Soy Milk, Grain Milk	Fish, Poultry, Meat, Skim Cheese, Eggs, Legumes, Nut Butter, Seeds	Oils and Fats, Parmesan Cheese
Serving Size ►	½ cup	½ cup cut up or 1 small or ¾ cup juice	½ cup cooked, 1 cup raw or ¾ cup vegetable juice	1 cup or ½ cup cottage or ricotta cheese	1 ounce fish, poultry, meat, or skim cheese or 1 egg or ½ cup legumes or 2 T. nut butter	1 teaspoon oils/fats or 2 T. Parmesan cheese

Daily Calories ▼	Number of Servings ►					
2,000	8	5½	9	1½	6½	1½
1,800	7½	5	8½	1½	6	1½
2,200	9	6⅓	10⅓	1¾	7½	1¾
2,400	10	6¾	11¼	2	8	2
2,600	10¾	7½	12	2	8¾	2
2,800	11	8	13	2¼	9½	2¼

Note: To calculate the amount you should put onto your plate, multiply the number of servings by the serving size. For example, for a 2,000-calorie diet, 7 servings times ½ cup serving size equals 3½ cups.

Note that the number of calories in this sample is 2,000. That's the number of calories that would be required by a man who is 5 feet, 11 inches tall, weighs 180 pounds, has a low activity level, and a body mass index (BMI) of 25. This is a high number, indicating that this man has more fat to lean muscle than is ideal for his frame and activity level. Ideally he should weigh 158 pounds, giving him a BMI of 22. He might easily achieve this goal by reducing his daily caloric intake to 2,000 calories.

To find out how many calories you should be eating, you can go to my Web site, www.thenutritionsolution.com/quiz. You will find that the number of calories you should be eating depends on these factors:

- your height and weight
- your activity level
- your BMI

Go to the page entitled "Nutritional Quiz" and enter your personal data.

Activity Level and Age

You no doubt know your activity level and whether you are active or sedentary. Naturally we slow down as we age and will need fewer calories. However, we don't need a special allowance for age as long as activity level is considered. (Some nutritionists calculate a decrease in daily calories for every ten years of age.) As long as we allow for an increasingly sedentary lifestyle (lower activity level), we automatically allow for advancing age. An allowance for your activity level is one of the questions you will be asked if you log on to my Web site.

Note that for calorie counts in the food plan, all starchy vegetables have the same nutritional composition as grains and are listed with them. When you are selecting which color vegetables to eat, you will be getting the phytochemicals that account for a particular color, regardless of how you account for its calories. If you do move one of your vegetable choices into the grains column because it's starchy, just replace one grain serving with your starchy vegetable and add another non-starchy vegetable to your intake for the day.

Now we will consider the daily menu plan for combination-type women. This plan maintains the percentages of total calories from carbohydrates, proteins, and fats, just as the men's plan does. For women the percentages are 55 percent for carbohydrates, 20 percent for proteins, and 24 percent for fat.

Daily Meal Plan for Combination-Type Women

Food Group ▶	Cereals, Grains, Breads, Starchy Vegetables	Fruit and Fruit Juice	Non-starchy Vegetables	Yogurt, Kefir, Soy Milk, Grain Milk	Fish, Poultry, Meat, Skim Cheese, Eggs, Legumes, Nut Butter, Seeds	Oils and Fats, Parmesan Cheese
Serving Size ▶	½ cup	½ cup cut up or 1 small or ¾ cup juice	½ cup cooked, 1 cup raw, or ¾ cup vegetable juice	1 cup or ½ cup cottage or ricotta cheese	1 ounce fish, poultry, meat, or skim cheese or 1 egg or ½ cup legumes or 2 T. nut butter	1 teaspoon oils/fats or 2 T. Parmesan cheese

Daily Calories ▼	Number of Servings ▶					
1,800	9	3½	4½	2	6	1
1,200	6	2½	3	1½	4	1
1,400	7¼	2¾	3⅔	1⅔	4¾	1
1,600	8¼	3¼	4	1¾	5½	1
2,000	10¼	4	5	2⅓	6¾	1
2,200	11¼	4½	5⅔	2½	7½	1¼
2,400	12⅓	4¾	6	2¾	8¼	1½

Note: To calculate the amount you should put onto your plate, multiply the number of servings by the serving size. For example, for a 2,000-calorie diet, 7 servings times ½ cup serving size equals 3½ cups.

This plan is suitable for a woman 5 feet 5 inches tall, weighing 135 pounds, and having a low activity level. By low activity level, I mean a woman who works out two or three times a week and has a desk job. The weight-to-height ratio of this woman yields an ideal BMI of 22. Women who are pregnant should increase their daily calorie intake by 20 percent. Lactating women should increase their intake by 30 percent. Use your nonpregnant weight to calculate your base calories. If you were overweight when you got pregnant, you may want to modify your base calories intake. Work with your physician to determine what number of base calories you should use.

Again, we find that for calorie-counting purposes, starchy vegetables that you choose would be subtracted from your grain servings. Remember to replace them in the vegetable column with a leafy green vegetable. Now that we have established how many servings of each food you will need to eat, let's see how you might plan your daily menus.

Daily Menu Plans for Combination Types

Ideally, you should eat one main and two smaller meals each day. You will be the best judge of which meal is to be your largest. You may find it convenient to rotate the time of day you eat this meal. For example, if you eat a large meal fairly late at night, you may not be hungry until midday the next day.

Most people do best if they do not eat a large meal past 6 or 7 P.M. You will notice that I don't include desserts in any of my meal plans. That's because you should reserve them for special occasions only. It's best not to eat them after a heavy meal. In some countries, this plan is worked out with tea and sweets in the afternoon and dinner is served later.

I suggest you keep a supply of herbal teas at work and make yourself a cup around 4 P.M. Take a little break and then return to finish up your day's work. Ginseng tea, of which there are several kinds, will enliven you. Korean and

Chinese ginseng are invigorating and strengthening. Siberian and American ginseng are balancing and help relieve stress. If you want to try ginseng, buy only the best-quality tea because the active constituents will be better balanced.

Avoid drinking sodas. They may contain high levels of sugars or artificial sweeteners and phosphates. The latter compounds interfere with calcium uptake and utilization. These drinks are acidic and weaken digestion.

Basic Meal Plan and Options

These meal plans allow for 2,000 calories. You can adjust up or down on servings, depending on which plan you're following (men's or women's) and the number of calories you should be eating.

Breakfast

1 cup of oil-free granola; or 1½ cups of cooked cereal; or 2 cups of unsweetened cereal (2 grain)

1 cup of milk or yogurt (1 dairy)

½ large banana or ½ cup of berries (1 fruit)

6 oz. of tomato vegetable juice (1 vegetable)

Lunch

Large vegetable salad: 2 cups of dark mixed greens (2 vegetable) with 1 hard-boiled egg (1 meat)

2 T. of albacore tuna, water packed (2 meat)

1 cup of assorted vegetables, jicama, radishes, or daikon, leftover vegetables from dinner (1 vegetable, if raw, 2, if cooked)

Snack (either in the A.M. or P.M.):

¼ cup of mixed nuts (2 fat, 1 meat)

½ cup of grapes (1 fruit)

Dinner

Option One

2 cups penne pasta with arugula, goat cheese (recipe below)

1 cup apple salad (chopped apples, celery, and walnuts or raisins, dressed with yogurt and lemon juice)

Option Two

2 cups chicken and shiitake soup (recipe below)

1 cup mandarin salad (sections of mandarin oranges, ¼ cup pomegranate seeds on a bed of bitter greens, yogurt and chutney dressing)

Option Three

2 cups seafood and lemon risotto (recipe below)

1 cup mixed steamed vegetables (onions, carrots, kale, garlic)

2 cups of mixed greens, ½ cup cucumber; avocado; olive oil and balsamic or rice vinegar; cracked pepper

I prefer to use plain dressings of olive oil and lemon juice or mild vinegar from cruets. Rotate the oil taste by using canola or flaxseed oils. Lemon juice, balsamic and rice vinegars are milder than red wine vinegar. I use yogurt for creamy dressings and add green goddess herbs, horseradish and pepper, or chutney for flavoring. When making cheese-type dressings, choose feta or goat cheese because these agree with all types.

You can also add variety to your meals by offering the following sauce. Combination types can also use any of the sauces suggested for Yellows, Reds, or Greens.

✍ Sesame Tahini Sauce for All Types

This sauce is a good source of calcium. If you add 1 T. of parsley, you will add phytochemicals called phthalides *as well. This is a great dipping sauce, a wonderful salad dressing, and adds zest to baked fish.*

2 to 3 cloves of garlic, crushed	4 T. lemon juice
¼ cup sesame tahini	¼ tsp. sea salt (optional)
	3 T. spring water

1. Crush or mash the garlic cloves into a smooth paste, add the tahini and beat until well blended.

2. Beat in the lemon with a wire whisk. Add the salt and mix it in thoroughly.

3. Add the water, mixing, a little at a time. A blender can also be used to prepare this sauce.

Now here are three recipes to try. Two are main dishes and the third is a delicious soup.

✒ Penne Pasta with Arugula, Zucchini, Walnuts, and Peppered Goat Cheese

6 cups penne pasta, cooked	1 onion, diced and sautéed in
3 T. extra virgin olive oil	olive oil until soft
3 cloves garlic, minced	½ cup walnuts, toasted
1½ cups chicken stock	½ cup peppered goat cheese,
1 bunch arugula or mixed cook-	crumbled
ing greens, washed	2 T. Italian parsley, minced
3 zucchini, cut to matchstick size	Sea salt and pepper to taste

1. To toast the walnuts, spread them on a cookie sheet and cook them in a 400°F oven for 5 minutes.

2. Gently heat the olive oil in a large skillet or pan and sauté the garlic, onion, and zucchini until tender.

3. Add the arugula and sauté until barely wilted.

4. Add the walnuts and goat cheese and the cooked penne pasta and cook 2 minutes.

5. Add sea salt and pepper and garnish with parsley.

Makes 8 servings

Nutrition information: Serving size: 1 cup; calories per serving: 203; servings per of food groups: grains, 1½; fruit, 0; vegetables, ¾; meat, ¼; fat, 1¼; milk,0

The peppered goat cheese lends a savory character to the pasta and vegetables. It doesn't taste at all "goaty" for those of you who might be skeptical! Finish this meal with an apple, berry (or grape), and chopped celery salad. Add apple pie or pumpkin pie spice to yogurt and use this to dress your salad.

✒ Chicken, Shiitake, and Bok Choy Soup

3 cups thinly sliced bok choy	4 tsp. rice vinegar
6 oz. fresh shiitake mush-	8 cups chicken broth
rooms, stemmed, caps	2 T. minced peeled fresh
diced	ginger
3 T. fish sauce (bottled oys-	1 T. low-salt tamari or soy
ter sauce or fish bouillon	sauce
will work)	¼ tsp. chili or hot pepper oil
1 T. sesame oil	2 green onions, sliced

1. In a saucepan, bring chicken broth, mushrooms, and ginger to a boil.
2. Reduce heat and simmer 3 minutes.
3. Add fish sauce, tamari or soy sauce, sesame oil and chili oil; simmer 2 minutes.
4. Add bok choy; simmer until tender.
5. Stir in vinegar, season soup to taste and ladle into bowls.
6. Sprinkle with green onions and serve.

Makes 4 servings

Nutrition information: Serving size: 2 cups; calories per serving: 146; servings per food group: grains, 0; fruit, ¼; vegetables, 1; meat, 2; fat, ¾; milk, 0

This soup is delicious and nourishing. There's something about chicken soup that warms the soul and heals the body! The zestiness of bok choy and polysaccharides in shiitake are healing. Serve the soup with a mandarin, jicama, and kiwi salad on a bed of dark greens. Use miso dressing on the fruit or yogurt mixed with mango chutney.

❧ Seafood and Lemon Risotto

1 medium leek, sliced	½ medium yellow bell pepper, chopped
1 cup arborio rice	
2 cups chicken or vegetable broth, to be added in divided portions	3 T. Parmesan cheese
	2 cloves of garlic, minced
	1 cup dry white wine
8 oz. of medium shrimp, rinsed, peeled, and deveined	8 oz. of bay scallops, rinsed
½ medium red bell pepper, chopped	¼ lb. snow pea pods, trimmed and halved crosswise
	2 T. chopped fresh basil
	2 T. lemon rind

1. Cook leek and garlic over medium-low heat until leek is tender, 5 minutes.
2. Add rice and 1½ cups chicken or vegetable broth, bringing to a boil, reduce heat and let simmer uncovered for 5 minutes. Stir occasionally to mix vegetables and rice.
3. Add remaining broth and wine. Increase heat to medium and cook for several minutes stirring constantly, until liquid is almost all absorbed.
4. Add scallops, shrimp, pea pods, and bell peppers.
5. Cook and continue stirring until liquid is reduced but rice is still very moist and saucy.

6. Stir in Parmesan, basil, and lemon rind.
7. Heat through and serve.

Makes 8 servings

Nutrition information: Serving size: 1 cup; calories per serving: 105; servings per food group: grains, ½; fruit, 0; vegetables, ⅓; meat, 0; fat, 1⅓; milk, 0

This is an elegant main course. Arborio rice makes its own sauce as it cooks. Serve this dish with a steamed vegetable medley and a dark green salad with lemon and pepper dressing or a low-fat dressing.

Food Selections for Combination Types

Now you'll need a personalized shopping list for foods, beverages, spices, and condiments. I am listing your foods by category, first by where they fit into your daily menu plan—grains, vegetables, fruits, dairy, meat, or oils— then by food color. In the third column are comments about each food to guide you in shopping and preparing them.

The food selections listed here can be eaten by any type. These foods won't upset any color, but they also aren't as therapeutic as the specific foods listed for Yellows, Reds, and Greens. You might consider these the "safe" foods that you can serve anyone in your family or dinner guests.

Fresh produce is one of your best food investments. You can fill up your shopping cart with produce and spend a small portion of your grocery budget. Skip the middle aisles of the market where items that are nutrient depleted and most costly are stocked. Begin shopping in the produce section and fill in with staples such as grains, pasta, flours, legumes, spices, and high-quality oils. Finish up with fresh dairy products and a little fish or poultry.

Eat Your Colors **Vegetables: Combination Types**

Vegetable Color	Description	Suggestions for Use
Green	aduki sprouts	sprout in 3 days, use in salads, snacks, stir fries
Green	artichoke, globe	steamed, hot or cold, hearts in salads, casseroles
Green	artichoke, Jerusalem	use instead of potatoes, steamed, cold on salads
Green	arugula	zesty dark green on salads, with fruit or steamed vegetables
Green	asparagus	lightly steamed, hot or cold
Green	baby green mix (mesclun)	mix of bitter, astringent leaves, salad or steamed
Green	bok choy	best in stir fries or steamed with other vegetables
Green	broccoli sprouts	highest in sulforaphane, steamed or raw
Green	broccoli, broccoli rabe	steamed or raw, snacks, salads
Green	cilantro	"Chinese parsley," also common in Mexican dishes
Green	collards	steamed or added to soups, stews, casseroles

Vegetable Color	Description	Suggestions for Use
Green	dandelion greens	tender spring variety in salads, steamed
Green	grape leaves	usually wrapped around rice, snack, or side dish
Green	green beans	lightly steamed, cold on salads
Green	iceberg lettuce	least nutritive of greens, source of vitamin K
Green	kale	highest in lutein and zeaxanthin for eyes
Green	leafy green and red lettuces	best lettuces for salads, sandwiches
Green	leeks	steamed in vegetable medleys, soups, stews
Green	parsley	flat or Italian, raw, steamed or added to any dish
Green	parsnips	steamed, very sweet and tasty
Green	turnip greens	steamed, adds zest to vegetables, soups, stews
Green	watercress	raw or steamed, salads, vegetable combinations
Green	zucchini	versatile, raw sticks, grilled, stir fries, salads
Orange	bell peppers, orange	sweeter than other bell peppers, raw or cooked
Orange	carrots	best steamed, 36% more carotene yield
Yellow	bell peppers, yellow	sweeter than other bell peppers, raw or cooked
Yellow	corn, fresh	steam, eat hot/cold, on/off cob, add to any dish
Yellow	daikon	peel and eat raw, salads, milder than radishes
Yellow	jicama	peel and eat raw, salads, can steam with veggies
Yellow	mushrooms, any kind	shiitake are healing, others best steamed
Yellow	onions, yellow	sauté or steam
Yellow	potatoes, yellow	steam or boil, use sparingly, not every day
Yellow	squash, yellow	summer varieties, steamed or grilled

Eat Your Colors Fruits: Combination Types

Most people don't eat enough fruit. You should make sure to have at least one whole fruit or six ounces of fruit juice a day. Vitamin C and other water-soluble phytochemicals in fruit wash out of the system in a day, so it's important to supply fruit daily. Some people find it easy to ensure they are getting the proper weekly servings of fruit by having a "fruit day" when the emphasis for that day is to eat several servings of fruit. Minerals and carotenoids that fruits provide will also be stored in the body from day to day. It's best to eat fruit that is in season and grown locally, if at all possible. In some places, fresh fruit is not as readily available during some seasons. During this time, frozen fruit can be an acceptable substitute. Be sure to add variety to your fruit choices and try the bottled apricot, pear, and tropical fruit juices. Read labels to make sure your selection is pure juice and not just sweetened water flavored with juice.

Fruit Color	Description	Suggestions for Use
Green	cherimoya	tropical fruit, good for salads or snacking
Green	grapes, green	in salads, snacks, baked with chicken
Green	guava, fruit and juice	tropical fruit, good for salads or snacking
Green	kiwi, fruit and juice	rich in vitamin C, scoop out or peel and slice
Green	tamarind	available in Indian stores, condiment

Orange	apricots, fresh, frozen, juice	rich in carotene, enjoy all year-round
Orange	mangos, fresh, juice, chutney	rich in carotene, enjoy all year-round
Orange	orange, navel, fresh, juice	most popular juice, best in winter months, vitamin C
Orange	tangerines, fresh, juice	mandarins are favorite snack
Red, Blue, Purple	blueberries, fresh, frozen	high in antioxidants, use all year
Red, Blue, Purple	boysenberries, fresh, juice	best in summer, local crop
Red, Blue, Purple	grapes, red, purple	in salads, snacks, raisins
Red, Blue, Purple	marion berries	best in summer, local crop
Red, Blue, Purple	oranges, blood	extra sweet, best in fall
Red, Blue, Purple	pears, red Bosc, Comice, etc.	fall and winter, raw or baked
Red, Blue, Purple	pomegranate, seeds, juice	fall and winter, raw or baked
Red, Blue, Purple	raspberries, fresh, frozen	raw in summer, in sauces, dressings
Red, Blue, Purple	strawberries, fresh, frozen	raw in summer, in sauces, dressings
Yellow	apples, yellow	raw or in salads
Yellow	cherries, Rainier	spring, very sweet
Yellow	grapes, yellow/green	in salads, snacks, baked with chicken, raisins
Yellow	lemons, fresh, juice	good substitute for vinegar, marinades, at table
Yellow	pears, yellow Anjou or Bartlett	fall and winter, raw or baked

Eat Your Colors Tan Foods: Combination Types

Foods in this group are very important. However, in *Eat Your Colors* plans, they are considered complementary colors in order to emphasize the importance of eating colorful fruits and vegetables. Tan foods occupy the second most important place in your meal plans. These foods supply a rich assortment of phytochemicals, particularly if they are not highly processed. Unfortunately, most people rely heavily on tan foods that have been stripped of most nutrients and then mixed with sugar, fats, artificial colors, and flavors. Baked goods, most chips, crackers, and snack foods fall into this category. We are also seeing increasing numbers of tan foods enriched with phytochemicals and classified as functional foods. Your best bet is to stick with a variety of whole grains, whole-grain pasta, whole-grain flours, brown and white rice and beans, dried peas and lentils. These foods are packed with valuable, naturally occurring phytochemicals. They are also cost-effective foods for those who are budget-minded.

Type of Food	Description	Suggestions for Use
Breads	biscuits	baked, hot or cold for snacks, sandwiches
Breads	bread, white, or French, sweet	plain or toasted
Breads	muffin, English; white, whole grain	warmed or toasted
Breads	muffin, bran or whole grain	plain or warmed
Breads, baked goods	pita or flat bread, white, whole grain	plain or warmed
Breads, croutons	stuffing, bread	baked or filling, stove top or salad topping
Breads, chips	tortillas, white flour	plain, in casseroles, plain chips
Breads	waffles and pancakes, any grain	hot with real maple syrup, crushed fruit
Grains	basmati rice, white or brown	steamed
Grains, cereals	corn grits	steamed, hot or cold
Grains	cornmeal	steamed, hot or cold
Grains	couscous	steamed, hot or cold
Grains	mochi	baked, served as dessert or snack
Cereals	oat bran	sprinkle on food, in cereals or baked goods
Cereals	oats	cooked, in baked goods
Grains, pasta	pasta, basil	cooked, serve with vegetables, in casseroles
Grains, pasta	pasta, spinach	cooked, serve with vegetables, in casseroles
Grains, pasta	pasta, white	cooked, serve with vegetables, in casseroles
Grains, pasta	pasta, whole grain	cooked, serve with vegetables, in casseroles
Grains	rice; white, arborio, jasmine, etc.	steamed, casseroles, stuffing
Grains, pasta	udon noodles	boiled, in casseroles, with stir fries
Cereals	wheat bran	added to cooked cereals, baked goods
Legumes (pulses)	aduki bean	cooked or sprouted
Legumes (pulses)	mung bean	cooked or sprouted
Legumes (pulses)	urad dhal	a kind of black bean, available whole, which takes longer to cook, or split with or without skin (quick cooking). Serve well cooked with vegetables, grains

Eat Your Colors White Foods: Combination Types

Dairy products, cow's milk, buttermilk, and cheeses are a significant cause of allergies in some people. Goat, sheep's milk and cheese don't seem to cause the same problems and are acceptable for all types. Being a combination type, you will have to assess the effects of dairy products on you. Weight gain, congestion, and sinus problems may result from consumption of dairy products.

Naturally cultured dairy products, including cottage cheese, kefir, and yogurt, are good for all types. Soured products such as sour cream and buttermilk are not acceptable substitutes. Look for cultured products that contain live cultures, are low-fat and unsweetened. Most kefir is flavored with fruit, is unsweetened and is good for you. You can add your own fruit or vegetables to cottage cheese and yogurt.

As for meeting your daily calcium requirement, you will get plenty of calcium if you eat all the vegetables in your daily meal plan. Soy milk contains the same amount of calcium as cow's milk and is an acceptable replacement. For many people, taking dietary supplements that combine calcium and magnesium is a good idea.

You have probably found that I discourage eating red meat throughout *Eat Your Colors*. This is consistent with the recommendations of leading authorities. You can enjoy red meat on occasion especially if you choose lean cuts and grill or bake them. Be sure to read over the section in chapter 9 (page 122) that discusses how to reduce your intake of heterocyclic amines that form on meat, poultry, and fish when they are cooked over high heat.

Type of Food	Description	Suggestions for Use
Dairy	cottage cheese	salads, pureed; use in place of cheese
Dairy	eggs	not fried, as a garnish, whites OK for most
Dairy	kefir	liquid yogurt, beverage, dressing
Dairy	yogurt	snack, topping, make soft cheese
Fish	bass, sea, lake	sauté or bake
Fish	cod	breaded, sautéed, baked (no added oil)
Fish	haddock	breaded, sautéed, baked (no added oil)
Fish	halibut	grilled or baked
Fish	orange roughy	breaded, sautéed, baked (no added oil)
Fish	scrod	breaded, sautéed, baked (no added oil)
Fish	sole, English and petrale or flounder	breaded, sautéed, baked (no added oil)
Fish	squid	breaded, sautéed, and in stews
Fish	trout	sautéed, grilled (no added oil)
Fish	white fish	breaded, sautéed, baked (no added oil)
Meat	beef, lamb	lean cuts only, grilled, baked, stews
Poultry	chicken	baked or grilled
Poultry	turkey	baked or grilled
Oils	black currant	no heat, dietary supplements
Oils	borage	no heat, dietary supplements
Oils	canola, regular or super	reg., dressings, medium heat; super, high heat
Oils	evening primrose	no heat, dietary supplements
Oils	flaxseed	no heat, for sunshine butter, dressings
Oils	ghee (clarified butter)	cooking and at table
Oils	grape seed	high heat
Oils	pumpkin seed	no heat, dietary supplement
Oils	rice bran	high heat
Oils	safflower, regular, high oleic	medium-high heat

Type of Food	Description	Suggestions for Use
Oils	sunflower, regular, high oleic	medium heat
Seeds	poppy seeds	sprinkle on salads, baked goods
Seeds	psyllium seed	add to beverages, dietary supplement
Seeds	pumpkin seeds	snack, sprinkle on salads
Seeds	sunflower seeds	same, use sunflower seed butter in place of peanut butter

Gold Foods: Combination Types

Beverages, condiments, and spices are precious. You use them in small quantities and they modify the nature of what you're eating. Hot and pungent spices such as ginger, cayenne, mustard, and pepper stimulate digestion and help boost a sluggish metabolism. Because of this, they are sometimes referred to as "thermogenic," which means generating heat or speeding metabolism. These are popular spices for weight loss for this reason.

Herbal teas and the beverages you'll find in this table contain phytochemicals that can calm you down, wake you up, improve your digestion or help detoxify your body. They are an important part of your plan. You may find some you've never heard of, and I urge you to try them. You may be pleasantly surprised. Many people are trying herbal chai for the first time and finding it a welcome substitute for coffee.

You will also find natural sweeteners in this table that are much better for you than white sugar. You have probably noticed that more products are sweetened with fruit juice concentrate, barley malt syrup, molasses, or maple sugar. Most supermarkets now stock raw sugar and some offer Sucanat, maple or other natural sugars. Stevia is an herb that is sold as a dietary supplement and also has an intensely sweet flavor. You can use it instead of sugar or artificial sweeteners added to foods or in baking.

Food Type	Description	Suggestions for Use
Beverages	almond milk	delicious substitute for dairy, alone or in baking
Beverages	aloe vera	small amount can be added to any juice
Beverages	amasake	sweet rice milk, drink as is or use instead of milk
Beverages	apricot juice	use on hot cereal or in baking instead of milk
Beverages	berry juice	use on hot cereal or in baking instead of milk
Beverages	carob drinks	use instead of cocoa in drinks
Beverages	mango juice	drink or cook with it, good for sauces
Beverages	mineral water	drink instead of distilled water
Beverages	peach nectar	use the same as the other fruit juices

Beverages	pomegranate juice	use the same as the other fruit juices
Beverages	soy milk	natural flavors for drinking, plain in place of milk
Beverages	spring water	non-bubbly water better than distilled
Condiments	carob	use in place of chocolate in baking, reduce sugar
Condiments	lemon juice	dressings, marinades, sprinkled on food
Herbal Teas	alfalfa	nutritive, phytoestrogens
Herbal Teas	bancha	invigorating and cleansing
Herbal Teas	chamomile	calming, upset stomach
Herbal Teas	comfrey	calming; not for pregnancy
Herbal Teas	fennel	digestive aid
Herbal Teas	hops	sedative, sleep aid
Herbal Teas	jasmine	aromatic, energizing
Herbal Teas	lemon balm (melissa)	sedative, reduces anxiety, hyperactivity
Herbal Teas	lemon grass	source of vitamin A
Herbal Teas	marshmallow	upset stomach, expectorant
Herbal Teas	passionflower	sedative, sleep aid
Herbal Teas	peppermint	heartburn, nasal congestion
Herbal Teas	raspberry leaf	relieves nausea, uterine tonic
Herbal Teas	rose hips	astringent, high in vitamin C
Herbal Teas	sarsaparilla	anti-rheumatic
Herbal Teas	spearmint	colds, relieves congestion, anti-inflammatory
Herbal Teas	wintergreen	gargle for sore throats, pain reliever, antiseptic
Seasonings	allspice	baking
Seasonings	basil	baking
Seasonings	black pepper	cooking, at table
Seasonings	caraway	baking, cooking
Seasonings	cardamom	baking, cooking, tea
Seasonings	cilantro	raw and cooking
Seasonings	cinnamon	baking and at table
Seasonings	cloves	baking
Seasonings	coriander	cooking and baking
Seasonings	curry powder	cooking
Seasonings	dill weed and seed	fresh dill, marinades, cooking
Seasonings	fennel	cooking and at table
Seasonings	garam masala	cooking
Seasonings	ginger, fresh, powder, crystallized	fresh in tea, powder, crystallized on/in food
Seasonings	mint	fresh and in cooking, fruit salads, beverages
Seasonings	nutmeg	baking, cooking at table
Seasonings	peppermint	fresh or in cooking
Seasonings	saffron	cooking, rice, stews; baking
Seasonings	spearmint	fresh, cooking
Seasonings	turmeric	in cooking, curries
Sweeteners	barley malt, syrup or crystals	beverages, baked goods, at table
Sweeteners	brown rice syrup	beverages, baked goods, at table
Sweeteners	date sugar	baking, at table
Sweeteners	fruit sugar or fruit juice concentrates	beverages, baking, at table

Food Type	Description	Suggestions for Use
Sweeteners	maple syrup or sugar (real maple)	baking, at table
Sweeteners	*Stevia*	baking, at table

Now that you know your personal foods, mark your shopping list for what to buy at the grocery store.

Food Group	Food Color	Food
Vegetables	yellow	fresh corn, daikon, yellow squash, sweet potatoes, onions, parsnips, potatoes
	red	radicchio
	orange	carrots, winter squash
	green	artichokes, asparagus, cruciferous vegetables, green beans, mustard greens, parsley, spinach, sprouts, summer squash, watercress
Fruit (fresh, dried, juice)	yellow	yellow grapes, lemons, mango
	red	berries, pomegranate, apples, red grape raisins
	orange	apricots, peaches
	green	guava, cherimoya, limes, kiwi
Grains	tan	couscous, rice, oats, quinoa, wild rice
Breads	tan	flour tortillas, white and whole grain bread
Cereals	tan	barley, corn grits, Kashi, millet, oat
Legumes	tan	aduki, mung, tofu, urad dhal
Dairy	white	cottage cheese, kefir, yogurt
Dairy	white	eggs
Dairy	white	soy milk
Oils	white	canola, sunflower
Seeds	white	pumpkin, sunflower, soy nuts
Fish	white	trout, all white-flesh fish, tuna
Poultry	white	chicken, turkey
Seasonings	gold	black pepper, cinnamon, cilantro, dill, garlic, ginger, mint, nutmeg, parsley, turmeric
Beverages	gold	herbal teas, amasake

part four

Harmonize
Your Colors

❖

16

Signs and Symptoms Specific to Your Color

Eat Your Colors has shown you what color you are and how to use diet to strengthen your primary color and balance your complementary colors. You have read about the protective power of natural constituents called phytochemicals in several groups of foods and learned how they help prevent disease. In this chapter, we are going to take a closer look at how you can recognize when your colors are out of balance and what to do to restore harmony and prevent serious problems.

I have stressed throughout this book that most people are a blend of Yellow, Red, and Green. Now, I'm going to show you what Ayurveda teaches about the patterns of disharmony that may arise from each color. To enjoy vibrant health you will be on the alert for signs of imbalance for your primary color. However, you will also need to be aware of the symptoms of disharmony associated with your complementary colors.

It's important to study all the colors. Equilibrium between your three colors must constantly be maintained to keep all systems running smoothly. Your body is a dynamic system whose forces are in constant flux. When out of balance, these forces, which are your three colors, will send signals that you will learn to recognize. Your body has a remarkable ability to heal itself if you give it the chance by adjusting your diet and lifestyle. Biologists call this homeostasis, defined as "the ability or tendency of an organism or cell to maintain internal equilibrium by adjusting its physiological processes."

Conditions by Body Type

Maintaining homeostasis is the primary concern of Ayurvedic medicine and diseases are treated according to what's out of balance, not what the disease might be. The same disease can occur in different types, but will be treated differently. For example, allergies can be of Yellow origin (inhalant allergies, hay fever), Red (skin rashes, psoriasis), or Green (sinusitis, lung congestion). These are all allergic reactions, but in each of these cases the symptoms are different and the treatment will also be different. Let's see how this works.

Let's suppose Yellow is your primary color and Green is a complementary color. You are bothered by chronic sinus congestion and would like to correct it. Moreover, your sinus congestion has now taken a nasty turn and progressed to a sinus infection. Sinus congestion is a Green condition, as described in chapter 3. However, if you are a Yellow type, your sinuses may have become aggravated by congestion in your intestines. This results in an inability to clear inhaled allergens from your respiratory membranes. When the congestion in your sinuses did not drain, bacteria set up housekeeping, your sinus cavities became inflamed, and you got an infection (Red condition). It does seem odd from the modern medical perspective that the whole process began in your colon and that this affected such a distant part of your body. However, keep in mind that the primary source of aggravation in Yellow types is the colon. The important thing to note from this discussion is the progression of a condition from one that was minor and occurring on the surface (the colon) to a systemic condition (toxic buildup in body fluids) and congestion. It finally progressed to the third and deeper level, sinusitis. The suffix -itis indicates inflammation and involvement of your third color— Red. Anytime you encounter a condition with this suffix, you know you're dealing with a third-level condition, and one that may well require medical attention. We can now visualize a scenario of how sinus congestion in Yellows arises from the colon.

- Poor diet, little intake of fluids, daily coffee consumption, have led to digestive problems and stagnation in the colon. The dietary transgressions at first produced intestinal gas and other signs. This was followed by an accumulation of toxins in the body and impaired absorption of nutrients, further weakening the body.
- Increased sensitivity to inhaled substances such as smog and other environmental pollutants followed, and this was complicated by an abrupt change in the weather.
- The tongue has a peculiar thick white coating and the condition has gotten worse.
- The sinuses became increasingly congested and now there is a significant pain and pressure in the sinus cavities in the temples and cheekbones.
- The coating on your tongue has changed to yellow and there are red spots on its tip. You feel chilled and tired all over.

What should you do?

First—Adhere strictly to your Yellow-type diet. Eat light warm foods and drink lots of warm fluids. Brew some fresh ginger tea and sip it throughout the day. Put several thin slices of washed fresh ginger root into a pot, cover with one or two cups of spring water and boil for at least ten minutes. Rest. You might consider a three-day cleanse eating only your color vegetables and vegetable juices. However, this will have to wait until you have the infection under control. Anytime you are in a stressful situation, wait until you can take some time to relax and pay attention to your body before undertaking a cleanse.

Second—Inhale moist heat such as a sauna or rising steam from a kettle for immediate pain relief. Ayurvedic healers use a nasal wash of herbs to reduce the swelling and promote drainage.

Third—Check the list of foods that aggravate your Green color that you'll find at the end of chapter 7. You should eliminate whole-wheat cereals and baked goods, dairy products, oily foods, very sweet fruit, and fruit juices for three or four days if your symptoms are minor, otherwise continue to avoid them for a week or two until your symptoms clear. Normally, these foods are good for Yellows but not for Greens, and you're dealing with a Green condition. Make sure also to eliminate highly acidic foods and beverages such as citrus juices, vinegar, and pickled foods. Coffee will aggravate sinus conditions, even though Green types can drink small amounts of it. You will find these condiments and coffee discussed in chapter 10.

Fourth—Stick to ginger tea until the infection has cleared and then add hot pungent spices such as cayenne and pepper or add an Ayurvedic formula called *trikatu,* available by mail order and in some stores, to your food. You can also add peppermint tea. As your sinuses drain, your stomach will likely be upset. You may also find massaging your neck, shoulders, throat, and temples with sesame oil and warming spices such as cajeput and menthol helpful.

Fifth—Add medicinal herbs and other supplements for one month to clear your sinuses, remove toxins, and rebalance your system:

Triphala: one capsule three times a day with meals. Continue until digestive complaints and sinus drainage disappear. This may take up to three months.

Amla: two capsules morning and evening with meals. Repeat at first signs congestion is accumulating in your digestive system.

Ashwagandha: one capsule morning and evening before meals. Repeat when under stress.

Probiotic: acidophilus and bifido cultures, 10,000 units per day

Prebiotic: arabinogalactans, 500 mg per day

Zinc monomethionine: 50 mg of elemental zinc per day

Vitamin A: 20,000 IU per day

Vitamin C: 1,000 mg per day with bioflavonoids, including quercetin, 500 mg per day

If this situation just described were a repeating pattern of illness, it would be a good idea to begin the therapeutic program at the first sign of trouble, when digestion and elimination appear to be impaired. You can also anticipate the situations or times of year when your symptoms are most likely to appear and cleanse beforehand. For Yellows, autumn would be the season to prepare for ahead of time.

For any condition you are experiencing, you might go through the steps below as you work through your health challenge. The sample responses are from the above example; you should insert your own responses. Understand that this method is for minor disturbances only. If you have a serious condition, you must seek medical advice.

- Describe your condition (sinus congestion, pain).
- Identify your color and the organ associated with it (Yellow, colon).
- Match your symptoms with the information located on page 246 in this chapter so that you can better interpret what's going on. (Sinus congestion is a Green condition, sinusitis is Red.) The symptoms you first describe may not be your color. (They're not.) However, they started because your primary color was out of balance. (Yellow, digestive complaints and sluggish colon.)
- What season of the year and time of day do your symptoms occur? (autumn, early morning headaches, begins between 2 and 6 A.M., returns around 4 P.M.)
- How old are you? (early forties—the Red years, prime time to progress to a sinus infection, a Red complication)
- What is the color of the condition you have identified most strongly associated with? (Green, the white-coated tongue further confirms this)

Remedy (using the suggestions on pages 247–48)

Analyze your diet and eliminate anything that aggravates your primary color.

Study the list of aggravating foods and beverages for the complementary color associated with the symptoms you have identified (listed below).

Add herbs and spices strengthening for that complementary color (listed below).

Use therapeutic herbal combinations to help clear the condition (listed below).

By following these steps, you will most likely resolve the imbalance. For most of us, a path of weakness will follow a similar course. You will no doubt see familiar conditions arise repeatedly. You may find that seasonal changes or your work environment are contributing to your symptoms. Therefore, you will learn to head off your symptoms by adopting your nutritional healing plan sooner. In most cases, this will be sufficient to alleviate the symptoms. For acute conditions, the remedies suggested in this chapter may be of additional help.

Pulse and Tongue Diagnosis

Traditional medicine systems including Ayurvedic and Chinese evaluate the pulse and tongue as part of the medical exam. You probably noticed that I listed a white tongue coating in the symptoms above. Pulse diagnosis takes years of practice and is more difficult than tongue diagnosis. However, you may be aware of your own pulse and it can further help you identify your color. You will need to be resting when you time the number of beats per minute for your pulse. This is a simple description of normal pulse rates for each color.

- *Yellow*—fast pulse, 80 to 100 beats per minute
- *Red*—moderate pulse, 70 to 80 beats per minute
- *Green*—slow pulse, 60 to 70 beats per minute

The skilled practitioner can detect subtle changes in your pulse and is able to derive a lot of information about your condition.

Tongue diagnosis is easier. Develop the habit of checking your tongue in the mirror in the morning when you first arise. Soon you will become accustomed to what your normal tongue condition looks like—that is, when you're healthy. If you are out of balance, your tongue will give you clues as to which of your colors is out of balance. Here's what to look for:

- *Yellow*—dark coloration, brownish to blackish
- *Red*—yellow coating, perhaps with red spots toward the tip
- *Green*—white coating with excess mucus

An additional sign, especially in menstruating women, is a pale tongue, likely due to anemia. The skilled practitioner will notice other clues to your condition such as cracks, where spots or coating is located, scallops along the edge, or location of lines.

Conditions According to Your Environment

In the following discussions, I will use the term *dosha* more frequently than *type*. The word dosha is more convenient to use when discussing the changing environment within your body and the dynamic equilibrium between your colors. In Part Three of *Eat Your Colors,* I discussed the time of year when you are most vulnerable to symptoms. I also discussed the time of day and night when you will be most challenged. All of these factors should be taken into consideration when assessing what's going on in your body. You must also realistically assess your work and home environment. Our bodies are extremely sensitive to our surroundings, but we choose to ignore this most of the time. Any adjustments you can make in your lifestyle to accommodate your health will pay dividends down the line.

Conditions According to Your Age

As part of the natural world, your life will follow a natural pattern, or cycle. The cycle is divided into thirds, each governed by a particular color. Ayurveda teaches that your age is a factor in determining which symptoms will likely occur. This will aid in interpreting signals your body is sending. Let's explore the human life cycle a little further to aid your understanding.

The Human Life Cycle

Green is the color that predominates during childhood and through the teen years. This is the time of life when all types are most prone to Green-type conditions such as colds and congestion. You may remember having frequent upper respiratory infections when you were very young and these seemed to diminish as you got older. Anyone who is around children knows colds are a common occurrence. This period of life is when the structure of the body is determined. Bones and muscles grow, reproductive organs mature, the distribution of fat to lean muscles changes and the body takes on the characteristics of adulthood. Children display Green personality characteristics—loving, forgiving, and willing to go with the flow. They can also be stubborn, self-centered, neglectful, greedy, and attached, all signs of Green imbalance. Children also have excellent memories—a Green characteristic—and one that parents may often lament.

A transition period occurs between the ages of fourteen and the late twenties, as one progresses through puberty and into adulthood. As we pass through this stage, symptoms begin to shift toward those typical of Red types. The increased desire for independence that's typical of teen years is one way we know this is happening. Another symptom is skin problems—teenage acne is a characteristic Red condition. Digestive complaints such as stomach pains, vomiting, or eating disorders also may appear at this time. And of course, we begin to take control of our lives: getting an education, planning and starting a career all pertain to the organizational and planning skills of the Red constitution.

Red is associated with adulthood—from twenty to fifty-five or sixty. We are more aggressive, take charge of our lives and spend on luxuries, according to our means. We get better organized, learn to adapt to changes in work or home environment, define who we are and what we do best. This period of life, which is marked by drive, success and personal ambition, also gives rise to Red conditions. These include heartburn, hyperacidity, asthma, stiffness or rheumatism, bleeding disorders, and chronic headaches. Eye and hearing problems are common Red conditions and we certainly see our vision changing as we get older. Weight gain, especially in the upper body, occurs at this time. Sleep may become more difficult and dreams are often violent and full of action and color. Red personality changes that are seen include quick temper, increased anger, combativeness, impatience, and intolerance of others.

As we reach the age of fifty, various body functions begin to change. Women go through menopause and men's libido decreases. Hair begins to turn gray and may fall out. For many, this is when years of imbalance begin to take their toll and Yellow symptoms begin to appear. These include depression, mood swings, constipation, dryness, flatulence, arthritis, nervous indigestion, lack of appetite, heart arrhythmia, sciatica, and reduced energy levels.

Yellow becomes more pronounced after the age of fifty-six, and this is the time when you will most likely have Yellow-type conditions. Neurological conditions such as nervousness, anxiety, memory loss, and neuralgia may occur. The ability to digest certain foods and the quantity of food one needs are reduced, and the ability to bounce back from stress lessens. Stamina is not what it used to be and insomnia increases.

Years of wear and tear begin to take their toll as structural components of the body give way. Rheumatoid conditions may creep into joints and flexibility decreases. Elderly people often have a weakened voice and may have reduced lung capacity as well. However, most of these conditions can be alleviated—particularly in the early stages—by a change in lifestyle, resetting your goals and priorities and following your eating plan more closely.

None of us like to think of a time when we don't have robust health. Yet we must be realistic and recognize that ill health will result if we don't pay attention to how we are living our lives, regardless of our biological age. As for the Yellow years, it's a time of life to relish one's accomplishments and set more realistic goals for the future. It's also a time when many people are finally able to enjoy the small pleasures of life as the need to "drive and provide" diminishes. And, if you heed the lessons in this book, the Yellow years can be a time of excellent health.

Now let's examine some of the finer points concerning how to recognize signs of imbalance in your body.

Ayurveda Assessment Tools

There are many tools Ayurveda provides to assess one's condition. Learning to access all of these tools takes considerable study and practice and is best left in the hands of physicians skilled in the practice of Ayurveda. However, I am including in my discussions some of the simpler ones that are easier to understand and use. There are two ways you can categorize physical changes you observe in your body:

1. *Characteristics of Each Color* The first category defines symptoms by color—each color being concerned with one aspect of your anatomy and physiology.

- Yellow is movement—it's concerned with all bodily movement, including the flow of body fluids, secretions, and nerve transmission. *Its primary location is the colon.*
- Red is metabolic processes—concerned with all cellular, tissue, organ, and body functions; in other words, metabolism. *Its primary location is the small intestine.*
- Green is structure and substance—all body structures, secretions, and fluids. *Its primary location is the stomach.*

This first category is used to identify the nature of imbalance based on the body part affected and the nature of the symptoms: whether movement is limited, an organ is malfunctioning, or there is something wrong with a structural component of the body. You will begin understanding any symptoms you have by closely studying your color. Subtle signs of imbalance usually precede obvious symptoms. Symptoms related to each of the three colors will occur in parts of the body that are not the primary location of that color. Ayurveda provides a second system for identifying five specific areas of the body that are affected by each color. These are subdivisions that fine-tune the characteristics of each color.

2. *Divisions of Color* The second category divides each color—yellow, red, and green—into five divisions or shades. Each shade corresponds to a specific area of the body where a symptom can occur. Consequently, this second system provides for the characteristics of each color in all parts of the body. Let's move on to discuss how imbalance or disharmony in each color affects the other two.

Yellow Disharmony and How to Rebalance

Perhaps it isn't surprising that 60 percent of disease conditions are due to imbalance of the Yellow dosha. This seems logical since this color predominates later in life when chronic conditions are most likely to occur. Remember that Yellow characteristics involve movement—of muscles, organs, bones, energy, circulation of vital fluids, digestive enzymes, lubricating fluids, semen, menstrual blood, breath, nervous impulses, and elimination of wastes. Any blockage or reduction in flow of these substances will ultimately affect the structures (Green) and functions (Red) of the body.

Slowdown in the movement of any substance in the body can therefore be considered the primary cause of conditions that we experience. For example, blood becomes "sticky" and its movement is impeded because of biochemical changes induced by diet. Debris carried within the blood is deposited onto arterial walls and plaque builds up, further impeding blood flow. From this emerges atherosclerosis: a breakdown in vascular structure (Green) and function (Red). The process takes years to unfold and can be at least partially reversed along the way by a change of diet and lifestyle.

Reduced elimination of body waste, urine, feces, perspiration, or expelled air results in buildup of mucus, toxins, and poisons within the body. The most common cause is poor elimination due to eating the wrong foods, too little intake of fluids and withholding urination or evacuation. Until proper elimination of waste is restored, good health will not return.

According to Ayurveda, the Yellow dosha governs the other two because it bridges the gap between what's inside the body and the external environment. It's the Yellow dosha that regulates what moves into our body and what flows out of it. The Yellow dosha also links the structural components of the body with its various functions. Clearly body structures must move in order to function. That's why movement controls the other two. Now, let's get some more detail on exactly how the five divisions work for the Yellow type.

The Yellow Divisions

The first two yellow divisions are concerned with the upper body between the navel and the brain. The first of these concerns downward movement and the second controls upward movement.

The first Yellow division includes brain activity and nerve impulses that travel from the brain downward through nerves to the face, throat, chest, and diaphragm. It is concerned with your senses, mind, and heart and controls such processes as inhaling, swallowing, and sneezing. The senses of smell, hearing, and taste all occur in this first Yellow division. In the brain, this division controls acquisition of new information, wisdom, and spiritual and intellectual insight. The movement of food down the alimentary tract (swallowing) is a property of this division. The flow of impulses in nerves and the flow of fluids in the heart, arteries, veins, and lymph vessels are also controlled by this division. Examples of conditions associated with this subdivision include asthma, anxiety, insomnia, hiccups, and tinnitus (ringing in the ears). Yellow-type allergies occur in this division and involve a hypersensitive reaction to something in your environment (allergen) that provokes an allergic response. Typical symptoms for this type of allergy would be hay fever, sneezing, and dry sensitive nasal membranes.

The second Yellow division is concerned with movement upward from the navel through the lungs, throat, and nose. It concerns clearing carbon dioxide and waste products from the lungs and inhaling oxygen and moisture. This division controls inhalation, exhalation, vomiting, speaking, enthusiasm, and memory. In the brain, acquired information is processed, catalogued, and stored. This second division also controls speech and voice control in speaking or signing. On the psychological level, this division controls the enthusiasm with which one greets new adventures and a general zest for life. Typical conditions associated with this yellow subdivision are sore throat, weak voice, laryngitis, tonsillitis, and coughing.

The third Yellow division maintains cardiovascular and nervous response to stress throughout the body. It is concerned with the heart and regulates blood pressure and heart rhythm. This division also controls muscle and limb movement, plus movement of nerve impulses between the brain and other parts of the body. It involves the response to pain, yawning, blinking, opening and closing one's eyelids. Nerve impulses flowing through the heart and blood vessels are part of this subdivision and imbalances that might occur are high blood pressure, vascular and lymphatic stagnation, and heart arrhythmia. On the psychological level, this division supports compassion and accommodation to change and the needs of others.

The fourth Yellow division maintains enzymatic function in the stomach, small and large intestines, and liver. The secretions it moves are digestive enzymes and bile. Imbalance in this subdivision might involve nervous indigestion, diarrhea, constipation, poor digestion and absorption. Stress and rushed eating habits play a big role in this division because stress and eating on the run reduce the flow of digestive enzymes.

The fifth Yellow division maintains elimination of feces, urine, sweat, menstrual blood, and production of sperm, ovum, and fetus. This subdivision is located in the colon and regulates the elimination of all substances from the lower body. It includes bowel movement, urination, ejaculation, menstruation, passing gas, and childbirth. It also maintains the lining of the colon and preserves its ability to eliminate toxins and absorb nutrients produced by friendly bacteria. This division also maintains the fluid surrounding the fetus in the uterus. Not eating a varied diet with lots of whole grains and vegetables has a significant impact on this Yellow division. Disorders in the sub-dosha are extremely common and lead to functional disturbances such as chronic constipation, diarrhea, diverticulitis, appendicitis, irritable bowel syndrome, and development of colorectal polyps. Sexual and reproductive dysfunction and menstrual disorders all stem from this division.

Here is a summary table of Yellow conditions, their location and typical symptoms. Notice that Yellow color covers very general body location and conditions while the shades of Yellow are more specific.

Summary of Yellow Symptoms and Their Location

Color and Divisions:	Body Location	Actions	Symptoms
Yellow	small intestine, colon	separate waste, eliminate	flatulence, constipation or diarrhea
First	brain to navel—downward movement, throat, chest, diaphragm	acquisition of new information, senses, heart rhythm, inhalation, swallowing, sneezing	hiccups, asthma, anxiety, insomnia, tinnitus, difficulty swallowing, dry mouth and tongue
Second	navel to brain—upward movement	exhalation, resistance to allergens, voice and breathing, enthusiasm, memory	vomiting, weak speech, reduced lung capacity, sore throat, dry cough, tonsillitis
Third	heart—movement from inside to outside of body	maintains blood pressure, muscle movement, extremities, nerve transmission	yawning, eyelid movement, irregular heart beats, high blood pressure
Fourth	small intestine—movement from outside to inside the body	digestive enzyme and bile secretion	indigestion, diarrhea, constipation, malabsorption
Fifth	large intestine	elimination, urine, feces, menses, semen, childbirth, gas	constipation, miscarriage, amenorrhea, hemorrhoids, irritable bowel, sexual dysfunction, incontinence

In Yellow types, the colon and pelvic cavity is the part of the body that is most vulnerable to imbalance. Therefore, your symptoms of imbalance will most likely begin here. Your constitutional type controls the movement of bodily secretions (not the secretions themselves), nerve system communication, excretion, and birthing (for females). When your constitution is weak, you will have difficulty digesting foods and assimilating nutrients. You may also have central nervous system problems such as headache, stiff neck, back, or shoulders.

The first strategy in dealing with any of these or any other Yellow conditions is to adhere strictly to the Yellow meal plans. This is usually enough to relieve these symptoms. However, if they have been occurring over a long period of time or are more serious in nature, it may be helpful to add dietary supplements. Following is a list of Yellow symptom categories and suggested supplements to overcome imbalances indicated by the cause. I will begin by giving you a basic supplement plan for Yellows.

Primary Colors

Carotenoids—Use natural carotenoid mixes only. These will be soft gelatin capsules.
Carotene mix: alpha, beta, gamma carotenes, lycopene; 1 capsule daily
Astaxanthin, 2 mg daily
Lutein, 6 mg daily

Complementary Colors

Vitamin C and Flavonoids:
1,000 mg vitamin C with 500 mg bioflavonoids

Vitamin E, CoEnzyme Q_{10}, Lipoic Acid:
Mixed tocopherols, 200 IU daily
CoQ_{10}, 30 mg daily
Lipoic acid, 50 mg daily

Essential Fatty Acids:
Flaxseed oil, or DHA (docosahexaenoic acid) capsules, 200 mg daily

B-Vitamins:
25–50 mg of each B vitamin, 800 mcg of folic acid, daily

Minerals:
Calcium and magnesium—amino acid chelated, 750–1,000 mg of each daily
Zinc—amino acid chelated, 30 mg daily
Trace mineral amino acid chelated complex—manganese, selenium, chromium, molybdenum, vanadium, 1 tablet or capsule daily

Remedies for Your Color Yellow

The following table lists indications of Yellow-type imbalance and suggested remedies. Add these to your basic program and continue the therapy for at least one month. Depending on the condition, you may need to continue for longer periods of time. Suggested total daily amounts for each remedy are given and you should use these in divided doses preferably with meals. If you are taking medications or are pregnant or lactating, consult your health care provider before following these suggestions.

Yellow Divisions: Indications and Remedies

Division—location body system	Indications	Herbal Remedies Amounts per day, take in divided doses
First—upper body, downward direction brain and CNS, sympathetic	headaches, hiccups, asthma, tinnitus, swallowing, fear, anxiety, nervousness, scattered, depression, insomnia, poor memory	*anxiety:* Kava (*Piper methysticum,* 70% ext) 200 mg *depression:* St. John's wort (*Hypericum perforatum,* 0.2% ext) 500 mg *memory:* Bacopa (*Bacopa monniera,* 20% ext) 300 mg *migraine:* Feverfew (*Tanacetum parthenium,* 0.2% ext) 125 mg *insomnia:* Valerian (*Valeriana officinalis,* 0.5% ext) 300 mg *asthma:* Coleus (*Coleus forskohlii,* 10% ext) 350 mg
Second—upper body, upward direction respiratory system, parasympathetic	inhalant allergies, hay fever, sneezing, sore throat, dry cough, laryngitis, lung capacity, tonsillitis, vomiting, weak speech, energy, stamina	*stamina:* Ashwaganda (*Withania somnifera,* 1.5% ext) 600 mg *allergies:* Amla (*Emblica officinalis,* 30% ext) 500 mg, (*Tylophora asthmatica,* 0.1% ext) 120 mg, Holy basil (*Ocimum* sp.) 250 mg *sore throat, etc.:* Ginger (*Zingiber officinalis,* 5% ext) 500 mg, gargle and sip fresh ginger tea *absorption:* Digestive enzyme formula, two capsules with each meal
Third—heart blood and lymph vessel circulation, musculoskeletal, skin	yawning, blinking, varicose veins, lymphadenopathy, high blood pressure, arrhythmia, angina, eczema, thin skin, stiff neck and shoulders, backache, sciatica, arthritis	*high blood pressure:* (*Coleus forskohlii* 1% ext) 350 mg *angina:* (*Terminalia arjuna,* 1% ext) 400 mg *arthritis:* (*Boswellia serrata,* 65%, ext) 600 mg *eczema:* (*Evening primrose oil,* 45 mg/cap) 1,500 mg *inflammation:* Turmeric (*Curcumin longa,* 95% ext) 750 mg *pain, topical:* Capsaicin cream (0.025%) 4 times daily on painful area *skin:* Gotu Kola (*Centella asiatica,* 8% ext) 75 mg
Fourth—small intestine upper GI	indigestion, malabsorption, dry mouth, irritable bowel syndrome, bile and digestive enzyme secretion	*absorption:* Turmeric (*Curcumin longa,* 95% ext) 750 mg *digestion/absorption:* Trikatu (blend of 3 peppers) 1 cap with each meal

Division—location body system	Indications	Herbal Remedies Amounts per day, take in divided doses
		peristalsis: Triphala (Ayurvedic formula) 90 mg with each meal
		digestion: Digestive enzymes formula, 2 caps before every meal
Fifth—large intestine lower GI, urogenital, elimination	diarrhea, constipation, flatulence, miscarriage, amenorrhea, childbirth, hemorrhoids, poor sex drive/function, incontinence, ejaculation, aging	*colon function:* Acidophilus sp. 5–10 billion units per day Arabinogalactans or FOS; 500 mg *PMS, menopause:* soy isoflavones, 60 mg; trans-resveratrol, 10 mg *prostate:* Saw palmetto (*Serenoa repens,* 90% ext) 320 mg *libido:* (*Mucuna pruriens,* 10% ext) 350 mg *anti-aging/impotence:* (*Tribulus terrestris,* 20%) 600 mg *aphrodisiac:* Amla (*Emblica officinalis,* 30% ext) 500 mg

Red Disharmony and How to Rebalance

Red color is concerned with bodily functions and 30 percent of conditions arise from it. The drive that characterizes this color can easily push the other colors out of balance, affecting numerous metabolic processes. It is extremely important to reduce the aggravation to the Red dosha by reassessing priorities and paying attention to your diet. The Red dosha, like the others, is divided into five divisions, each regulating a specific area of the body.

The Red Divisions

The first Red division is located in the stomach and small intestine. This is where digestive functions take place. In the stomach, food is churned and mixed with gastric juice to begin protein breakdown. In the small intestine, food is neutralized by pancreatic juice and mixed with bile and enzymes to further digest proteins, carbohydrates, and fats. Absorption also occurs in the small intestine. Digestive and absorptive efficiency depends on the function of the stomach, intestines, liver, gallbladder, and pancreas. How well these organs function determines the strength of one's digestive "fire." However, all colors contribute to digestive fire, and consequently indigestion can come from a deficiency of any of them. While the functional strength of these organs is determined by Red, the digestive fluids and their composition, plus the organs themselves, are determined by Green. And, as we saw above, the flow of digestive juices and peristalsis are Yellow functions. All bodily functions depend upon the nutrient processing and absorption that occurs in the stomach, small and large intestines. That's why digestive function is the first condition to be addressed in the discussion of symptoms. The first symptom that this Red division is weakened may be lack of energy, mental clarity, and immune dysfunction. Other symptoms that commonly occur are nausea, vomiting, malabsorption syndromes, heartburn, gastric burning, gastritis, and ulcers.

The second Red division regulates liver, gallbladder, spleen, and bone marrow function. As I mentioned earlier, the liver processes everything we eat, drink, and breathe. In addition, metabolic enzymes in the liver detoxify the body and process vitamins, minerals, hormones, cholesterol, fat, medications, alcohol, and other substances. The liver produces bile, a product of cholesterol metabolism, and stores it in the gallbladder. It's the liver that gives bile its yellowish green color—derived from carotenes. The liver also serves as a storage site for fat-soluble vitamins and glycogen, a storage form of sugar. This second Red subdivision is responsible for the formation and breakdown of red blood cells. It also controls the bone marrow. Conditions that arise when this division is out of balance include bilious conditions (jaundice, gallstones), anemia, leukemia, lethargy, skin disorders, and excessive anger or combativeness.

The third Red division is located in the brain and heart. It controls the power of communication, awareness of our environment, judgment, and discrimination. On the subconscious level, this division interprets sensory input and decides on appropriate responses. It is the Red shade most closely associated with attention, learning, reasoning, remembering, organizing, and sensory integration. These skills, sometimes referred to as "executive skills," are highly refined in Red types and are one of their outstanding characteristics. Emotions, material and spiritual goals are centered in the heart and depend on heart function, the role of this division. Conditions that arise when this division is out of balance include selfishness, aggressiveness, depression, confusion, indecisiveness, and low self-esteem.

The fourth Red division is located in the eyes and is concerned with eye function and vision. It maintains lens and corneal function, ability to focus, the humors of the eye, function of the retina, ocular muscles, and function of the tear ducts. When this Red shade malfunctions, vision problems such as near- or farsightedness occur. The sclera (white of eye) reddens, and cataracts, glaucoma, astigmatism, and disorders of the tear ducts occur.

The fifth Red division is located in the skin and maintains its elasticity, function of oil and sweat glands, and surface temperature. It maintains scalp and follicle functions and hair growth. This sub-dosha regulates the elimination of waste and absorption of nutrients through the skin. Disorders of this sub-dosha result in rashes, boils, acne, dermatitis, eczema, psoriasis, and skin cancer.

We can now summarize the symptoms of Red disharmony using Western systems to categorize them.

Summary of Red Symptoms and Their Location

Color and Divisions	Body Location	Actions	Symptoms
Red	small intestine	all metabolic functions	digestive disturbances, relieved by eating
First	stomach, duodenum, pancreas, small intestine	digestion, absorption, assimilation, immunity, mental assimilation and clarity, discrimination	nausea, vomiting, malabsorption, pharyngitis, heartburn, duodenal ulcers, fatigue, gastritis, epigastric reflux, T-cell dysfunction, immune problems
Second	liver, spleen, stomach	formation of blood cells, bile/stool color, liver and spleen metabolism, emotions: maintains calmness, general well-being	anemia, jaundice, hepatitis, lethargy, fever, skin disorders, bone marrow diseases, excessive anger, aggressiveness
Third	brain, heart	emotional balance, cognitive function, brain metabolism, communication, awareness, discrimination, thinking, learning, sensory integration, goal setting	selfish, indecisive, confused, low self-esteem, neuropsychological and learning disorders, functional heart and venous disorders
Fourth	eyes	maintains eye function, vision, emotions: intuition, creativeness, pliability	astigmatism, bloodshot eyes, near/far-sightedness, cataracts, glaucoma, tear duct/gland disorders
Fifth	skin	complexion, skin luster and color, resiliency, skin temperature, sweat/oil glands, skin absorption and elimination	acne, allergic dermatitis, boils, rashes, psoriasis, skin infections, skin cancer

There is a basic supplementation program for Red types that you should follow and it is based on your primary and complementary colors:

Primary Colors

Carotenoids and Vitamin A—Use natural carotenoid mixes only. These will be soft gel capsules. Red types do not do well with tomatoes, yet lycopene is an important carotene for the skin. You should consider using lycopene supplements that contain seed oils and are not acidic.

Carotene mix: alpha, beta, gamma carotenes, lycopene,
1 capsule daily
Lycopene, 1 capsule daily
Vitamin A, 10,000 IU per day

Vitamin C and Anthocyanidins
Pycnogenol or grape seed OPCs, 250 to 1,000 mg daily
Resveratrol, 10 mg daily
Vitamin C with bioflavonoids, 1,000 mg daily

Vitamin E Tocotrienols, CoQ$_{10}$
Vitamin E, 400 to 800 IU daily
Tocotrienols, 5–10 mg daily
CoQ$_{10}$, 60–120 mg daily

Essential Fatty Acids
Fish oil capsules, 2,000–3,000 mg daily
Evening primrose oil, 180 mg daily

Complementary Colors
B-Vitamins
25–50 mg of each B vitamin, 400 mg of folic acid, daily

Minerals
Calcium and magnesium—amino acid chelated, 1,000 mg calcium and
750 mg magnesium
Zinc—amino acid chelated, 30 mg
Trace mineral complex—manganese, selenium, chromium, molybde-
num, vanadium, 1 tablet or capsule daily

Remedies for Your Color

The following table lists indications of Red-type imbalance and suggested
remedies. Add these to your basic program and continue the therapy for at
least one month. Depending on the condition, you may need to continue for
longer periods of time. Suggested total daily amounts for each remedy are
given and you should use these in divided doses, preferably with meals. If you
are taking medications or are pregnant or lactating, consult your health care
provider before following these suggestions.

Red Divisions: Indications and Remedies

Division—location body system	Indications	Herbal Remedies Amounts per day, take in divided doses
First—small intestine, stomach	nausea, vomiting, malabsorption, pharyngitis, heartburn, duodenal ulcers, irritable bowel syndrome, fatigue, gastritis, epigastric reflux, T-cell dysfunction, immune problems, weight gain	*heartburn:* Ginger (*Zingiber officinalis,* 5% ext) 500 mg with meals *ulcers:* DGL licorice (*Glycyrrhiza glabra,* 3% ext) 600 mg *weight management:* Coleus (*Coleus forskohlii,* 1% ext) 350 mg; Citrin or citrimax (*Garcinia cambogia,* 50% HCA) 1,500 mg *diuretic:* Guduchi (*Tinospora cordifolia,* 2.5%) 600 mg *digestion and absorption:* Digestive enzymes, 2 caps with meals *immune:* Ashwaganda (*Withania somnifera,* 1.5% ext) 250–500 mg
Second—spleen, liver, pancreas, stomach	anemia, jaundice, hepatitis, cholesterol problems, lethargy, fever, bone marrow diseases, excessive anger, aggressiveness	*cholesterol:* Turmeric (*Curcuma longa,* 95% ext) 500 mg; Soy isoflavones, 60 mg; Guggula (*Commiphora mukul,* 2.5% ext) 500 mg *liver toxicity:* Milk thistle (*Silybum marianum,* 80% ext) 300 mg; Bhoonimb *(Andrographis paniculata,* 10% ext) 750 mg *hepatitis:* Bhumyaamlaki (*Phyllanthus amarus,* 0.02% ext) 600 mg; Picroliv (*Picrorhiza kurroa,* 4% ext) 500 mg *bruising:* Arjuna (*Termalia arjuna,* powder) 500 mg
Third—brain and heart	selfish, indecisive, confused, low self-esteem, neuropsychological and learning disorders	*depression:* St. John's wort (*Hypericum perforatum,* 0.2% ext) 500 mg; (*Mucuna pruriens,* 20%) 350 mg *detox:* Amla (*Emblica officinalis,* 30% ext) 120 mg; Barberry (*Berberis vulgaris,* powder) 500 mg *tonic:* Morinda (*Morinda citrifolia,* powder) 350 mg *learning:* DHA, 200 mg *heart:* Green tea (*Camellia sinensis,* 40% ext) 200 mg; trans-resveratrol, 10 mg

Fourth—pupils of the eyes	astigmatism, bloodshot eyes, near/farsightedness, cataracts, glaucoma, tear duct/gland disorders	*vision:* Astaxanthin, 4 mg; Grape seed (95% ext) 200 mg; DHA, 200 mg
Fifth—skin	acne, allergic dermatitis, boils, rashes, psoriasis, vitiligo, skin infections, skin cancer	*acne:* (*Rubia cordifolia,* 4:1 ext) 250 mg; Gotu kola (*Centella asiatica,* 8% ext) 75 mg; (*Inula racemosa,* 2% ext) 300 mg *vitiligo:* Pantothenic acid, 500 mg; Raw adrenal complex, 500 mg

Green Disharmony and How to Rebalance

Only 10 percent of disease conditions are due to body structures, according to Ayurveda. This may surprise you since most of us refer to various conditions as something wrong with a part of our body. This idea is firmly rooted in Western medical thinking that seeks to isolate the part that is diseased and treat or remove it. This is appropriate for trauma where the body is injured and immediate steps are needed to repair it. However, there is a growing realization among physicians that the disease process may be more important to intercept. This can most easily be done through dietary change. The earlier a disease process is detected, the easier it is to correct.

Yet we have a long way to go before the subtle signs of disharmony get the attention of most doctors. Western-trained physicians have not been taught to look for subtle signs of imbalance, which represents the greatest departure from traditional medical practice. Ayurvedic physicians, on the other hand, attribute few diseases to body structures. In most cases, they will assess their patients for functional disorders long before they diagnose a problem in an affected body structure. This is assuming, of course, that the physician sees the patient on a regular basis. This is problematic, given the current health care system in the United States. Consequently you will have to take charge of your own health and find a physician who practices complementary medicine—combining the best of mainstream and alternative therapies.

The Green Divisions

The first Green division is located in the stomach and upper gastrointestinal tract: esophagus and sphincters that close off both ends of the stomach. This subdivision is concerned with maintaining the protective mucosal lining of these structures. It prevents the stomach from digesting itself with its own gastric fluids and prevents partially digested food from washing back into the esophagus (epigastric reflux). This Green subdivision forms the sticky bolus of food that is swallowed and the slurry of digested food that passes into the intestines from the stomach. When this subdivision is out of balance, the tongue will be coated white, one will experience fatigue, especially after eating, and nausea and vomiting may occur. Conditions associated with this subdivision are peptic ulcers, epigastric reflux, lack of appetite, anorexia, bulimia, obesity, diabetes, and food allergies.

The second Green subdivision is located in the chest and lower back. It controls the lungs, alveoli, lining of the heart (pericardium), heart muscle, and lining of the chest cavity. The moisture and lubrication of these organs are controlled by this subdivision. An early sign of imbalance is low back pain. Conditions that occur later include cardiac arrhythmia, congestive heart failure, wheezing, asthma, or emphysema.

The third Green subdivision is located in the mouth, tongue, teeth, and salivary glands and governs the sense of taste. Salivary amylase begins the breakdown of starches in the mouth and these glands also secrete the sticky substance that coats the food bolus mentioned above. This subdivision protects the lining of the mouth, gums, and teeth. Conditions associated with an imbalance in this subdivision include bad breath and salivary gland disorders such as "dry mouth." Other conditions are poor sense of taste and various gum diseases.

The fourth Green subdivision is located in the brain, spinal fluid, and sinuses. It controls memory as it pertains to the physical way information is stored and retrieved. This subdivision also governs the genetic information that is passed from one generation to another. In animal species, this would also include "instinct." Conditions associated with imbalance in this subdivision are poor memory recall, sinus congestion, sinusitis, and diseases of the brain such as tumors.

The fifth Green subdivision is located in the joints and it maintains joint lubricants including synovial fluid. An imbalance in this subdivision results in various forms of joint dysfunction, bursitis, and loose, swollen, or painful joints.

Summary of Green Symptoms and Their Location

Color and Divisions	Body Location	Actions	Symptoms
Green	stomach	all body structures, secretions, fluids	congestion, benign tumors
First	stomach, esophagus	maintains the secretory and protective lining of the stomach, mucus, emotions: maintains compassion, groundedness	peptic ulcers, vomiting, fatigue, coated tongue, eating disorders, obesity, food allergies

Second	chest, lower back	maintains the linings of the heart and lungs, alveoli, pericardium, pleural cavity, heart muscle	wheezing, asthma, cardiac arrhythmia, congestive heart failure, low back pain, emphysema
Third	mouth, salivary glands	maintains the linings and secretions of the mouth, tongue, salivary glands, begins breakdown of starch in the mouth	poor sense of taste, bad breath, gum disease, salivary gland disorders
Fourth	brain, spinal fluid, sinuses	maintains the brain, spinal fluid, sinuses, memory, genetic memory emotions: emotional stability, calmness, contentment	upper respiratory and sinus congestion, colds, flu, pneumonia, runny nose, rhinitis, brain tumors
Fifth	joints, synovial fluid	maintains joint fluids	loose, painful swollen joints, rheumatoid arthritis, edema, bursitis, TMJ

In Greens, the upper respiratory and upper GI tracts are the most vulnerable to imbalance. Therefore, your symptoms will most likely begin here. Your constitutional type controls fluid balance in the body, all of the body fluids, secretions, and protective mucus. It also controls bodily structures such as bones, muscles, tendons, organs, brain, and all tissues. The physical structures of the body are the last to be harmed, except in cases of trauma and that's why the Green dosha is least responsible for diseases. However, there are two major problems that arise from Green imbalance: obesity and diabetes. Both of these conditions have their root in accumulation of body fluids and mucus. This leads to functional disorders.

The first strategy for dealing with these and other Green disorders is to adhere strictly to the Green meal plans and get daily exercise. This is the only way you can win the battle against obesity. You may need some help to achieve your health goals and the following supplements are suggested to overcome green conditions.

Primary Colors

Herbs

Garlic—standardized garlic extract capsules, 400 mg per day
Green tea—standardized extract capsules, 250–500 mg daily
Cayenne—standardized extract capsules, 100,000 Scoville units per
  day

Minerals

Calcium and magnesium—amino acid chelated, 1,000 mg and 500 mg, respectively

Zinc—amino acid chelated, 30 mg

Trace mineral complex: amino acid chelated, copper, manganese, selenium, molybdenum, vanadium bis-glycinate, 5 mg daily

Chromium polynicotinate, 200 mcg daily

Carotenoids

Natural carotene mix—delivering 25,000 IU beta, alpha, gamma carotenes

Antioxidants

Vitamin E complex with tocotrienols, 400 IU

Alpha lipoic acid, 300 mg daily

CoQ_{10}, 60 mg daily

Probiotics, Prebiotics (Immune Enhancers)

Acidophilus cultures, 5–10 billion units daily

Arabinogalactans, 1,000 mg daily

Green Divisions: Indications and Remedies

Division—location body system	Indications	Herbal Remedies Amounts per day, take in divided doses
First— upper gastrointestinal tract	peptic ulcers, vomiting, fatigue, coated tongue, eating disorders, obesity, food allergies, diabetes	*eating disorders:* Bioperine (*Piper nigrum*, 95% ext) 1 cap with meals *ulcers:* DGL Licorice (*Glycyrrhiza glabra*, 3% ext) 750 mg *obesity:* Citrin or citrimax (*Garcinia cambogia*, 50% ext) 1,500 mg; Chitosan, one capsule before meals containing fat; Bitter orange (*Citrus aurantium*, 3% ext) 250 mg; Curcumin (*Curcuma longa*, 95% ext) 750 mg *diabetes:* Bitter melon (*Mormordica charantia*, 7.5% ext) 75 mg; Gudmar (*Gymnema sylvestre*, 25% ext) 500 mg; Fenugreek fibers (*Trigonella-foenum-graecum*) or flaxseed fibers (*Linum usitatissimum*) 1 heaping teaspoon per day

Second— chest, lower back	wheezing, asthma, cardiac arrhythmia, congestive heart, low back pain, emphysema	*asthma:* Coleus (*Coleus forskohlii,* 10 % ext) 30 mg; Vasa (*Adhatoda vasica,* 2% ext) 100 mg; Capsaicin (*Capsicum anuum,* 75% ext) 100,000 Scoville units/day; Country mallow (*Sida cordifolia,* 0.8% ext) 300 mg (don't use if you have arrhythmia); Ginger (*Zingiber officinalis,* 20% ext) 500 mg
Third— mouth, salivary glands	poor sense of taste, bad breath, gum disease, salivary gland disorders	*taste insensitivity:* Amla (*Emblica officinalis,* 30% ext) 500 mg; Bioperine *(Piper nigrum,* 95% ext) 1 cap with meals *gum disease:* CoQ_{10}, 60 mg; Triphala (Ayurvedic formula, 45% ext) 90 mg with each meal
Fourth— brain, spinal cord, sinuses, nose	upper respiratory and sinus congestion, colds, flu, pneumonia, runny nose, rhinitis, brain tumors	*colds:* Vasa (*Adhatoda vasica,* 2% ext) 100 mg *rejuvenation:* Arjun (*Terminalia belerica,* 35%) 300 mg *allergic rhinitis:* Anthrapachaka (*Tylophora asthmatica,* 0.1% ext) 120 mg
Fifth— joints, synovial fluid	loose, painful swollen joints, rheumatoid arthritis, edema, bursitis, TMJ, gout, carpal tunnel syndrome	*arthritis, gout:* Fish oil caps, 2,500 mg; Glucosamine HCL, N-Acetyl Glucosamine complex, 1,500 mg; Boswellia (*Boswellia serrata,* 65% ext) 600 mg; Curcumin (*Curcuma longa,* 95% ext) 750 mg *diuretic:* Guduchi (*Tinospora cordifolia,* 2.5% ext) 600 mg

Take Charge of Your Health!

We all experience times when we get sick, and not surprisingly it often occurs when we have been under an unusual amount of stress. We may have been pushing to the limit and finally, our body says, "Enough!"—and we get the rest we should have taken long ago.

It takes many years for the body to get so overwhelmed. It succumbs to chronic illness, and as a chronic illness progresses, it becomes increasingly difficult to treat. Initially, it takes very little to heal yourself. But as one becomes increasingly ill, healing becomes more difficult.

Traditional medical healers recognize three levels of symptoms. The first level is exterior or surface and occurs on the outside of the body or on the surface of the respiratory or gastrointestinal tracts. The second level involves penetration into the deeper layers of the body. This is indicated by chronic disease involving tissues. The third and deepest level involves the structures of the body, organs, bones, and muscles. Here is another illustration of what I mean.

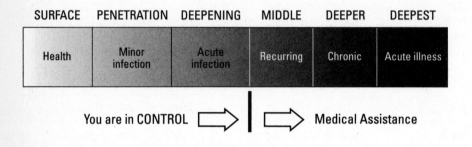

Notice that during the first three stages of the chart, you are in charge of your health. The third stage may involve a visit to a health care provider. It depends on how early you detect the symptoms and how resilient your body is. Take some time to realistically assess where you fit on the chart. At any time along the way, you can reverse disease processes, but it's much easier to catch it before it occurs. Many people are walking around with third- and fourth-stage illnesses. Are you one of them? Apply the principles in this book and take charge of your life.

What About the Future and Phytochemical Research?

We might wish that we understood exactly how phytochemicals work and which to load up on to prevent specific conditions. That's what scientists might ultimately hope to do. In the meantime, the ancient healing systems provide a better solution. By understanding the three body types and the particular path of disharmony in each, traditional healers are better able to predict which nutrients will be protective. Without identifying specific phytochemicals, Ayurvedic healers have effectively treated conditions with foods and herbs. By studying their practices, we now have a system that identifies which foods are important for each body type and its corresponding color. All you have to do to maintain robust health is follow their guidelines and *Eat Your Colors!*

References

1: What Is a Nutraceutical?

International Food Information Council, *Functional Foods Now* (Washington, D.C.: International Food and Nutrition Council, 1999).

United States Department of Agriculture, *Beltsville Human Nutrition Center Report*, 2 Apr. 2000.

Hasler, C. M., "Functional Foods: Their Role in Disease Prevention and Health Promotion," *Food Technology* 52 (1998): 52–70.

Sloan E., "The Top Ten Up-and-Coming Nutraceutical Markets," www.nutraceuticalsworld. com, 1 Apr. 2000.

Spiessbach, K., "Are Nutraceuticals the Future of Food?" *Reuters Health eLine*, www.medscape. com, 1998.

Neporent, L., "Checkups: Food Containing Many Promises," *New York Times*, 13 June 1999.

Hankinson, S. E., Stampfer, M.J., "All That Glitters Is Not Beta Carotene," *JAMA* 272 (18) (1994): 1455–56.

The Foundation for Innovation in Medicine (FIM), www.fimdefelice.org, 25 Feb. 2000.

Klausner, R.D., et al., "Beta Carotene and Vitamin A Halted in Lung Cancer Prevention Trial," *National Institutes of Health*, 18 Jan. 1996.

Gershoff, S., ed., "The Trials of Beta-Carotene: Is The Verdict In?" *Tufts University Diet & Nutrition Letter*, 14 (1) (Mar. 1996): 4–6.

Block, G., "Fruit, Vegetables, and Cancer Prevention: A Review of the Epidemiological Evidence," *Nutrition and Cancer* 18 (1994): 1–29.

Svoboda, R., *Prakruti: Your Ayurvedic Constitution* (Albuquerque, N.M.: Geocom, 1989).

Bhagvat Sinh Jee, H. H., *A Short History of Aryan Medical Science*, 2nd ed. (Gondal, India: Shree Bhagvat Sinh Jee Electric Printing Press, 1927), p. 123.

2: The Ancient Wisdom of *Eat Your Colors*

Bhagvat Sinh Jee, H. H., *A Short History of Aryan Medical Science*, 2d ed. (Gondal, India: Shree Bhagvat Sinh Jee Electric Printing Press, 1927).

Basham, A.L., "The Practice of Medicine in Ancient and Medieval India," in Leslie Charles, ed., *Asian Medical Systems: A Comparative Study* (Berkeley: University of California Press, 1976).

Srinivasamurti, G., "The Science and Art of Indian Medicine," in *Theories and Philosophies of Medicine,* 2d ed. (New Delhi, India: Institute of History of Medicine and Medical Research, 1973).

Sharma, H., *The Body's Healing Intelligence: Awakening Nature's Healing Intelligence* (Twin Lakes, Wisc.: Lotus Press, 1997), pp. 21–28.

Tarabilda, E. F., *Ayurveda Revolutionized: Integrating Ancient and Modern Ayurveda* (Twin Lakes, Wisc.: Lotus Press, 1997), pp. 11–22.

3: What Defines Your Color?
4: What Is My Type?

Encyclopedia Britannica, 2001, www.britannica.com.

Bolonchuk, W. W., et al., "The Association of Dominant Somatotype of Men with Body Structure, Function During Exercise and Nutritional Assessment," *U.S. Agricultural Research Service,* 8 Aug. 1998.

Svoboda, R. E., *Prakruti: Your Ayurvedic Constitution* (Albuquerque, N.M.: Geocom, 1989), pp. 35–54.

Tarabilda, E. F., *Ayurveda Revolutionized: Integrating Ancient and Modern Ayurveda* (Twin Lakes, Wisc.: Lotus Press, 1997), pp. 17–22.

Lad, V., *Ayurveda: The Science of Self-Healing* (Wilmot, Wisc.: Lotus Light, 1990), pp. 31–36, 38–39, 64–68.

Lad, U., Lad., V., *Ayurvedic Cooking for Self-Healing* (Albuquerque, N.M.: The Ayurvedic Press, 1994).

Tiwari, M., *Ayurveda, A Life in Balance* (Rochester, Vt.: Healing Arts Press, 1995), pp. 43–55.

Tirtha, S. S., *The Ayurveda Encyclopedia* (Bayville, N.Y.: Ayurvedic Holistic Center Press, 1998).

5: Yellow Foods

Khachick, F., "Carotenoids in Fruits, Vegetables, and Human Blood and Their Role in Nutritional Prevention of Cancer, Heart Disease, and Cataract," *Nutrient in Composition Laboratory Report* (Beltsville, Md.: BHNRC, ARA, USDA, 1998).

Woodall, A. A., et al., "Carotenoids and Protection of Phospholipids in Solution or in Liposomes Against Oxidation by Peroxyl Radicals: Relationship Between Carotenoid Structure and Protective Ability," *Biochimica et Biophysica Acta* 1336 (1997): 575–86.

Tinkler, J. H., et al., "Dietary Carotenoids Protect Human Cells from Damage," *Journal of Photochemistry and Photobiology* 26 (1994): 283–85.

Miki, W., "Biological Functions and Activities of Animal Carotenoids," *Pure and Applied Chemistry* 63 (1) (1991): 141–46.

Jorgensen, K., "Carotenoid Scavenging of Radicals: Effect of Carotenoid Structure and Oxygen Partial Pressure on Antioxidative Activity," *Zeitschrift Lebensm Unters Forsch* 196 (5) (May 1993): 423–29.

Britton, G., "Structure and Properties of Carotenoids in Relation to Function," *FASEB Journal* 9 (1995): 1551–58.

Pool-Zobel, B. L., et al., "Mechanisms by Which Vegetable Consumption Reduces Genetic Damage in Humans," *Cancer Epidemiology, Biomarkers and Prevention* 7 (10) (Oct. 1998): 891–99.

Sheng, Y., et al., "DNA Repair Enhancement by a Combined Supplement of Carotenoids, Nicotinamide and Zinc," *Cancer Detection and Prevention* 22 (4) (1998): 284–92.

Zhang, L.-X., Cooney, R. V., Bertram, J. S., "Carotenoids Enhance Gap Junctional Communication and Inhibit Lipid Peroxidation in C3H/10T1/2 Cells: Relationship to Their Cancer Chemopreventive Action," *Carcinogenesis* 12 (11) (1991): 2109–14.

Palozza, P., et al., "Canthaxanthin Induces Apoptosis in Human Cancer Cell Lines," *Carcinogenesis* 19 (2) (Feb. 1998): 373–76.

Murakoshi, M., et al., "Potent Preventive Action of α-Carotene Against Carcinogenesis: Spontaneous Liver Carcinogenesis and Promoting Stage of Lung and Skin Carcinogenesis in Mice

Are Suppressed More Effectively by α-Carotene Than by ß-Carotene," *Cancer Research* 52 (Dec. 1992): 6583–87.

Ford, E. S., Giles, W. H., "Serum Vitamins, Carotenoids, and Angina Pectoris: Findings from the National Health and Nutrition Examination Survey III," *Annals of Epidemiology* 10 (2) (Feb. 2000): 106–16.

Stahl, W., et al., "Carotenoids and Carotenoids Plus Vitamin E Protect Against Ultraviolet Light-induced Erythema in Humans," *American Journal of Clinical Nutrition* 71 (3) (Mar. 2000): 795–98.

Frieling, U. M., et al., "A Randomized, 12-Year Primary-Prevention Trial of Beta Carotene Supplementation for Nonmelanoma Skin Cancer in the Physician's Health Study," *Archives of Dermatology* 136 (2) (Feb. 2000): 179–84.

Okai, Y., Higashi-Okai, K., "Possible Immunomodulating Activities of Carotenoids in *In Vitro* Cell Culture Experiments," *International Journal of Immunopharmacology* 18 (12) (Dec. 1996): 753–58.

Jyonouchi, H., et al., "Effects of Various Carotenoids on Cloned, Effector-Stage T-Helper Cell Activity," *Nutrition and Cancer* 26 (1996): 313–24.

Jacques, P. F., "The Potential Preventive Effects of Vitamins for Cataract and Age-Related Macular Degeneration," *International Journal for Vitamin and Nutrition Research* 69 (3) (May 1999): 198–205.

Sommerburg, O. G., "Lutein and Zeaxanthin Are Associated with Photoreceptors in the Human Retina," *Current Eye Research* 19 (1999): 491–95.

Bone, R. A., "Preliminary Identification of the Human Macular Pigment," *Vision Research* 25 (1995): 1531–35.

Landrum, J. T., Bone, R. A., "Carotenoid Nutrition and the Human Retina," *International Journal of Integrative Medicine* 2 (3) (May/June 2000): 28–33.

Khachik, F., et al., "Identification of Lutein and Zeaxanthin Oxidation Products in Human and Monkey Retinas," *Investigative Ophthalmology and Visual Science* 38 (9) (Aug. 1997): 1802–11.

Bates, C. J., et al., "Quantitation of Vitamin E and a Carotenoid Pigment in Cataractous Human Lenses, and the Effects of a Dietary Supplement," *International Journal for Vitamin and Nutrition Research* 66 (4) (1996): 316–21.

Seddon, J. M., et al., "Dietary Carotenoids, Vitamins A, C, and E, and Advanced Age-Related Macular Degeneration," *JAMA* 272 (2) (Nov. 1994): 1413–20.

Jacques, P. F., Chylack, L. T., "Epidemiologic Evidence of a Role for the Antioxidant Vitamins and Carotenoids in Cataract Prevention," *American Journal of Clinical Nutrition* 53 (1 Suppl.) (Jan. 1991): 352S–355S.

Jacques, P. F., Chylack, L. T., "The Potential Preventive Effects of Vitamins for Cataract and Age-Related Macular Degeneration," *International Journal for Vitamin and Nutrition Research* 69 (3) (May 1999): 198–205.

Slattery, M. L., et al., "Carotenoids and Colon Cancer," *American Journal of Clinical Nutrition* 71 (2) (Feb. 2000): 575–82.

Gerster, H., "The Potential Role of Lycopene for Human Health," *Journal of the American College of Nutrition* 16 (2) (Apr. 1997): 109–26.

Stahl, W., Sies, H., "Lycopene: A Biologically Important Carotenoid for Humans?" *Archives of Biochemistry and Biophysics* 336 (1) (Dec. 1996): 1–9.

Clinton, S. K., et al., "Cis-trans Lycopene Isomers, Carotenoids, and Retinol in the Human Prostate," *Cancer Epidemiology, Biomarkers and Prevention* 5 (10) (Oct. 1999): 823–33.

Gann, P. H., et al., "Lower Prostate Cancer Risk in Men with Elevated Plasma Lycopene Levels: Results of a Prospective Analysis," *Cancer Research* 59 (6) (Mar. 1999): 1225–30.

Giovannucci, E., "Tomatoes, Tomato-Based Products, Lycopene, and Cancer: Review of the Epidemiologic Literature," *Journal of the National Cancer Institute* 91 (4) (Feb. 1999): 317–31.

Clinton, S. K., "Lycopene: Chemistry, Biology, and Implications for Human Health and Disease," *Nutrition Reviews* 56 (2 Pt.) (Feb. 1998): 35–51.

Levy, J., et al., "Lycopene Is a More Potent Inhibitor of Human Cancer Cell Proliferation than Either Alpha Carotene or Beta Carotene," *Nutrition and Cancer* 24 (3) (1995): 257–66.

Riso, P., et al., "Does Tomato Consumption Effectively Increase the Resistance of Lymphocyte DNA to Oxidative Damage?" *American Journal of Clinical Nutrition* 69 (4) (Apr. 1999): 712–78.

Kohlmeier, L., et al., "Lycopene and Myocardial Infarction Risk in the EURAMIC Study," *American Journal of Epidemiology* 146 (8) (Oct. 1997): 618–26.

Dugas, T. R., et al., "Dietary Supplementation with Beta-Carotene, But Not Lycopene, Inhibits Endothelial Cell-Mediated Oxidation of Low-Density Lipoprotein," *Free Radical Biology and Medicine* 26 (9–10) (May 1999): 1238–44.

Fuhrman, B., et al., "Hypocholesterolemic Effect of Lycopene and Beta-Carotene Is Related to Suppression of Cholesterol Synthesis and Augmentation of LDL Receptor Activity in Macrophages," *Biochemical and Biophysical Research Communications* 233 (3) (Apr. 1997): 658–62.

Porrini, M., et al., "Absorption of Lycopene from Single or Daily Portions of Raw and Processed Tomato," *British Journal of Nutrition* 80 (4) (Oct. 1998): 353–61.

Jorgensen, K., Skibsted, L. H., "Carotenoid Scavenging of Radicals: Effect of Carotenoid Structure and Oxygen Partial Pressure on Antioxidative Activity," *Zeitschrift Lebensm Unters Forsch* 196 (5) (May 1993): 423–29.

Terao, J., "Antioxidant Activity of ß-Carotene Related Carotenoids in Solution," *Lipids* 24 (1989): 659–61.

O'Connor, I., O'Brien, N., "Modulation of UVA Light-Induced Oxidative Stress by Beta-Carotene, Lutein and Astaxanthin in Cultured Fibroblasts," *Journal of Dermatological Science* 16 (3) (Mar. 1998): 226–30.

Miki, W., "Biological Functions and Activities of Animal Carotenoids," *Pure and Applied Chemistry* 63 (1) (1991): 141–46.

Chew, B. P., et al., "A Comparison of the Anticancer Activities of Dietary Beta-Carotene, Canthaxanthin and Astaxanthin in Mice *In Vivo*," *Anticancer Research* 19 (3A) (May–June 1999): 1849–53.

Woodall, A. A., et al., "Carotenoids and Protection of Phospholipids in Solution or in Liposomes Against Oxidation by Peroxyl Radicals: Relationship Between Carotenoid Structure and Protective Ability," *Biochimica et Biophysica Acta* 1336 (1997): 575–86.

Jyonouchi, H., et al., "Immumomodulating Actions of Carotenoids: Enhancement of *In Vivo* and *In Vitro* Antibody Production to T-Dependent Antigens," *Nutrition and Cancer* 21 (1994): 47–58.

Jyonouchi, H., et al., "Astaxanthin, a Carotenoid Without Vitamin A Activity, Augments Antibody Responses in Cultures Including T-helper Cell Clones and Suboptimal Doses of Antigen," *Journal of Nutrition* 125 (1995): 2483–92.

Jyonouchi, H., et al., "Studies of Immunomodulating Actions of Carotenoids. II. Astaxanthin Enhances *In Vitro* Antibody Production to T-dependent Antigens Without Facilitating Polyclonal B-Cell Activation," *Nutrition and Cancer* 19 (1993): 269–80.

Jyonouchi, H., et al., "Studies of Immunomodulating Actions of Carotenoids. I. Effects of ß-Carotene and Astaxanthin on Murine Lymphocyte Functions and Cell Surface Marker Expression in *In Vitro* Culture System," *Nutrition and Cancer* 16 (1991): 93–105.

Malmsten, C., "Dietary Supplementation with Astaxanthin-rich Algal Meal Improves Muscle Endurance: A Double Blind Study on Male Students," unpublished study from the Karolinska Institut, Gustavsberg, Sweden, 1998.

Kurashige, M., et al., "Inhibition of Oxidative Injury of Biological Membranes by Astaxanthin," *Physiological Chemistry, Physics and Medical NMR* 22 (1) (1999): 27–38.

Woodall, A. A., et al., "Oxidation of Carotenoids by Free Radicals: Relationship Between Structure and Reactivity," *Biochimica et Biophysica Acta* 1336 (1997): 33–42.

Tso, M., et al., "Method of Retarding and Ameliorating Central Nervous System and Eye Damage," Washington D.C., U.S. Patent and Trademark Office Patent No. 5,527,544, 18 June 1996.

Stahl, W., Spies, H., "Uptake of Lycopene and Its Geometric Isomers Is Greater from Heat-Processed than from Unprocessed Tomato Juice in Humans," *Journal of Nutrition* 112 (1992): 2161–66.

Erdman, J. W., et al., "Absorption and Transport of Carotenoids," *Annals of the New York Academy of Sciences* 691 (Dec. 1993): 76–85.

6: Red Foods

Hollman, P. C., Katan, M. D., "Dietary Flavonoids: Intake, Health Effects and Bioavailability," *Food and Chemical Toxicology* 37 (9–10) (Sept./Oct. 1999): 937–42.

Sakagami, H., et al., "Methionine Oxidation and Apoptosis Induction by Ascorbate, Gallate and Hydrogen Peroxide," *Anticancer Research* 17 (4A) (July/Aug. 1997): 2565–70.

Ribéreau-Gayon, P., "The Tannins," in *Plant Phenolics* (Edinburgh: Oliver & Tweed, 1972), p. 169.

al-Sereiti, M. R., et al., "Pharmacology of Rosemary (*Rosmarinus officinalis* L.) and Its Therapeutic Potentials," *Indian Journal of Experimental Biology* 37 (2) (Feb. 1999): 124–30.

Nardini, M., et al., "Effects of Caffeic Acid on Tert-butyl Hydroperoxide-Induced Oxidative Stress in U937," *Free Radical Biology and Medicine* 25 (9) (Dec. 1998): 1098–1105.

Natella, F., et al., "Benzoic Acid and Cinnamic Acid Derivatives as Antioxidants: Structure-Activity Relation," *Journal of Agricultural and Food Chemistry* 47 (4) (Apr. 1999): 1453–59.

Nardini, M., et al., "Inhibition of Human Low-Density Lipoprotein Oxidation by Caffeic Acid and Other Hydroxycinnamic Acid Derivatives," *Free Radical Pathology and Medicine* 19 (5) (Nov. 1995): 541–52.

Yamanaka, N., et al., "Prooxidant Activity of Caffeic Acid, Dietary Non-Flavonoid Phenolic Acid, on Cu^{+2}-Induced Low Density Lipoprotein Oxidation," *FEBS Letters* 405 (2) (Mar. 1997): 186–90.

Satoh, K., et al., "Copper, But Not Iron, Enhances Apoptosis-Inducing Activity of Antioxidants," *Anticancer Research* 17 (4A) (July/Aug. 1997): 2487–90.

Barch, D. H., et al., "Structure-Function Relationships of the Dietary Anticarcinogen Ellagic Acid," *Carcinogenesis* 17 (2) (Feb. 1996): 265–69.

Stoner, G. D., Mukhtar, H., "Polyphenols as Cancer Chemopreventive Agents," *Journal of Cellular Biochemistry* (Suppl. 22) (1995): 169–80.

Kuzminski, L. N., et al., "Cranberry Juice and Urinary Tract Infections: Is There a Beneficial Relationship?" *Nutrition Reviews* 54 (11, pt. 2) (1996): S87–S90.

Avorn, J., et al., "Reduction of Bacteriuria and Pyuria After Ingestion of Cranberry Juice," *JAMA* 271 (1994): 751–54.

Zafrini, D., et al., "Inhibitory Activity of Cranberry Juice on Adherence of Type I and Type P Fimbriated Escherichia coli to Eucaryotic Cells," *Antimicrobial Agents and Chemotherapy* 33 (1) (Jan. 1989): 92–98.

Habash, M. D., et al., "The Effect of Water, Ascorbic Acid, and Cranberry Derived Supplementation on Human Urine and Uropathogen Adhesion to Silicone Rubber," *Canadian Journal of Microbiology* 45 (10) (Oct. 1999): 691–94.

Sobota, E. E., "Inhibition of Bacterial Adherence by Cranberry Juice: Potential Use for the Treatment of Urinary Tract Infections," *Urology* 32 (Suppl.) (1988): 9–11.

Walker, E. B., et al., "Cranberry Concentrate: UTI Prophylaxis," *Journal of Family Practice* 45 (1997): 167–68.

Weiss, E. B., et al., "Inhibiting Interspecies Coaggregation of Plaque Bacteria with a Cranberry Juice Constituent," *Journal of the American Dental Association* 130 (1) (Jan. 1999): 36.

Raloff, J., "Berry Promising Anticancer Prospects," *Science News* 157 (10) (2000).

Aviram, M., et al., "Pomegranate Juice Consumption Reduces Oxidative Stress, Atherogenic Modifications to LDL, and Platelet Aggregation: Studies in Humans and in Atherosclerotic Apolipoprotein E-deficient Mice," *American Journal of Clinical Nutrition* 71 (5) (May 2000): 1062–76.

Schubert, S. Y., et al., "Antioxidant and Eicosanoid Enzyme Inhibition Properties of Pomegranate Seed Oil and Fermented Juice Flavonoids," *Journal of Ethnopharmacology* 66 (1) (July 1999): 11–17.

Butland, B. K., et al., "Diet, Lung Function, and Lung Function Decline in a Cohort of 2,512 Middle Aged Men," *Thorax* 55 (2) (Feb. 2000): 102–6.

Raloff, J., "Well-Done Research: New Recipes for Making Seriously Browned Meats Less of a Cancer Risk," *Science News* 155 (Apr. 1999): 264–66.

Wang, H., et al., "Antioxidant Polyphenols from Tart Cherries (Prunus cerasus)," *Journal of Agricultural and Food Chemistry* 47 (3) (Mar. 2000): 840–44.

Balough, Z., Gray, J. I., et al., "Formation and Inhibition of Heterocyclic Aromatic Amines in Fried Ground Beef Patties," *Food and Chemical Toxicology* 38 (5) (May 2000): 395–401.

Abu-Amsha, R., et al., "Phenolic Content of Various Beverages Determines the Extent of Inhibition of Human Serum and Low-Density Lipoprotein Oxidation In Vitro: Identification and Mechanism of Action of Some Cinnamic Acid Derivatives from Red Wine," *Clinical Science* 91 (4) (Oct. 1996): 449–58.

Leger, A. S., et al., "Factors Associated with Cardiac Mortality in Developed Countries with Particular Reference to the Consumption of Wine," *Lancet* 1 (8124) (May 1979): 1017–20.

Demrow, H. S., et al., "Administration of Wine and Grape Juice Inhibits *in vivo* Platelet Activity and Thrombosis in Stenosed Canine Coronary Arteries," *Circulation* 91 (4) (Feb. 1995): 1182–88.

Ferrero, M. E., et al., "Activity *In Vitro* of Resveratrol on Granulocyte and Monocyte Adhesion to Endothelium," *American Journal of Clinical Nutrition* 68 (6) (Dec. 1998): 1208–14.

Jang, M., et al., "Cancer Chemopreventive Activity of Resveratrol, a Natural Product Derived from Grapes," *Science* 275 (5297) (Jan. 1997): 218–20.

Scott, B. C., et al., "Evaluation of the Antioxidant Actions of Ferulic Acid and Catechins," *Free Radical Research Communications* 19 (4) (1993): 241–53.

Bagchi, D., *Green Tea: Antioxidant Power to Fight Disease* (Los Angeles: Keats Publishing, 1999), p. 7.

Taylor, N., *Green Tea: The Natural Secret for a Healthier Life* (New York: Kensington Publishing, 1988), pp. 1–2.

Hara, Y., "Multifunctional Activities of Tea Polyphenols," Food Research Laboratories, Mitsui Norin Co., Ltd., Fujieda-city, Japan, unpublished, 1993.

Brown, M. D., "Green Tea (Camilla sinensis) Extract and Its Possible Role in the Prevention of Cancer," *Alternative Medicine Review* 4 (5) (1999): 360–70.

Dulloo, A. G., et al., "Efficacy of a Green Tea Extract Rich in Catechin Polyphenols and Caffeine in Increasing 24-h Energy Expenditure and Fat Oxidation in Humans," *American Journal of Clinical Nutrition* 70 (1999): 1040–45.

Katiyar, S. K., et al., "Green Tea and Skin," *Archives of Dermatology* 136 (8) (Aug. 2000): 989–94.

Mukhtar, H., Ahmad, N., "Tea Polyphenols: Prevention of Cancer and Optimizing Health," *American Journal of Clinical Nutrition* 71 (6 Suppl.) (June 2000): 1698S–1702S.

Ren, F., et al., "Tea Polyphenols Down-Regulate the Expression of the Androgen Receptor in LNCaP Prostate Cancer Cells," *Oncogene* 19 (15) (Apr. 2000): 1924–32.

Nakachi, K., et al., "Influence of Drinking Green Tea on Breast Cancer Malignancy Among Japanese Patients," *Japanese Journal of Cancer Research* 89 (3) (Mar. 1998): 254–61.

Hegarty, V. M., et al., "Tea Drinking and Bone Mineral Density in Older Women," *American Journal of Clinical Nutrition* 71 (4) (Apr. 2000): 1003–7.

Harvey, P., "Cup of Tea Can Cut the Risk of Heart Attack," *NNFA Today* 13 (10) (Nov. 1999): 9.

Middleton, E., "Biological Properties of Plant Flavonoids: An Overview," *International Journal of Pharmacognosy* 34 (5) (1996): 344–48.

7: Green Foods

Raloff, J., "Fighting Cancer—If You Don't Like Broccoli," *Science News* 152 (1997):183.

McKechnie, J. L, ed., *Webster's New Universal Unabridged Dictionary*, 2nd ed. (New York: Simon & Schuster, 1987), p. 438.

Michaud, D. S., et al., "Fruit and Vegetable Intake and Incidence of Bladder Cancer in a Male Prospective Cohort," *Journal of the National Cancer Institute* 91 (7) (1999): 605–13.

Walaszek, Z., et al., "Reduced Levels of D-Glucaric Acid in Mammary Tumor-Bearing Hosts and the Effect of Its Supplementation During Estrogen Replacement and Tamoxifen Therapy," *Proceedings of the Annual Meeting of the American Association for Cancer Research* 37 (1996): A1254.

Hecht, S. S. "Chemoprevention of Cancer by Isothiocyanates, Modifiers of Carcinogen Metabolism," *Journal of Nutrition* 129 (Mar. 1999): 768S–774S.

Hecht, S. S., "Tobacco and Cancer: Approaches Using Carcinogen Biomarkers and Chemoprevention," *Annals of the New York Academy of Sciences* 833 (Dec. 1997): 91–111.

Hecht, S. S., "Chemoprevention of Lung Cancer by Isothiocyanates," *Advances in Experimental Medicine and Biology* 401 (1996): 1–11.

Jiao, D., et al., "Thiol Conjugates of Isothiocyanates as Chemopreventive Agents of Tobacco Nitrosamine-Induced Lung Cancer (Meeting abstract)," *Proceedings of the Annual Meeting of the American Association for Cancer Research* 38 (1997): A2423.

Shapiro, T. A., et al., "Human Metabolism and Excretion of Cancer Chemoprotective Glucosinolates and Isothiocyanates of Cruciferous Vegetables," *Cancer Epidemiology, Biomarkers and Prevention* 7 (12) (Dec. 1998): 1091–100.

Stoner, G. D., et al., "Isothiocyanates and Freeze-Dried Strawberries as Inhibitors of Esophageal Cancer," *Toxicology Science* 52 (2 Suppl.) (Dec. 1999): 95–100.

Cover, C. M., Firestone, G. L., "Indole-3-Carbinol and Tamoxifen Cooperate to Arrest the Cell Cycle of MCF-7 Human Breast Cancer Cells," *Cancer Research* 59 (6) (1999): 1244–51.

Cover, C. M., "Long-Term Responses of Women to Indole-3-Carbinol or a High Fiber Diet," *Cancer Epidemiology, Biomarkers and Prevention* 3 (7) (1994): 591–95.

Sarne, D., "Effects of the Environment, Chemicals and Drugs on Thyroid Function," *Thyroid Disease Manager,* University of Illinois College of Medicine, Chicago (1999): www.thyroidmanager.org.

Hashim, S., et al., "Chemoprevention of DMBA-Induced Transplacental and Translactational Carcinogenesis in Mice by Oil from Mustard Seeds," *Cancer Letters* 134 (2) (1998): 217–26.

Lust, K. D., "Maternal Intake of Cruciferous Vegetables and Other Foods and Colic Symptoms in Exclusively Breast-Fed Infants," *Journal of the American Dietetic Association* 96 (1) (1996): 46–48.

Koch, H. P., Lawson, L. D., "The Composition and Chemistry of Garlic Cloves and Processed Garlic," in *Garlic: The Science and Therapeutic Application of Allium sativum L. and Related Species* (Baltimore, Williams & Wilkins, 1996), pp. 1–11, 38, 41, 68.

Lawson, L., "Garlic Oil for Hyperlipidemia: Analysis of Recent Negative Results," *Quarterly Review of Natural Medicine* (Fall 1998): 187–89.

Warshafsky, S., et al., "Effect of Garlic on Total Serum Cholesterol," *Annals of Internal Medicine,* 119 (1993): 599–605.

Silagy, C. A., Neil, A. N., "A Meta-Analysis of the Effect of Garlic on Blood Pressure," *Journal of Hypertension* 12 (1994): 463–68.

Adler, A. J., Holub, B. J., "Effect of Garlic and Fish Oil Supplementation on Serum Lipid and Lipoprotein Concentrations in Hypercholesterolemic Men," *American Journal of Clinical Nutrition* 65 (2) (1997): 445–50.

Saradeth, S., et al., "Does Garlic Alter the Lipid Pattern in Normal Volunteers?" *Phytomedicine* 1 (1994): 183–85.

Rendu, F., et al., "Ajoene, the Antiplatelet Compound Derived from Garlic, Specifically Inhibits Platelet Release Reaction by Affecting the Plasma Membrane Internal Micro Viscosity," *Biochemical Pharmacology* 38 (8) (1989): 1321–28.

Goldman, I. L., et al., "Antiplatelet Activity in Onion (*Allium cepa*) Is Sulfur Dependent," *Thrombosis and Haemostasis* 76 (3) (1997): 450–52.

Das, I., et al., "Potent Activation of Nitric Oxide Synthase by Garlic: A Basis for Its Therapeutic Applications," *Current Medical Research and Opinion* 13 (5) (1995): 257–63.

Lau, B. H., et al., "*Allium sativum* (Garlic) and Cancer Prevention," *Nutrition Research* 10 (1990): 937–48.

8: Tan Foods

Rimm, E. F., et al., "Vegetable, Fruit, and Cereal Fiber Intake and Risk of Coronary Heart Disease Among Men," *Journal of the American Medical Association* 275 (6) (Feb. 1996): 447–51.

Liu, S., et al., "Whole Grain Consumption and Risk of Ischemic Stroke in Women: A Prospective Study," *Journal of the American Medical Association* 284 (12) (Sept. 2000): 1534–40.

Meyer, K. A., et al., "Carbohydrates, Dietary Fiber, and Incident Type 2 Diabetes in Older Women," *American Journal of Clinical Nutrition* 71 (4) (Apr. 2000): 921–30.

Schatzkin, A., et al., "Lack of Effect of a Low-Fat, High-Fiber Diet on the Recurrence of Colorectal Adenomas: Polyp Prevention Trial Study Group," *New England Journal of Medicine* 342 (16) (Apr. 2000): 1149–55.

Alberts, D. S., et al., "Lack of Effect of a High-Fiber Cereal Supplement on the Recurrence of Colorectal Adenomas," *New England Journal of Medicine* 342 (16) (Apr. 2000): 1156–62.

Challier, B., et al., "Garlic, Onion and Cereal Fibre as Protective Factors for Breast Cancer: A French Case-Controlled Study," *European Journal of Epidemiology* 14 (8) (Dec. 1998): 737–47.

Liljeberg, H. G., et al., "Effect of the Glycemic Index and Content of Indigestible Carbohydrates of Cereal-Based Breakfast Meals on Glucose Tolerance at Lunch in Healthy Subjects," *American Journal of Clinical Nutrition* 69 (4) (Apr. 1999): 647–55.

Holt, S. H., et al., "The Effects of High-Carbohydrate vs. High-Fat Breakfasts on Feelings of Fullness and Alertness, and Subsequent Food Intake," *International Journal of Food Sciences and Nutrition* 50 (1) (Jan. 1999): 13–28.

Bruce, B., et al., "A Diet High in Whole and Unrefined Foods Favorably Alters Lipids, Antioxidant Defenses and Colon Function," *Journal of the American College of Nutrition* 19 (1) (Feb. 2000): 61–67.

Zielinski, H., Kozlowska, H., "Antioxidant Activity and Total Phenolics in Selected Cereal Grains and Their Different Morphological Fractions," *Journal of Agricultural and Food Chemistry* 48 (6) (June 2000): 2008–16.

Hill, M. J., "Cereals, Cereal Fibre and Colorectal Cancer Risk: A Review of the Epidemiological Literature," *European Journal of Cancer Prevention* 6 (3) (June 1997): 219–25.

Slavin, J., et al., "Whole-Grain Consumption and Chronic Disease: Protective Mechanisms," *Nutrition and Cancer* 27 (1) (1997): 14–21.

Johnson, I. T., "Antioxidants and Anticarcinogens," *European Journal of Cancer Prevention*, 7 (Suppl. 2) (May 1998): S55–62.

Nair, P. P., et al., "Diet, Nutrition Intake, and Metabolism in Populations at High and Low Risk for Colon Cancer: Dietary Cholesterol, Beta-sitosterol, and Stigmasterol," *American Journal of Clinical Nutrition* 40 (4 Suppl.) (Oct. 1984): 927–30.

Moghadasian, M. H., Frohlich, J. J., "Effects of Dietary Phytosterols on Cholesterol Metabolism and Atherosclerosis: Clinical and Experimental Evidence," *American Journal of Medicine* 107 (1999): 588–94.

Koide, T., et al., "Antitumor Effect of Hydrolyzed Anthocyanin from Grape Rinds and Red Rice," *Cancer Biotherapy and Radiopharmaceuticals* 11 (4) (Aug. 1996): 273–77.

Fuller, R., Gibson, G. R., "Modification of the Intestinal Microflora Using Probiotics and Prebiotics," *Scandinavian Journal of Gastroenterology* 32 (Suppl. 222) (1997): 28–31.

Hauer, J., Anderer, F. A., "Mechanism of Stimulation of Human Natural Killer Cytotoxicity by Arabinogalactan from *Larix occidentalis*," *Cancer Immunology and Immunotherapy* 36 (1993): 237–44.

Luettig, B., et al., "Macrophage Activation by the Polysaccharide Arabinogalactan Isolated from Plant Cell Cultures of Echinacea Purpurea," *Journal of the National Cancer Institute* 81 (1989): 669–75.

De Francischi, M. L., et al., "Chemical, Nutritional and Technological Characteristics of Buckwheat and Non-Prolamine Flours in Comparison to Wheat Flour," *Plant Foods and Human Nutrition* 46 (4) (Dec. 1994): 323–29.

Shils, Maurice, et al., *Modern Nutrition in Health and Disease,* 8th ed. (Philadelphia: Lea & Febiger, 1994).

Messina, M. J., "Legumes and Soybeans: Overview of Their Nutritional Profiles and Health Effects," *American Journal of Clinical Nutrition* 70 (3 Suppl.) (1999): 439S–450SS.

Persky, V., "Soy and Cancer Risk: Epidemiological Studies" (Meeting abstract), First International Symposium on the Role of Soy in Prevention and Treatment of Chronic Disease, Mesa, Arizona, 20–23 February 1994.

Moyad, M. A., "Soy, Disease Prevention, and Prostate Cancer," *Seminars in Urology and Oncology* 17 (2) (1999): 97–102.

Tham, D. M., et al., "Clinical Review 97: Potential Health Benefits of Dietary Phytoestrogens: A Review of the Clinical, Epidemiological, and Mechanistic Evidence," *Journal of Clinical Endocrinology and Metabolism* 83 (7) (1998): 2223–35.

Messina, M., "Hypothesize Health Benefits of Soybean Isoflavones," *Fundamentals of Applied Toxicology* 30 (1) (1996): 87.

Cline, J. M., "Phytochemicals for the Prevention of Breast and Endometrial Cancer," *Cancer Treatment Research* 94 (1998): 107–34.

Katare, M., et al., "Inhibition of Aberrant Proliferation and Induction of Apoptosis in Preneoplastic Human Mammary Epithelial Cells by Natural Phytochemicals," *Oncology Reports* 5 (2) (1998): 311–15.

Capone, S. L., Bagga, D., Heber, D., Glaspy, J., "Effect of Low-Fat Diet with Fish Oil and Soy Supplementation on Composition of Body Fat in High-Risk Breast Cancer Patients" (Meeting abstract), *Proceedings of the Annual Meeting of the American Society of Clinical Oncology* 15 (1996): 1408.

Bagga, D., et al., "Effects of a Very Low-Fat, High-Fiber Diet on Serum Hormones and Menstrual Function: Implications for Breast Cancer Prevention," *Cancer* 76 (12) (Dec. 1995): 2491–96.

Margolis, S., et al., "Coronary Heart Disease," *Johns Hopkins White Papers*. Baltimore, Md., 2000.

Komaroff, A. L., ed., "A New Theory of Heart Attack," *Harvard Health Letter* 25 (2) (Dec. 1999): 1–2.

Anderson, J. W., et al., "Meta-Analysis of the Effects of Soy Protein Intake on Serum Lipids," *New England Journal of Medicine* 333 (5) (Aug. 1999): 276–82.

Wong, W. W., "Cholesterol-Lowering Effect of Soy Protein in Normocholesterolemic and Hypercholesterolemic Men," *American Journal of Clinical Nutrition* 68 (6 Suppl.) (Dec. 1998) 1285S–1389S.

Grundy, S. M., Abrams, J. J., "Comparison of Actions of Soy Protein and Casein on Metabolism of Plasma Lipoproteins and Cholesterol in Humans," *American Journal of Clinical Nutrition* 38 (2) (Aug. 1983): 245–52.

Jenkins, D. J., et al., "Combined Effect of Vegetable Protein (Soy) and Soluble Fiber Added to a Standard Cholesterol-Lowering Diet," *Metabolism* 48 (6) (June 1999): 809–16.

Potter, S. M., et al., "Soy Protein and Isoflavones: Their Effects on Blood Lipids and Bone Density in Postmenopausal Women," *American Journal of Clinical Nutrition* 68 (6 Suppl.) (Dec. 1998): 1375S–1379S.

Lo, G. S., Cole, T. G., "Soy Cotyledon Fiber Products Reduce Plasma Lipids," *Atherosclerosis* 82 (1–2) (May 1999): 59–67.

Baum, J. A., et al., "Long-Term Intake of Soy Protein Improves Blood Lipid Profiles and Increases Mononuclear Cell Low-Density-Lipoprotein Receptor Messenger RNA in Hypercholesterolemic, Postmenopausal Women," *American Journal of Clinical Nutrition* 68 (3) (Sept. 1998): 545–51.

Potter, J. M., Nestel, P. J., "Greater Bile Excretion with Soy Protein than with Cow Milk in Infants," *American Journal of Clinical Nutrition* 20 (5) (May 1976): 546–51.

Knight, D. C., Eden, J. A., "A Review of the Clinical Effects of Phytoestrogens," *Obstetrics and Gynecology* 87 (5 Pt. 2) (May 1996): 897–904.

Duncan, A. M., et al., "Modest Hormonal Effects of Soy Isoflavones in Postmenopausal Women," *Journal of Clinical Endocrinology and Metabolism* 84 (10) (Oct. 1999): 3479–84.

Setchell, K. D., "Soybean Isoflavones: Metabolism and Physiology" (Meeting abstract), *First International Symposium on the Role of Soy in Preventing and Treating Chronic Disease*, Mesa, Arizona, 1994.

Stephens, F. O., "Breast Cancer Aetiological Factors and Associations: A Possible Protective Role of Phytoestrogens," *Australian and New Zealand Journal of Surgery* 67 (11) (Nov. 1997): 755–60.

Washburn, "Effect of Soy Protein Supplementation on Serum Lipoproteins, Blood Pressure and Menopausal Symptoms in Perimenopausal Women," *Menopause* 6 (1) (Spring 1999): 7–13.

Crouse, J. R., "A Randomized Trial Comparing the Effect of Casein with That of Soy Protein Containing Varying Amounts of Isoflavones on Plasma Concentrations of Lipids and Lipoproteins," *Archives of Internal Medicine* 159 (17) (Sept. 1999): 2070–76.

Scheiber, M. D., et al., "Isoflavones and Postmenopausal Bone Health: A Viable Alternative to Estrogen Therapy?" *Menopause* 6 (3) (Fall 1999): 223–41.

Potter, S. M., "Soy Protein and Isoflavones: Their Effects on Blood Lipids and Bone Density in Postmenopausal Women," *American Journal of Clinical Nutrition* 68 (6 Suppl.) (Dec. 1998): 1375S–79S.

Ishimi, Y., et al., "Selective Effects of Genistein, a Soybean Isoflavone on B-Lymphopoiesis and Bone Loss Caused by Estrogen Deficiency," *Endocrinology* 140 (4) (Apr. 1999): 1893–1900.

Head, K. A., "Ipriflavone: An Important Bone-Building Isoflavone," *Alternative Medicine Reviews* 4 (1) (Feb. 1999): 10–22.

Cassidy, A., et al., "Biological Effects of a Diet of Soy Protein Rich in Isoflavones on the Menstrual Cycle of Pre-Menopausal Women," *American Journal of Clinical Nutrition* 60 (3) (Sept. 1994): 333–41.

Xu, X., et al., "Effects of Soy Isoflavones on Estrogen and Phytoestrogen Metabolism in Pre-Menopausal Women," *Cancer Epidemiology Biomarkers* 7 (12) (Dec. 1998): 1101–8.

Jerman, R., "Diet High in Soy Benefits Fetus," *Medical Tribune* (1999).

Willard, S. T., et al., "Phytoestrogens Have Agonistic and Combinational Effects on Estrogen Responsive Gene Expression in MCF-7 Human Breast Cancer Cells," *Endocrine* 8 (2) (Apr. 1998): 117–21.

Helferich, W. G., "Food Phytoestrogens: An Abundance of Weak Estrogen Agonists" (Meeting abstract), *Fundamental and Applied Toxicology* 30 (1) (Feb. 1996): 87.

Wang, C., Kurzer, M. S., "Effects of Phytoestrogens on DNA Synthesis in MCF-7 Cells in the Presence of Estradiol or Growth Factors," *Nutrition and Cancer* 31 (2) (1998): 90–100.

9: White Foods

"Intakes of 19 Individual Fatty Acids: Results from the 1994–96 Continuing Survey of Food Intakes by Individuals," *U.S. Department of Agriculture Food Surveys Group* (Beltsville, Md.: Beltsville Human Nutrition Research Center, Dec. 1997).

Simopolous, A. P., "Is Insulin Resistence Influenced by Dietary Linoleic Acid and Trans Fatty Acids?" *Free Radical Biology and Medicine* 17 (4) (1994): 367–72.

Ponte, E., et al., "Cardiovascular Disease and Omega-3 Fatty Acids," *Minerva Medical* 88 (9) (1997): 343–53.

Bowman, S. A., et al., "The Healthy Eating Index: 1994–96," *U.S. Dept. of Agriculture, Center for Nutrition Policy and Promotion,* Washington, D.C., 1998, p. 3.

Nelson, C. J., "Dietary Fat, Trans Fatty Acids, and Risk of Coronary Heart Disease," *Nutrition Reviews* 156 (8) (1998): 250–52.

Bell, R. A., et al., "An Epidemiologic Review of Dietary Intake Studies Among American Indians and Alaska Natives: Implications for Heart Disease and Cancer Risk," *Annals of Epidemiology* 7 (4) (1997): 229–40.

Feskens, E. J., Kromhout, D., "Epidemiologic Studies on Eskimos and Fish Intake," *Annals of the New York Academy of Science* 683 (1993): 9–15.

Mueller, B. A., Talbert, R. L., "Biological Mechanisms and Cardiovascular Effects of Omega-3 Fatty Acids," *Clinical Pharmacology* 7 (11) (1988): 795–807.

Mulvad, G., et al., "The Inuit Diet: Fatty Acids and Antioxidants, Their Role in Ischemic Heart Disease, and Exposure to Organochlorines and Heavy Metals: An International Study," *Arctic Medical Research* 55 (Suppl. 1) (1996): 20–24.

Hansen, J. C., et al., "Fatty Acids and Antioxidants in the Inuit Diet: Their Role in Ischemic Heart Disease (Ihd) and Possible Interactions with Other Dietary Factors," *Arctic Medical Research* 53 (1) (1994): 4–17.

Menotti, A., et al., "Food Intake Patterns and 25-year Mortality from Coronary Heart Disease: Cross-Cultural Correlations in the Seven Countries Study," *European Journal of Epidemiology* 15 (6) (1999): 507–15.

Ambrosone, C. B., et al., "Breast Cancer Risk Associated with Meat, Fish, and Chicken Consumption," *FASEB Journal* 9 (3) (1995): A579.

Caygill, C. P., Hill, M. J., "Fish, N-3 Fatty Acids and Human Colorectal and Breast Cancer Mortality," *European Journal of Cancer Prevention* 4 (4) (1995): 329–32.

Calder, P. C., "N-3 Polyunsaturated Fatty Acids in Cytokine Production in Health and Disease," *Annals of Nutrition and Metabolism* 41 (1997) (4): 203–34.

Calder, P. C., "N-3 Polyunsaturated Fatty Acids and Immune Cell Function," *Advances in Enzyme Regulation* 37 (1997): 197–237.

Kremeer, J. M., et al., "Effects of High-dose Fish Oil on Rheumatoid Arthritis After Stopping Nonsteroidal Antiinflammatory Drugs: Clinical and Immune Correlates," *Arthritis and Rheumatism* 38 (8) (1995): 1107–14.

Gallai, V., et al., "Cytokine Secretion and Eicosanoid Production in the Peripheral Blood Mononuclear Cells of MS Patients Undergoing Dietary Supplementation with N-3 Polyunsaturated Fatty Acids," *Journal of Immunology* 56 (2) (Feb. 1995): 143–53.

Sugano, M., et al., "Health Benefits of Rice Bran Oil," *Anticancer Research* 19 (5A) (Sept./Oct. 1999): 3651–57.

Rukmini, C., Raghuram, T. C., "Nutritional and Biochemical Aspects of the Hypolipidemic Action of Rice Bran Oil: A Review," *Journal of the American College of Nutrition* 10 (6) (Dec. 1993): 593–601.

Nicolosi, R. J., et al., "Rice Bran Oil Lowers Serum Total and Low Density Lipoprotein Cholesterol and Apo B Levels in Non Human Primates," *Atherosclerosis* 88 (2–3) (June 1991): 133–42.

Qureshi, A. A., et al., "Isolation and Identification of Novel Tocotrienols from Rice Bran with Hypocholesterolemic, Antioxidant, and Antitumor Properties," *Journal of Agricultural and Food Chemistry* 48 (8) (Aug. 2000): 3130–40.

Kagan, V. E., Packer, L., et al., "Recycling of Vitamin E in Human Low Density Lipoproteins," *Journal of Lipid Research* 33 (3) (Mar. 1992): 385–97.

Tomeo, A. C., et al., "Antioxidant Effects of Tocotrienols in Patients with Hyperlipidemia and Carotid Stenosis," *Lipids* 30 (12) (Dec. 1995): 1179–83.

Bartoli, R., et al., "Effect of Olive Oil on Early and Late Events of Colon Carcinogenesis," *Gut* 46 (Feb. 2000): 191–99.

Stoneham, M., et al., "Olive Oil Has Protective Effect on Colorectal Cancer Development," *Reuters Medical News* (Sept. 2000). As reported in *Journal of Epidemiological Community Health* 54 (Sept. 2000): 756–60.

Lopez, L. R., et al., "Monounsaturated Fatty Acid (Avocado) Rich Diet for Mild Hypercholesterolemia," *Archives of Medical Research* 27 (4) (Winter 1996): 519–23.

Carranza, J., et al., "Effects of Avocado on the Level of Blood Lipids in Patients with Phenotype II and IV Dyslipidemias," *Archivos del Instituto de Cardiologia de Mexico* 65 (4) (July/Aug. 1995): 342–48.

Raloff, J., "Better Butter? This One May Fight Cancer," *Science News* 156 (Dec. 1999): 375.

Salmon, C. P., et al., "Minimization of Heterocyclic Amines and Thermal Inactivation of *Escherichia coli* in Fried Ground Beef," *Journal of the National Cancer Institute* 92 (21) (Nov. 2000): 1773–78.

Hanif, R., et al., "Curcumin, a Natural Plant Phenolic Food Additive, Inhibits Cell Proliferation and Induces Cell Cycle Changes in Colon Adenocarcinoma Cell Lines by a Prostaglandin-Independent Pathway," *Journal of Laboratory and Clinical Medicine* 130 (6) (Dec. 1997): 576–84.

10: Herbs, Spices, Condiments, and Beverages

Aruoma, O. I., et al., "An Evaluation of the Antioxidant and Antiviral Action of Extracts of Rosemary and Provençal Herbs," *Food and Chemical Toxicology* 34 (5) (May 1996): 449–56.

Verma, S. K., Bordia, A., "Antioxidant Property of Saffron in Man," *Indian Journal of Medical Sciences* 52 (6) (May 1998): 205–207.

Kelm, M.A., et al., "Antioxidant and Cyclooxygenase Inhibitory Phenolic Compounds from Ocimum Sanctum Linn," *Phytomedicine* 7 (1) (Mar. 2000): 7–13.

Agrawal, P., et al., "Randomized Placebo-Controlled, Single Blind Trial of Holy Basil Leaves in Patients with Noninsulin-Dependent Diabetes Mellitus," *International Journal of Clinical Pharmacology and Therapeutics* 34 (9) (Sept. 1996): 406–9.

Arora, D. S., Kaur, J., "Antimicrobial Activity of Spices," *International Journal of Antimicrobial Agents* 12 (3) (Aug. 1999): 257–62.

Nair, S. C., et al., "Saffron Chemoprevention in Biology and Medicine: A Review," *Cancer Biotherapy* 10 (4) (Winter 1995): 257–64.

Kochhar, K. P., et al., "Gastro-Intestinal Effects of Indian Spice Mixture (Garam Masala)," *Tropical Gastroenterology* 29 (4) (Oct.–Dec. 1999): 170–74.

Shah, B. H., et al., "Inhibitory Effect of Curcumin, a Food Spice from Turmeric, on Platelet-Activating Factor and Arachidonic Acid-Mediated Platelet Aggregation Through Inhibition of Thromboxane Formation and CA2$^+$ Signaling," *Biochemical Pharmacology* 58 (7) (Oct. 1999): 1167–72.

Zava, D. T., et al., "Estrogen and Progestin Bioactivity of Foods, Herbs, and Spices," *Proceedings of the Society for Experimental Biology and Medicine* 217 (3) (Mar. 1998): 369–78.

Frawley, D., Lad, V., *The Yoga of Herbs* (Twin Lakes, Wisc.: Lotus Press, 1986), pp. 192–223.

Tirtha, S.S., *The Ayurveda Encyclopedia* (Bayville, N.Y.: Ayurveda Holistic Center Press, 1998), pp. 155–58.

Duke, J., *Handbook of Biologically Active Phytochemicals and Their Activities* (Boca Raton, Fla.: CRC Press, 1992).

Duke, J., *Handbook of Phytochemical Constituents of GRAS Herbs and Other Economic Plants* (Boca Raton, Fla.: CRC Press, 1992).

Quinlan, P. T., et al., "The Acute Physiological and Mood Effects of Tea and Coffee: The Role of Caffeine Level," *Pharmacology, Biochemistry and Behavior* 66 (1) (May 2000): 19–28.

Kindmarch, I., et al., "A Naturalistic Investigation of the Effects of Day-Long Consumption of Tea, Coffee and Water on Alertness, Sleep Onset and Sleep Quality," *Psychopharmacology* 149 (3) (Apr. 2000): 203–16.

Dager, S. R., et al., "Human Brain Metabolic Response to Caffeine and the Effects of Tolerance," *American Journal of Psychiatry* 156 (2) (Feb. 1999): 229–37.

Kendler, K. S., Prescott, C. A., "Caffeine Intake, Tolerance and Withdrawal in Women: A Population Based Twin Study," *American Journal of Psychiatry* 156 (2) (Feb. 1999): 223–28.

Grubben, M. J., et al., "Unfiltered Coffee Increases Plasma Homocysteine Concentrations in Healthy Volunteers: A Randomized Trial," *American Journal of Clinical Nutrition* 71 (2) (Feb. 2000): 480–84.

Ruiz del Castillo, M. L., et al., "Rapid Analysis of Cholesterol-Elevating Compounds in Coffee Brews by Off-Line High-Performance Liquid Chromatography/High-Resolution Gas Chromatography," *Journal of Agricultural and Food Chemistry* 47 (2) (Feb. 1999): 695–99.

Stolzenberg-Solomon, R. Z., et al., "Association of Dietary Protein Intake and Coffee Consumption with Serum Homocysteine Concentrations in an Older Population," *American Journal of Clinical Nutrition* 69 (3) (Mar. 1999): 467–75.

Zivkovic, R., "Coffee and Health in the Elderly," *Acta Medica Croatica* 54 (1) (2000): 33–36.

Rakic, V., et al., "Effects of Coffee on Ambulatory Blood Pressure in Older Men and Women: A Randomized Controlled Trial," *Hypertension* 33 (3) (Mar. 1999): 869–73.

Ellison, E. F., "Tea and Other Beverage Consumption and Prostate Cancer Risk: A Canadian Retrospective Cohort Study," *European Journal of Cancer Prevention* 9 (2) (Apr. 2000): 125–30.

Heliovaara, M., et al., "Coffee Consumption, Rheumatoid Factor, and the Risk of Rheumatoid Arthritis," *Annals of the Rheumatic Diseases* 59 (8) (Aug. 2000): 631–35.

Tomlinson, B. U., et al., "Dietary Caffeine, Fluid Intake and Urinary Incontinence in Older Rural Women," *International Urogynecology Journal of Pelvic Floor Dysfunction* 10 (1) (1999): 22–28.

Arya, L. A., et al., "Dietary Caffeine Intake and the Risk for Detrusor Instability: A Case-Control Study," *Obstetrics and Gynecology* 96 (1) (July 2000): 85–89.

Leitzmann, M. F., Giovannucci, E., et al., "A Prospective Study of Coffee Consumption and the Risk of Symptomatic Gallstone Disease in Men," *JAMA* 281 (22) (June 1999): 2106–12.

Post, S. M., et al., "Cafestol, the Cholesterol-Raising Factor in Boiled Coffee, Suppresses Bile Acid Synthesis by Downregulation of Cholesterol 7α-Hydroxylase and Sterol 27-Hydroxylase in Rat Hepatocytes," *Arteriosclerosis, Thrombosis, and Vascular Biology* 17 (1997): 3064–70.

Giovannucci, E., "Meta-Analysis of Coffee Consumption and Risk of Colorectal Cancer," *American Journal of Epidemiology* 147 (11) (June 1998): 1043–52.

Ross, G. W., et al., "Association of Coffee and Caffeine Intake with the Risk of Parkinson Disease," *JAMA* 283 (20) (May 2000): 2674–79.

Kiyohara, C., et al., "Inverse Association Between Coffee Drinking and Serum Uric Acid Concentrations in Middle-Aged Japanese Males," *British Journal of Nutrition* 82(2) (Aug. 1999): 125–30.

Hurrell, R. F., et al., "Inhibition of Non-Heme Iron Absorption in Man by Polyphenolic Containing Beverages," *British Journal of Nutrition* 81 (4) (Apr. 1999): 289–95.

Pittler, M. H., Ernst, E., "Peppermint Oil for Irritable Bowel Syndrome: A Critical Review and Meta Analysis," *American Journal of Gastroenterology* 93 (7) (July 1999): 1131–35.

Liu, J. H., et al., "Enteric-Coated Peppermint-Oil Capsules in the Treatment of Irritable Bowel Syndrome: A Prospective Randomized Trial," *Journal of Gastroenterology* 32 (6) (Dec. 1997): 765–68.

Madisch, A., et al., "Treatment of Functional Dyspepsia with a Fixed Peppermint Oil and Caraway Oil Combination Preparation as Compared to Cisapride: A Multicenter, Reference-Controlled Double-Blind Equivalence Study," *Arzneimittel-Forschung* 49 (11) (Nov. 1999): 925–32.

Tate, S., "Peppermint Oil: A Treatment for Postoperative Nausea," *Journal of Advanced Nursing* 26 (3) (Sept. 1997): 543–49.

16: Signs and Symptoms Specific to Your Color

Duke, J., *Handbook of Medicinal Herbs* (Boca Raton, Fla.: CRC Press, 1985).

Frawley, D., Lad, V., *The Yoga of Herbs* (Twin Lakes, Wisc.: Lotus Press, 1986).

Tirtha, Swami S. S., *The Ayurveda Encyclopedia*, 2d ed. (Bayville, N.Y.: Ayurveda Holistic Center Press, 1998).

Holmes, P., *The Energetics of Western Herbs*, vols. 1 and 2 (Boulder, Colo.: Artemis, 1989).

Brown, D., *Herbal Prescriptions for Better Health* (Rockland, Calif.: Prima Publishing, 1998).

Majeed, M., Badnaev, V., *Boswellin—The Antiinflammatory Phytonutrient* (Piscataway, N.J.: Nutriscience, 1996).

Majeed, M., Badnaev, V., *Turmeric and the Healing Curcuminoids* (New Canaan, Conn.: Keats, 1996).

Majeed, M., Badnaev, V., *Capsaicin: The Anti-Arthritic Phytochemical* (Piscataway, N.J.: Nutriscience, 1997).

Majeed, M., Badnaev, V., *Bioperine: Nature's Own Thermonutrient and Natural Bioavailability Enhancer* (Piscataway, N.J.: Nutriscience, 1999).

Acknowledgments

This book would never have been completed without the help and dedication of my husband, Jon Zimmerman. My agent Jenny Bent has once again guided me in presenting my ideas. My editor Deb Brody has been extremely understanding and patient as we navigated this journey together. Several people have given me valuable suggestions, connected me with those who could teach me about functional foods and Ayurveda and helped clarify my thinking. They are Vladimir Badmaev, M.D., Ph.D.; Alan Tillotson, Ph.D., AHG.; D. Ay; Dr. Shailinder Sodhi; P. K. Dave; Bill Helferich, Ph.D.; Claire Hasler, Ph.D.; Mindy Kurzer, Ph.D.; Mark Messina, Ph.D.; Ronald Pryor, Ph.D.; and David Kyle, Ph.D.

Index

About the Author

MARCIA ZIMMERMAN is one of the most highly respected researchers, authors, and lecturers within the natural medicine and health care arena. With more than twenty-seven years' experience in the nutrition field, she has helped thousands of people achieve a healthier nutritional status and lifestyle. *Eat Your Colors* is the culmination of more than ten years of research and lectures across the United States. She is the author of *The A.D.D. Nutrition Solution* and lives in Chico, California.